Head, Neck and Thyroid Surgery

AN INTRODUCTION AND PRACTICAL GUIDE

T0138767

Head, Neck and Thyroid Surgery

AN INTRODUCTION AND PRACTICAL GUIDE

Edited by

Neeraj Sethi PHD FRCS (ORL-HNS)
Consultant Otolaryngologist Head and Neck Surgeon
Queen's Medical Centre, Nottingham University Hospitals NHS Trust, UK

R. James A. England FRCS (ORL-HNS)
Consultant Otolaryngologist, Thyroid Surgeon, Honorary Senior Lecturer
Hull and East Yorkshire NHS Hospitals Trust & Hull University, UK

Neil de Zoysa MSc FRCS (ORL-HNS)
Consultant Otolaryngologist Head and Neck Surgeon
Poole Hospital, Dorset, UK

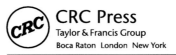

CRC Press
Taylor & Francis Group
Boca Raton London New York

CRC Press is an imprint of the
Taylor & Francis Group, an **informa** business

First edition published 2020
by CRC Press
6000 Broken Sound Parkway NW, Suite 300, Boca Raton, FL 33487-2742

and by CRC Press
2 Park Square, Milton Park, Abingdon, Oxon, OX14 4RN

© 2020 Taylor & Francis Group, LLC

CRC Press is an imprint of Taylor & Francis Group, LLC

This book contains information obtained from authentic and highly regarded sources. While all reasonable efforts have been made to publish reliable data and information, neither the author[s] nor the publisher can accept any legal responsibility or liability for any errors or omissions that may be made. The publishers wish to make clear that any views or opinions expressed in this book by individual editors, authors or contributors are personal to them and do not necessarily reflect the views/opinions of the publishers. The information or guidance contained in this book is intended for use by medical, scientific or health-care professionals and is provided strictly as a supplement to the medical or other professional's own judgement, their knowledge of the patient's medical history, relevant manufacturer's instructions and the appropriate best practice guidelines. Because of the rapid advances in medical science, any information or advice on dosages, procedures or diagnoses should be independently verified. The reader is strongly urged to consult the relevant national drug formulary and the drug companies' and device or material manufacturers' printed instructions, and their websites, before administering or utilizing any of the drugs, devices or materials mentioned in this book. This book does not indicate whether a particular treatment is appropriate or suitable for a particular individual. Ultimately it is the sole responsibility of the medical professional to make his or her own professional judgements, so as to advise and treat patients appropriately. The authors and publishers have also attempted to trace the copyright holders of all material reproduced in this publication and apologize to copyright holders if permission to publish in this form has not been obtained. If any copyright material has not been acknowledged please write and let us know so we may rectify in any future reprint.

Library of Congress Cataloging-in-Publication Data

Names: Sethi, Neeraj, editor. | England, R. James A, editor. | De Zoysa, Neil, editor.
Title: Head, neck and thyroid surgery : an introduction and practical guide / [edited by] Neeraj Sethi, R. James A. England, Neil De Zoysa
Description: Boca Raton : CRC Press, [2020] | Includes bibliographical references and index. | Summary: "This book covers the clinical approach to managing head and neck pathology as it presents to the otolaryngology department. Including cervical lymphadenopathy, salivary gland disease, oral, oropharyngeal, laryngeal and hypopharyngeal lesions as well as skin and thyroid tumours. Each chapter presents an evidence-based, practical, and user-friendly approach to assessing, investigating and managing these patients A practical, clinically applicable guide to managing head and neck pathology An evidence-based approach to the clear guidance provided in the book. Colour images and flow charts for quick reference Clear, concise and comprehensive, Head, Neck & Thyroid Surgery: An introduction and practical guide will be useful to trainees and clinicians in otolaryngology, maxillo-facial and plastic surgery"-- Provided by publisher.
Identifiers: LCCN 2019043915 (print) | LCCN 2019043916 (ebook) | ISBN 9780367855895 (hardback ; alk. paper) | ISBN 9781138035614 (paperback ; alk. paper) | ISBN 9781315266138 ebook
Subjects: MESH: Head--surgery | Neck--surgery | Thyroid Gland--surgery
Classification: LCC RF51 (print) | LCC RF51 (ebook) | NLM WE 700 | DDC 617.5/1059--dc23
LC record available at https://lccn.loc.gov/2019043915
LC ebook record available at https://lccn.loc.gov/2019043916

ISBN: 978-0-367-85589-5 (hbk)
ISBN: 978-1-138-03561-4 (pbk)
ISBN: 978-1-315-26613-8 (ebk)

Typeset in Minion Pro
by Nova Techset Private Limited, Bengaluru & Chennai, India

Visit the Taylor & Francis Web site at
http://www.taylorandfrancis.com

and the CRC Press Web site at
http://www.crcpress.com

CONTENTS

PREFACE

When searching the marketplace for books to help prepare the trainee attempting to manage patients with head and neck pathology in the clinic or ward we found a dearth of accessible texts. All the authors have, at some point in their lives, found themselves struggling to find easy-to-follow guidance and knowledge on the investigation, work-up and follow-up of patients with head and neck disease. With this in mind we set out to avoid an impenetrable, encyclopaedic tome and provide an easy-to-read, evidence-based introduction to this topic.

We have tried to set the scene for each subsite with a background of the clinically relevant anatomy and physiology before presenting the clinical manifestations of the more common head and neck pathologies in each area. In addition to evidence-based guidance on the work-up and management, we were determined to impart experience-based knowledge and tips on the same to help the trainee.

It is vital to acknowledge the contribution of all the authors who have given selflessly of their time and expertise. The driving enthusiasm and endless patience of the publishing team have kept this project moving forward towards a final product. Most importantly our families provide the love and support to be able to produce a worthy book.

This book is very much an introduction and practical guide. It will be invaluable for the trainee at the coalface, developing their approach for these patients. It should serve as a gateway to more heavyweight reference texts and in-depth literature searches, whilst equipping the trainee with confidence and practical knowledge.

Neeraj Sethi
R. James A. England
Neil de Zoysa

EDITORS

Neeraj Sethi has had a passion for head and neck surgery throughout his career. During his higher surgical training in otolaryngology, he completed a PhD in molecular biology in head and neck cancer, and has published and presented widely on many aspects of otolaryngology and head and neck surgery. After completing a fellowship in advanced head and neck surgical oncology and robotic surgery in Adelaide, he took up a consultant head and neck surgeon post at Queen Medical Centre, Nottingham. This book highlights his ongoing commitment to education and training in head and neck surgery.

R. James A. England has been a Consultant ENT Surgeon in Hull University Teaching Hospitals Trust for 20 years. His main interest is in thyroid/parathyroid surgery, and he is lead of the regional Thyroid MDT. He performs approximately 140 thyroidectomies and 80 parathyroidectomies annually. His main research interest is in the translational potential of microfluidic technologies in the personalised management of thyroid disease.

Neil de Zoysa trained at University College London and completed his higher specialist training at Guy's and St George's Hospitals. He completed dual fellowships in Head & Neck Surgery as part of the Royal College of Surgeons Interface Training Programme at Hull Royal Infirmary. He then went on to complete a fellowship in head, neck and skull base surgery at the Princess Alexandra Hospital in Brisbane, Australia. After having children, he moved to his wife's hometown in Poole, UK. He has an interest in thyroid cancer and HPV associated SCC. He also has an active interest in the career development and training of future surgeons.

CONTRIBUTORS

Shahzada Ahmed
Consultant ENT and Skull Base Surgeon
University Hospitals Birmingham NHS Trust
Birmingham, United Kingdom

Patrick J. Bradley
Emeritus Professor Head and Neck Oncologic
    Surgery
Nottingham, United Kingdom

Nick Brown
Consultant Oral and Maxillofacial Surgeon
York Teaching Hospital NHS Trust
York, United Kingdom

Mat Daniel
Consultant ENT Surgeon and Honorary Senior
    Lecturer
Nottingham University Hospitals NHS Trust
Nottingham, United Kingdom

Neil de Zoysa
Consultant Otolaryngologist Head and Neck Surgeon
Poole Hospital
Dorset, United Kingdom

R. James A. England
Consultant Otolaryngologist Head and
    Neck Surgeon
and
Honorary Senior Lecturer
Hull and East Yorkshire NHS Hospitals Trust
and
Hull University
Hull, United Kingdom

Andrew Foreman
Consultant Otolaryngologist and Reconstructive
    Head and Neck Surgeon
Royal Adelaide Hospital
Adelaide, South Australia

Jay Goswamy
Consultant Surgeon in Otorhinolaryngology
and
Clinical Lead for ENT Surgery
Manchester University NHS Foundation Trust
Manchester, United Kingdom

Jarrod J. Homer
Consultant Head and Neck/Thyroid Surgeon and
    Otolaryngologist
Manchester Royal Infirmary
Manchester, United Kingdom

Emma King
Consultant ENT Head and Neck Surgeon
Cancer Research UK Senior Lecturer Head and
    Neck Surgery
Poole Hospital
Poole, United Kingdom

Giri Krishnan
Surgical Registrar and Clinical Associate Lecturer
University of Adelaide
Adelaide, South Australia

Gordon A. G. McKenzie
Academic Clinical Fellow in Otolaryngology Hull
    Teaching Hospitals NHS Trust
and
Honorary Senior Clinical Lecturer
University of Bristol
Bristol, United Kingdom

James Moor
Consultant ENT Surgeon
Leeds Teaching Hospitals NHS Trust
Leeds, United Kingdom

Jiten D. Parmar
Department of Oral and Maxillofacial Surgery
Leeds Teaching Hospitals NHS Trust
Leeds, United Kingdom

Amit Prasai
Consultant ENT Surgeon
Leeds Teaching Hospitals NHS Trust
Leeds, United Kingdom

Salman Qureshi
Consultant Head and Neck/Neuro Radiologist
Hamad Medical Corporation
Doha, Qatar

Yujay Ramakrishnan
Consultant ENT and Skull Base Surgeon
Queen's Medical Centre
Nottingham University Hospitals NHS Trust
Nottingham, United Kingdom

Neeraj Sethi
Consultant Otolaryngologist Head and Neck
    Surgeon
Queen's Medical Centre
Nottingham University Hospitals NHS Trust
Nottingham, United Kingdom

David J. H. Shipway
Consultant Physician and Perioperative
    Geriatrician
North Bristol NHS Trust
and
Honorary Senior Clinical Lecturer
University of Bristol
Bristol, United Kingdom

Kishan Ubayasiri
Consultant Otolaryngologist/Head and Neck
    Surgical Oncologist
Nottingham University Hospitals NHS Trust
Nottingham, United Kingdom

Laura Warner
Consultant Otolaryngologist, Head and Neck
    Surgeon
Newcastle upon Tyne Hospitals NHS Foundation
    Trust
Newcastle upon Tyne, United Kingdom

ABBREVIATIONS

AJCC	American Joint Committee on Cancer	MEN	multiple endocrine neoplasia
CT	computerised tomography or computed tomography	MRI	magnetic resonance imaging
		PET	positron emission tomography
EBV	Epstein–Barr virus	RT	radiotherapy
ENT	ear, nose and throat	SCC	squamous cell carcinoma
FBC	full blood count	TNM	tumor, node, metastasis
FDG	fluorodeoxyglucose	UADT	upper aerodigestive tract
HPV	human papillomavirus	UICC	Union for International Cancer Control
IJV	internal jugular vein	US	ultrasound
IMRT	intensity-modulated radiotherapy	USS	ultrasound scan
MDT	multidisciplinary team		

1 ANATOMY AND DIFFERENTIAL DIAGNOSIS IN HEAD AND NECK SURGERY

Neeraj Sethi and Neil de Zoysa

INTRODUCTION

When assessing patients it is vital to formulate a differential diagnosis based on the initial history and examination. This guides decision-making in investigating patients swiftly and appropriately. Lack of investing thought into a differential diagnosis will lead to delays and unnecessary anxiety for the patient. Knowledge of the anatomy is essential to understanding what the pathology could possibly be. Whilst primary malignancy in neck lumps can occur (e.g. lymphoma, thyroid cancer or salivary gland cancer), the majority of malignant neck lumps are metastatic and immediate thought must be given to identifying the source of the primary tumour (which is likely to be in the upper aerodigestive tract).

Additionally, Occam's razor suggests a unifying diagnosis to be the most likely correct diagnosis.

This is often the case and makes sense in the setting of a patient with a sore throat, altered voice and a neck lump, where a differential diagnosis including hypopharyngeal carcinoma explains all symptoms. However, Hickam's dictum must be remembered which states 'a man can have as many diseases as he damn well pleases', and there will always be patients with multiple pathologies.

Whilst the anatomy for each subsite of the upper aerodigestive tract is considered in more detail in each specific chapter, here an overview will be provided to 'set the scene' for a general assessment of the patient referred to a head and neck surgery clinic. As well as anatomy, the patient's age, associated symptoms and risk factors for specific illnesses will guide differential formulation.

ANATOMY

▮ Triangles and levels

The neck is an anatomically complex but quite beautiful arrangement of vessels, cranial nerves, peripheral nerves, muscles and fascia.

For the purposes of clinical medicine and surgery, the neck can be broken down into triangles which are defined by palpable landmarks. This aids in both clinical examination and surgical planning.

From an operative point of view however it is equally important to understand the fascial planes of the neck. Generally speaking, these planes and their boundaries can be followed during surgery. By doing this, a clean operative field can be obtained ensuring complete and safe surgery via the relative ease at which important anatomy can be identified and preserved.

Important palpable bony landmarks are identified in **Figure 1.1**. These include the lower border of the mandible, the mastoid tip, the hyoid bone, the cricoid cartilage, the sternal notch, the clavicle and the anterior border of the trapezius muscle.

Using these landmarks, the neck can be divided into triangles as shown in **Figure 1.1**. The submandibular triangle has its superior border at the lower border of the mandible. It is then made up by the digastric muscle, which has two bellies running from the lesser cornu of the hyoid, one to the mastoid tip and one towards the digastric fossa of the mandible, just lateral to the symphysis (midpoint of the mandible).

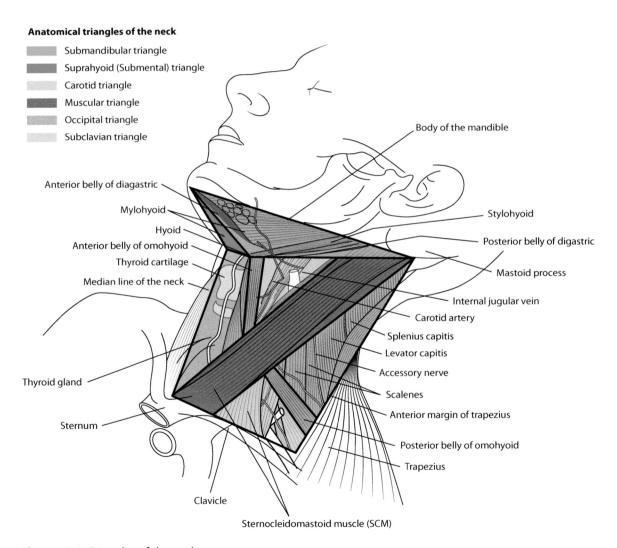

Anatomical triangles of the neck

- Submandibular triangle
- Suprahyoid (Submental) triangle
- Carotid triangle
- Muscular triangle
- Occipital triangle
- Subclavian triangle

Body of the mandible

Anterior belly of diagastric
Mylohyoid
Hyoid
Anterior belly of omohyoid
Thyroid cartilage
Median line of the neck

Stylohyoid
Posterior belly of digastric
Mastoid process
Internal jugular vein
Carotid artery
Splenius capitis
Levator capitis
Accessory nerve
Scalenes
Anterior margin of trapezius
Posterior belly of omohyoid
Trapezius

Thyroid gland

Sternum

Clavicle

Sternocleidomastoid muscle (SCM)

Figure 1.1 Triangles of the neck.

Between the two anterior bellies of the digastric muscle and the body of the hyoid is the suprahyoid (submental) triangle.

The carotid triangle runs from the posterior belly of the digastric muscle to its insertion at the mastoid tip, then down the posterior border of the sternomastoid muscle, then up along the omohyoid muscle towards the lesser cornu of the hyoid. The omohyoid muscle is palpable in slim or muscular patients. As a surrogate, a line can be made from the lower two-thirds of the sternomastoid muscle to the lesser cornu of the hyoid.

The muscular triangle runs below this line (the omohyoid), the remaining sternomastoid muscle and the midline.

The occipital triangle is bordered by the posterior border of the sternomastoid muscle towards the mastoid tip, then along the anterior border of the

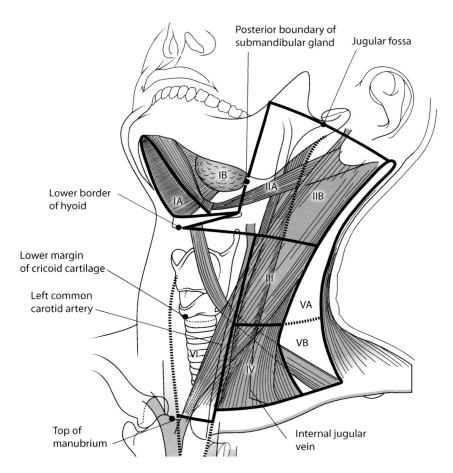

Figure 1.2 Levels of the neck. Level IA corresponds to the suprahyoid (submental) triangle. Level IB corresponds to the submandibular triangle. Level II corresponds to the upper half of the carotid triangle. Level III corresponds to the lower half of the carotid triangle. Level IV corresponds to the lateral half of the muscular triangle (lateral to the infrahyoid strap muscles or common carotid artery). Level V corresponds to the occipital triangle (it is divided into VA and VB by the spinal accessory nerve). Level VI is a rectangle in most patients, as it is in the midline, technically the area from inferior to the hyoid to the sternal notch, medial to the common carotid arteries. Level VII is mediastinal level relevant to thyroid and subglottic pathology. It is bordered by the sternal notch and the carotid arteries joining to the innominate or aortic arch.

trapezius, along the clavicle back to the sternomastoid. The subclavian (or supraclavicular triangle) is found within the posterior triangle, bounded by the inferior belly of omohyoid, the posterior border of sternocleidomastoid and the clavicle [1].

For the purposes of oncological description and axial imaging, the triangles are replaced by levels (see **Figure 1.2** and **Table 1.1**). Levels are a more reproducible way of describing the location of pathology and should be used in preference to

Table 1.1 Levels of the neck and contents.

Level	Contents
IA	Lymph nodes draining from the floor of mouth and lower lip. Thyroglossal and dermoid cysts can also be located here.
IB	Submandibular gland. Lymph nodes which drain the oral cavity, tongue and floor of mouth. Superficial to the submandibular gland; runs the marginal mandibular branch of the facial nerve. Deep to the gland lies the distal portion of the hypoglossal nerve, the mylohyoid muscle and deep to this the lingual nerve. The submandibular gland is supplied with blood by the facial artery, which can bleed briskly after trauma in this location.
II	Accessory nerve Upper end of internal jugular vein (IJV), both internal and external carotid arteries. The hypoglossal nerve crosses the external carotid artery here. The area is encircled by lymph nodes which drain the pharynx, larynx, face and skin. The internal jugular vein receives its major tributary, the common facial vein.
III	The internal jugular and common carotid artery (this bifurcates at the border of level II/III). The carotid sheath spans levels II to IV and contains the IJV and the carotid artery. The vagus nerve lies intimately with the carotid artery thus making its identification and preservation routine during neck dissection. Lymph nodes. Cervical plexus branches run along the floor of this level.
IV	Corresponds to the lateral half of the muscular triangle (lateral to the infrahyoid strap muscles or common carotid artery). It contains the roots of the carotid and internal jugular vein. At a variable height the subclavian vein and internal jugular vein form the origin of the superior vena cava. In some patients this can be just above the clavicle. In the left-hand side, the thoracic duct inserts posteriorly into the IJV which can be commonly injured in this location. Care should be taken in this area during neck dissection to avoid chylous leak. Cervical plexus branches also run through this level and the transverse cervical vessels.
V	Corresponds to the occipital triangle (it is divided into VA and VB by the spinal accessory nerve). This contains lymph nodes which drain the parotid area, the thyroid and skin of the face and neck. Transverse cervical vessels.
VI	This is a rectangle in most patients as it is in the midline, technically the area from inferior to the hyoid to the sternal notch, medial to the common carotid arteries. It contains the recurrent laryngeal nerves, thyroid and parathyroid glands, and trachea as well as vessels feeding and draining the thyroid.
VII	This is a mediastinal level relevant to thyroid and subglottic pathology. It is bordered by the sternal notch and the carotid arteries joining to the innominate or aortic arch. It is often cleared in cases of medullary thyroid cancer. It contains lymph nodes and thymus gland.

Table 1.2 Lymphatic levels drainage.

Level	Regions of drainage
IA	Floor of mouth, lower alveolus/gingiva, anterior and ventral tongue
IB	Tongue, oral cavity, buccal mucosa, lower alveolus/gingiva
II	Pharynx, larynx, posterior oral cavity
III	Oropharynx, larynx, hypopharynx, nasopharynx
IV	Hypopharynx, subglottis
V	Skin, parotid
VI	Thyroid, subglottis

triangles in documentation, correspondence and discussion. In addition, the lymphatic drainage at specific levels can help clinically identify the possible location of primary disease in the case of metastatic carcinoma.

The contents of these levels are shown in **Table 1.1** and the region of echelon drainage is shown in **Table 1.2**.

■ Fascial layers

A key area of understanding of applied surgical anatomy is of the deep cervical fascial planes (summarised by **Figure 1.3**). Note how the investing layer of cervical fascia is deep to the platysma. This is why subplatysmal skin flaps are elevated. This keeps skin flaps

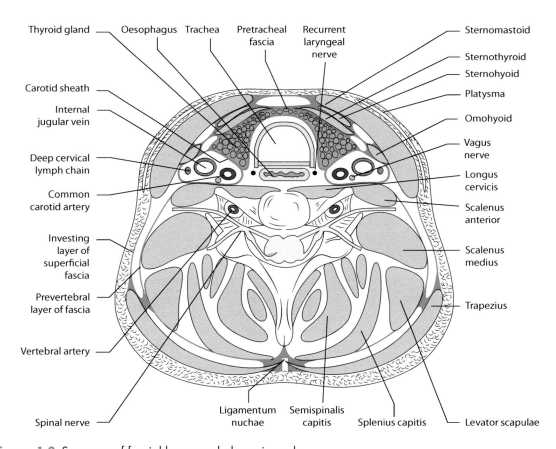

Figure 1.3 Summary of fascial layers and planes in neck.

well vascularised on a random pattern blood supply. In addition, for most neck surgeries, exposure can be gained to large areas of the neck without oncological compromise in the majority of cases. Special care should be taken in case of advance N3 nodal disease or indeed superficial tumours, especially in the parotid or submandibular gland where skin may need to be resected.

The investing layer of the deep cervical fascia can be followed in a relatively avascular fashion to expose the carotid sheath contents and indeed the superficial border of most neck dissections.

The pretracheal layer of the deep cervical fascia wraps the thyroid gland, the trachea and oesophagus/pharynx. The carotid sheath is part of the pretracheal fascia and connects it to the prevertebral and investing layer.

The prevertebral fascia is the deepest and forms an oncological barrier beyond which most tumours are considered unresectable. Beyond it lies the cervical spine, the paravertebral muscles including longus

cervicis (longus colli), the scalene muscles and levator scapulae. The brachial plexus, phrenic nerve and stellate ganglion lie within it.

A neck dissection can thus be conceptualised as a fascial dissection removing the envelope of investing cervical fascia and carotid sheath (although sparing all of the preservable contents).

The fascial planes have two main potential spaces which are clinically relevant: the parapharyngeal space and the retropharyngeal space (see **Figure 1.4**).

The parapharyngeal space

The parapharyngeal space can be conceptualised as an inverted pyramid with its base at the skull base and apex at the greater cornu of the hyoid. It is divided by the styloid process into post- and prestyloid spaces. Its medial margin is the middle (pretracheal) layer of the deep cervical fascia. Its lateral margin is the investing layer of deep cervical fascia. Its anterior margin is the investing fascia of the deep

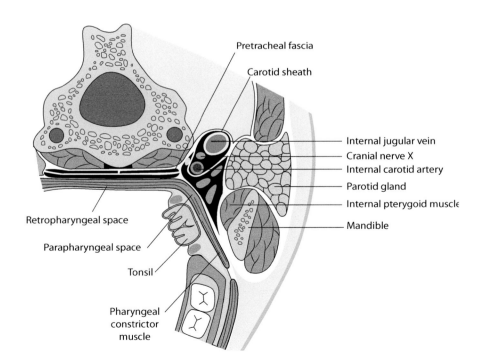

Figure 1.4 The retropharyngeal space in relation to the parapharyngeal space.

cervical fascia covering the medial pterygoid muscle. Its posterior margin is the prevertebral layer of the deep cervical fascia [1].

The retropharyngeal space

The retropharyngeal space runs from the base of skull to the thorax along the vertebra. It is anterior to the danger space. The space is directly posterior to the pharyngeal mucosal space. It lies anteromedial to the carotid space and posteromedial to the parapharyngeal space.

Its posterior margin is the alar fascia, which separates the retropharyngeal space from the danger space. The clinical relevance is that the danger space runs from the clivus to the mediastinum. This can result in infection spreading from the pharynx into the mediastinum leading to mediastinitis.

Further clinical relevance is that the space also contains nodal tissue, which can be a source of sepsis and also a site of cancer metastasis in the pharynx, particularly the posterior pharynx [1].

EMBRYOLOGY

The structures of the neck including the majority of relevant cranial nerves, vessels, muscles and bones are derived from the branchial (or Pharyngeal) arches.

These give rise to gills in fish embryos and are present from the fourth week of gestation onward.

The arches themselves are composed of mesoderm, which go on to form bone and cartilage within the neck (see **Table 1.3**).

This is often a confusing subject to learn and to teach. One approach is to understand the structure of the arches, which are mesoderm with an ectodermal and endodermal side. The endodermal side (which forms the pharyngeal pouches) go on to become glandular tissue. The ectodermal side (the branchial clefts) subsequently develop into sinuses, which in all cases bar the first branchial cleft (the external auditory canal) spontaneously obliterate [2].

Table 1.3 Pharyngeal arch and pouch derivatives.

Arch no.	Vascular	Nerve	Muscular	Skeletal	Pouch derivative
I (mandibular)	Maxillary artery	V	Muscles of mastication, tensor tympani, anterior belly digastric, tensor veli palatini	Malleus, incus, Meckel's cartilage	Middle ear Eustachian tube
II (hyoid)	Stapedial artery	VII	Muscles of facial expression, stapedius, stylohyoid, posterior belly digastric	Stapes, styloid process, body of hyoid	Supratonsillar fossa
III	Internal carotid artery	IX	Stylopharyngeus	Greater horn hyoid	Thymus, inferior parathyroid gland
IV	Right subclavian artery	X	Pharyngeal and laryngeal muscles	Laryngeal cartilage	Superior parathyroid gland

This first arch anomalies include accessory auricles, ear canal atresia and pre-auricular sinuses. The second branchial anomalies include the most common type of branchial cleft cyst (see Chapter 4) and can be branchial sinuses (ectoderm connected to mesoderm) or fistulae (from skin to tonsil). The third and fourth cleft anomalies are more rare but can present as cysts or abscesses of fistulae involving the parathyroid glands, thyroid and pharynx [2].

The first pouch forms the middle ear and Eustachian tube. The second pouch forms the palatine tonsil. The third pouch forms the thymus and inferior parathyroid glands due to the fact that the thymus descends into the mediastinum below the fourth pouch which become the superior parathyroid glands, i.e. they are superior in their anatomical location in a developed human. This also explains why inferior parathyroid glands can lie in the mediastinum and why thymectomy can revascularise the inferior parathyroid glands. The fifth pouch is the ultimobranchial body which gives rise to the C-cells of the thyroid gland [2].

The thyroid itself is not of branchial pouch origin and forms at 3–4 weeks gestation where it forms at the base of tongue as it descends through the developing neck leaving the foramen caecum. It descends and leaves behind it the thyroglossal duct as it passes through the developing hyoid bone into the neck where it fuses with the fifth pouch. This explains the rationale for the extent of surgery for thyroglossal duct cysts and indeed why it is impossible to develop medullary thyroid cancer within a thyroglossal duct cyst (though a papillary thyroid cancer within a thyroglossal duct cyst is possible) [2].

HISTORY

Effective history-taking is long-taught and emphasised throughout medical school and after. An accurate history guides differential diagnosis, and examination findings are often simply confirmatory of suspicions based on history. Details of the patient background, the history of presenting complaint and symptoms are essential.

▌ The patient

Patient age, ethnicity, occupation and sex all influence differential diagnosis. For example, malignant tumours are more common in older adults compared to children. However, thyroid masses are usually benign in adults but are more likely to be malignant in children. Similarly, lymph node swellings are more likely to be infective or inflammatory in children but would raise more suspicion of metastatic disease in adults.

Different ethnic groups should alert the clinician to different disease risk. Nasopharyngeal carcinoma is rare in the UK and Europe. It is common in certain areas of China (particularly in Guangdong) [3]. In India, head and neck cancer is the most common cancer. This is due to the cultural practice of chewing betel quid, which is highly carcinogenic. Though not common in the UK, this is a relevant question for a specific population.

Occupational exposure can trigger suspicion of different diseases such as hard-wood workers and an association with sinonasal carcinoma [4]. Dust exposure (sawdust, leather and metal) has been found to be associated with an increased risk of larynx cancer [5].

Though head and neck cancer is far more common in men compared to women (approximately 3:1) [6], thyroid lumps are more common in women but have a higher chance of being malignant in a man.

Lifestyle has a huge impact on differential diagnosis. The greatest risk factor for head and neck cancer is still smoking. Though alcohol is not directly a carcinogen on exposure to the mouth or pharynx, it appears to have a synergistic effect on the risk of head and neck cancer in smokers [7].

The problem

The length of time the presenting complaint has been present is a good indicator for the risk of malignancy. Symptoms present and unchanged for years are unlikely to be malignant. Recent symptoms that are evolving are a worrying concern, e.g. dysphagia progressing from solids to fluids over a period of 3 months is concerning for hypopharyngeal or cervical oesophageal carcinoma, whereas dysphagia to tablets present and unchanged for 2 years is more likely to represent benign pathology such as a pharyngeal pouch or web.

It is also important to remember the evolution of pathology that can provide a unifying diagnosis. For instance, a posterior triangle firm neck lump as a presenting symptom associated with a persistent ipsilateral otalgia should raise concern for a nasopharyngeal carcinoma that has metastasised to a cervical lymph node.

Red flags

There are signs that should raise concern for malignancy. These include:

- Persistent hoarseness
- Progressive high dysphagia
- Unexplained otalgia
- Persistent sore throat
- Tobacco use
- High alcohol intake
- Previous cancer
- Previous radiation exposure (particularly in thyroid malignancy)
- Family history of cancer

EXAMINATION

The examination should be stepwise and comprehensive in every patient.

The neck should be inspected and palpated.

All areas of the oral cavity and oropharynx should be examined directly and, if appropriate, bimanual palpation of the salivary glands and their ducts should be performed.

Anterior rhinoscopy and fibre nasendoscopy should be performed. Again this should be systematic and stepwise to ensure the nasal cavity, nasopharynx, oropharynx, larynx and hypopharynx are examined. This is a dynamic examination, and symmetry and mobility of the larynx should be noted.

CONCLUSION

Differential diagnosis is guided by the clinician's knowledge of the anatomy, embryology and disease processes that can occur in the head and neck. The patient leads the diagnostic process with their history and allows the clinician to perform an examination, which leads to findings to complete the journey.

REFERENCES

1 Brennan P, Mahadevan V, Evans B et al. *Clinical Head and Neck Anatomy for Surgeons.* CRC Press; 2015.

2 Shoenwolf G, Bleyl S, Brauer P, Francis-West P. *Human Embryology.* Churchill Livingstone; 2015.

3 Chang ET, Adami HO. The enigmatic epidemiology of nasopharyngeal carcinoma. *Cancer Epidemiol Biomarkers Prev.* 2006;15(10):1765–77.

4 Leclerc A, Martinez Cortes M, Gerin M, Luce D, Brugere J. Sinonasal cancer and wood dust exposure: Results from a case-control study. *Am J Epidemiol.* 1994;140(4):340–49.

5 Langevin SM, McClean MD, Michaud DS, Eliot M, Nelson HH, Kelsey KT. Occupational dust exposure and head and neck squamous cell

carcinoma risk in a population-based case-control study conducted in the greater Boston area. *Cancer Med*. 2013;2(6):978–86.

6 Bray F, Ren JS, Masuyer E, Ferlay J. Global estimates of cancer prevalence for 27 sites in the adult population in 2008. *Int J Cancer*. 2013;132(5):1133–45.

7 Dal Maso L, Torelli N, Biancotto E et al. Combined effect of tobacco smoking and alcohol drinking in the risk of head and neck cancers: A re-analysis of case-control studies using bi-dimensional spline models. *Eur J Epidemiol*. 2016;31(4):385–93.

2

IMAGING IN HEAD AND NECK SURGERY

Salman Qureshi

INTRODUCTION

Imaging is an important element within head, neck and thyroid surgery. This is part of a multimodality, multidisciplinary approach that is a crucial aspect of deciding management plans and surgical intervention.

Multidisciplinary team (MDT) meetings provide an excellent forum for reviewing imaging. The key principles which will help all clinicians within this setting will be discussed in this chapter.

IMAGING MODALITIES

Broadly speaking, the different imaging modalities commonly used by the head and neck surgeon are summarised in **Table 2.1**.

▓ Magnetic resonance (MR) sequences

In addition to T1-/T2-weighted images (see **Table 2.1**), there are other sequences available on magnetic resonance imaging (MRI). If fluid is bright and fat is dark, this suggests the images could also be T2 fat saturated or a short T1 inversion recovery (STIR) sequence. High-resolution T2 images ('heavily T2 weighted' sequences) can also mimic this, as everything is dark except fluid. Common uses for this sequence in head and neck are assessment of the internal acoustic meatus or MR sialography to assess for sialectasis.

ANATOMIC SUBSITES

▓ Pharynx/pharyngeal mucosal space radiologic anatomy

The head and neck cancer MDTs will generally include any extracranial or extraorbital head and neck malignancies. Much of the focus will be on squamous cell carcinoma of the upper aerodigestive tract, particularly the pharynx. This comes under the category of pharyngeal mucosal space when using the classical neck space radiological anatomy

Table 2.1 List of imaging modalities commonly used in head and neck surgery.

Modality	Advantages
Plain film	• Can be used in the acute setting to assess for foreign body.
Ultrasound	• Valuable tool for assessing neck lumps, particularly lymph nodes, thyroid and salivary glands. • Guides fine needle aspiration or core biopsies.
Computerised tomography (CT)	• Better for bony/cartilage detail. • In oncology, primarily used in laryngeal malignancies. • In the acute setting for infection or inflammation, intravenous contrast is given.
Magnetic resonance imaging (MRI)	• Constitutes the bulk of oncology work outside the larynx. • T1 imaging signal characteristics include hyperintense fat and hypointense fluid, whereas T2 imaging is hyperintense for both fat and fluid. • Intravenous gadolinium is routinely administered in oncology scans taken up by vascular tissues, such as tumours, and therefore improves delineation of tumour margins. The presence of contrast can be assessed by reviewing the mucosal margin. This is best seen in the nasal turbinates, which have a rich vascular supply.
Nuclear medicine	• A radioisotope is administered to the patient. The patient is then the source of the radiation, which can then be localised by the use of a gamma camera. However, the information obtained is primarily functional rather than anatomical (and may be supplemented by CT for localisation). • It is particularly useful in parathyroid localisation. • Positive emission tomography (PET) is used in oncology work, particularly for assessment of the unknown primary and recurrent disease.

as characterised by Harnsberger (see **Table 2.2**) [1]. An understanding of the normal imaging anatomy will help navigate this space. MRI scan is the key modality for this.

Nasopharynx

Anatomy

The anterior margin is demarcated by the posterior choanae. The posterior wall contains the adenoids as part of Waldeyer's lymphatic ring. This regresses with age. Posterolaterally, the pharyngeal recesses, also known as the fossa of Rosenmuller, can be a difficult region for clinical evaluation due to obscuration by the cartilaginous torus tubarius. However, this area can be readily reviewed by radiological cross-sectional evaluation. Anterolateral to the torus tubarius will be the opening of the Eustachian tube. Laterally are the veli palatini muscles, which are important demarcators for staging of nasopharyngeal tumours.

Imaging characteristics

Radiologically, the nasopharynx is best evaluated by MR scan (see **Figure 2.1**). The T2 sequence will demonstrate mild hyperintensity of the mucosal surfaces. Any thickening of this enhancement raises the possibility of a mucosal lesion. Extension through the veli palatini muscles and into parapharyngeal or retropharyngeal tissues can be demarcated on MR, particularly on the post contrast images using a combination of fat saturation and non-fat saturation.

Squamous cell carcinoma (SCC) will normally be centred on the fossa of Rosenmuller.

Oropharynx

Anatomy

The oropharynx contains continuation of Waldeyer's ring including the palatine tonsils and the lingual tonsil of the tongue base. These are separated by the anterior tonsillar pillar, which is formed by a projection of

Table 2.2 Harnsberger's radiologic neck spaces with contents and anatomic relations.

Neck space	Contents and relations
Parapharyngeal	Fat filled No foramina from skull base No muscle, mucosa or nodes Encroachment from adjacent spaces
Retropharyngeal	Fat and nodes – suprahyoid Fat only – infrahyoid Extends inferiorly into mediastinum Nodes drainage of naso/oropharynx
Perivertebral	Vertebral column, spinal canal Paraspinal muscles Nerves – phrenic, brachial plexus Vertebral artery
Posterior cervical	Between sternocleidomastoid and trapezius (level V) Accessory nerve
Parotid	Parotid gland Facial nerve and divisions via stylomastoid foramen ECA and retromandibular vein
Carotid	Carotid arteries and internal jugular vein (IJV) CN IX–XII (CN X only in infrahyoid) Jugular foramen/carotid canal – aortic arch
Masticator	4 muscles – masseter, temporalis, medial and lateral pterygoids CN V3 Foramen ovale and spinosum
Visceral	Infrahyoid Thyroid and parathyroid glands Cervical trachea and oesophagus CN X branches

the palatoglossus muscle. Whereas the palatine tonsil is separated from the posterior pharyngeal wall by the posterior tonsillar pillar, which is formed by a projection of the palatopharyngeus muscle.

Imaging characteristics

MR is the best modality due to greater soft tissue differential delineation. The mucosa has similar MRI characteristics as the nasopharynx. Lymphoid tissue in the palatine and lingual tonsils are mildly hyperintense on T2 with a dark band representing the tonsillar pillars (see **Figure 2.2**).

Tonsillar SCC will demonstrate avid enhancement allowing appreciation of tumour extension through pharyngeal walls. Nodal metastases can be evaluated on the MR scan (see **Figure 2.3**).

Hypopharynx

Three structures form the hypopharynx:

- *Pyriform sinus:* This is the anterolateral recess located posterolateral to the aryepiglottic fold, and the inferior apex is at the level of the true vocal cord.
- *Posterior pharyngeal wall:* Inferior continuation of the posterior oropharyngeal wall.
- *Post cricoid region:* Junction of pharynx and oesophagus.

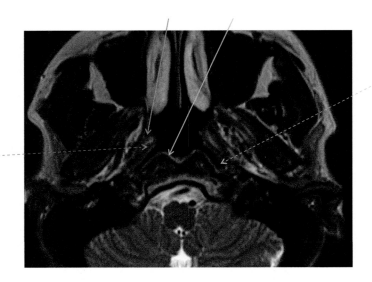

Figure 2.1 Axial T2 MRI neck showing the pertinent structures of the nasopharynx including the torus tubarius (dashed dark blue), Eustachian tube opening (dark blue) and fossa of Rosenmuller (dashed light blue). Note how the normal mucosal margin has a thin hyperintense line (light blue).

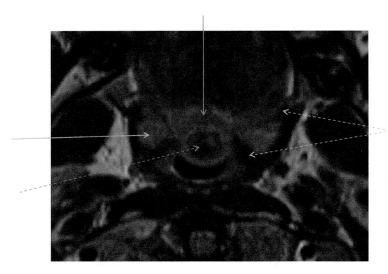

Figure 2.2 Axial T2 MRI neck demonstrating the normal oropharynx. The palatine tonsils (light blue) and lingual tonsil (dark blue) are mildly hyperintense with a darker band representing the tonsillar pillars (dashed light blue). The uvula (dashed dark blue) is also noted.

MRI is the preferred modality, but due to close proximity to the larynx, computerised tomography (CT) is also commonly used. The MRI mucosal characteristics are similar to the other pharyngeal subsites (see **Figure 2.4**).

Both MR and CT can assess expansion into the larynx and cartilage destruction as well as parapharyngeal or paraglottic fat involvement. However, decalcification associated with increasing age must be taken into account when considering cartilage destruction.

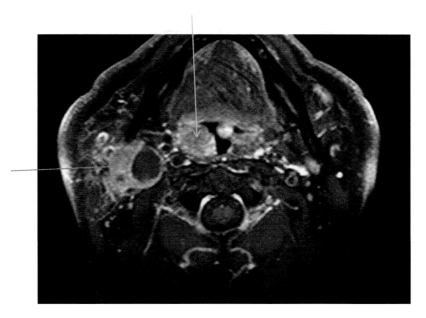

Figure 2.3 Axial T1 fat sat with contrast MRI neck demonstrating enlarged right palatine tonsil (light blue) with ipsilateral enlarged necrotic right level 2 node (dark blue) in keeping with squamous cell carcinoma and nodal metastases.

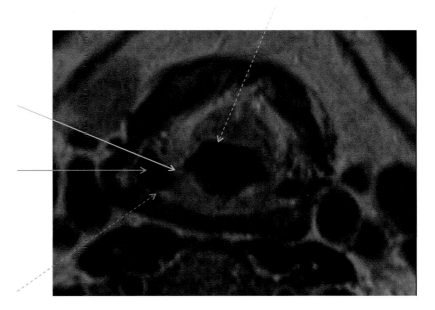

Figure 2.4 Axial T2 MRI neck demonstrating the hypopharynx posterior to the supraglottic larynx with epiglottis (dashed light blue). The pyriform sinus (dark blue) is posterolateral to the aryepiglottic fold (light blue) and anterior to the posterior pharyngeal wall (dashed dark blue).

CT is generally the preferred modality, primarily to counteract the effect of motion artefact due to breathing and swallowing. CT is sensitive for cartilage invasion, though the role of faster acquisition MR sequences is growing [2,3].

The supraglottis and subglottis are separated by the glottis (true vocal cords). All these subsections are appreciated well on CT with delineation of the appropriate cartilages (see **Figure 2.5**).

Formal staging of SCC cannot be based solely on radiology as vocal cord mobility has an implication. Impaired vocal cord mobility will upgrade localised tumours to T2 and similarly vocal cord fixation will upgrade to T3 (see **Figure 2.6**). Radiologically, the depth of thyroid cartilage involvement will differentiate between T3 and T4 tumours (see Chapter 11).

Supraglottic tumours tend to have a greater propensity for nodal metastases. This is primarily due to

the embryological origin from the buccopharyngeal analge, which is rich in lymphatics. This is opposed to the subglottis that is derived from the tracheobronchial buds, which have sparse lymphatics.

Neck spaces

Radiologically, the neck is subdivided into nine neck spaces commonly referred to as the Harnsberger neck spaces (see **Table 2.2** and **Figure 2.7**). The pharyngeal mucosal space has already been discussed in detail.

Cervical lymph nodes

To provide cross-speciality conformity, particularly in the setting of a multidisciplinary team, the standard cervical levels are used in radiology. Levels 1–6 are within the neck, with level 7 representing superior mediastinal nodes. Other groups of head and

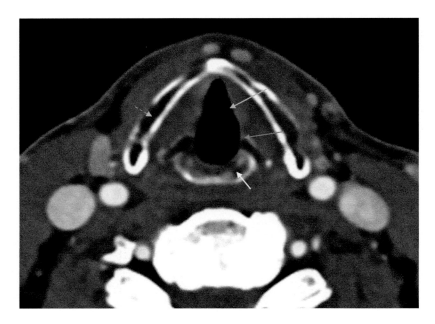

Figure 2.5 Contrast-enhanced axial CT demonstrating the normal position of the true cords (light blue). Note the vocal process of the arytenoid cartilage attached to the vocalis muscle (dark blue). The laryngeal cartilages are well demonstrated due to calcific high attenuation including the thyroid (dashed light blue) and cricoid (white) cartilages.

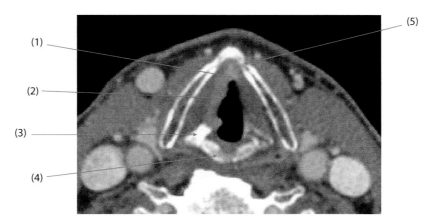

Figure 2.6 Axial CT neck with contrast neck demonstrating an exophytic lesion (2) emanating from the right vocal cord in keeping with squamous cell carcinoma. This extends to the anterior commissure (1) and the thyroid cartilage appears thinned on the contralateral side (5), however this is due to variable demineralisation rather than malignant encroachment. Cricoid cartilage (4) is intact though there is sclerosis of the ipsilateral arytenoid cartilage (3) which can be a sign of tumour infiltration.

Table 2.3 BTA thyroid nodules ultrasound classification.

Classification	Definition	Findings
U1	Normal	
U2	Benign	a. Halo, isoechoic/mildly hyperechoic b. Cystic change ± ring down sign (colloid) c. Microcystic/spongiform d. Peripheral eggshell calcification e. As (d) f. Peripheral vascularity
U3	Indeterminate	a. Homogeneous, markedly hyperechoic, solid, halo b. Hypoechoic, equivocal echogenic foci, cystic change c. Central/mixed vascularity
U4	Suspicious	a. Solid, hypoechoic b. Solid, very hypoechoic c. Disrupted peripheral calcification, hypoechoic d. Lobulated outline
U5	Malignant	a. Solid, hypoechoic, lobulated, irregular outline, microcalcification b. Solid, hypoechoic, lobulated, irregular outline, globular calcification c. Intranodular vascularity d. Taller than wide shape e. Associated lymphadenopathy

Source: Perros P et al. *Clin Endocrinol (Oxf)*. 2014;81 (Suppl 1):1–122.

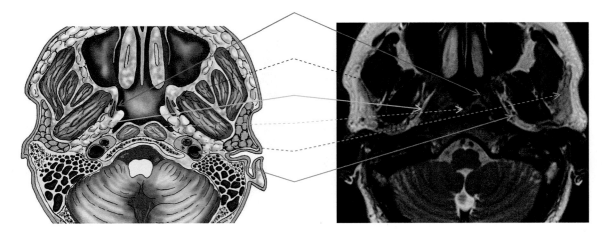

Figure 2.7 Graphic and axial T2 MRI scan demonstrating the major neck spaces. Pharyngeal mucosal space at the level of the nasopharynx (gray). Masticator space (dashed black) with the pterygoid musculature. Parapharyngeal space (light blue) containing hyperintense fat. Retropharyngeal space (dashed light blue). Parotid space (dashed dark blue). Carotid space (dark blue) containing vasculature and vagus nerve.

neck nodes not included in these levels include the parotid, facial and retropharyngeal [4].

Radiologically, both cross-sectional modalities provide similar sensitivities for evaluating cervical nodes. Identification of the hyoid bone will allow differentiation between levels I/VI and levels II/III. Identification of the cricoid cartilage will allow differentiation between levels III and IV. The posterior border of the sternocleidomastoid muscle allows differentiation between levels II, III, IV anteriorly and level V posteriorly.

Normal node characteristics

Normal nodes have a characteristic oval shape. Assessment of nodes involves measurement of the short axis and a general demarcation is 10 mm. Short axis enlargement beyond this suggests lymphadenopathy. However, this is variable at different levels. For example, a level 1a node measuring 9 mm in short axis

would be suspicious, whereas a slightly larger node measuring 12 mm in short axis in level 2 may still be within acceptable limits for this specific level.

Ultrasound can help in further evaluation of equivocal nodes (in all groups mentioned earlier except the retropharyngeal group). Sonographic appearances have the advantage of giving high-resolution internal architecture of the node. Typical benign ultrasound nodal characteristics include:

- Oval morphology
- Hyperechoic hilum
- Hilar vascularity
- Subcentimetre in short axis

Absence of these raises suspicion of lymphadenopathy. Ultrasound then has the further advantage of allowing direct sampling by fine needle aspiration or even core biopsy under imaging guidance.

POSITRON EMISSION TOMOGRAPHY (PET)

PET scanning utilises radiotracers to identify metabolic activity. Radiotracers are molecules labelled with a small amount of radioactive material to enable

identification on the scan. The most commonly used radiotracer is 18-fluorodeoxyglucose (18-FDG). This is essentially a radioactive glucose. It is taken up by cells and used as an energy source. Cells with an increased metabolic rate take up increased amounts of 18-FDG and appear avid on PET scans ('hot spots'). PET scanning has low resolution, but can be fused with CT scans so all them can be interpreted together. Hot spots on PET scans can be due to cancer (cancerous cells have increased metabolic rates and increased rates of glycolysis), infection or inflammation.

In head and neck cancer, PET scanning is used to assess response to non-surgical treatment (e.g. in oropharyngeal SCC treated with concurrent chemoradiotherapy), or to detect occult cervical lymph node metastases, distant metastases or synchronous primary tumour. It should be performed at least 3 months following treatment. Remnant activity in the primary site or nodal metastases treated raise suspicion for residual disease. The PET-NECK trial established the reliability of PET-CT-guided surveillance of patients following non-surgical treatment of oropharyngeal SCC [5]. Patients with a negative PET-CT scan can be reassured they have had a complete response to treatment (i.e. PET-CT has a high negative predictive value). Patients with equivocal

PET-CT scans of cervical lymph nodes post-treatment can either be treated with neck dissection or followed up with repeat PET-CT, or undergo ultrasound-guided fine needle aspiration cytology (USS FNAC) to try to confirm malignancy. The PET-NECK study (and others) suggest patients with equivocal post-treatment PET-CT scans have approximately 20% risk of residual carcinoma in the cervical lymph nodes [5,6]. This is similar to the standard risk threshold used elsewhere in head and neck cancer to decide whether to electively treat the neck [7].

▋ Practicalities

A period of 4–6 hours of fasting is required prior to PET scanning.

Strenuous exercise must be avoided for 24–48 hours prior to scanning.

A blood glucose of <200 mg/dL is also recommended at the time of scanning.

THYROID

The different histological subtypes of thyroid malignancy are covered in Chapter 6. Fundamental to the imaging characteristics of the different subtypes is an understanding of thyroid nodule evaluation. This is strongly dependant on the use of ultrasound. The British Thyroid Association (BTA) guidelines have developed a grading system based on ultrasound (see **Table 2.3**) [8].

Ultrasound also has the advantage of allowing concurrent fine needle aspiration. Traditionally, nuclear medicine has had a role in determining the presence of so-called 'hot' and 'cold' nodules (which still retain some role in medical management), but with the advent of the BTA guidelines, functional imaging has a limited role in the evaluation of potential malignancy [5]. The exception is incidental FDG avid thyroid nodules on PET. In some studies, these have up to 40% risk of malignancy and therefore these require formal evaluation including fine needle

aspiration and possible diagnostic hemithyroidectomy [9,10].

Cross-sectional imaging has limited role in evaluation of thyroid nodules. However, CT is useful in preoperative assessment of thyroid goitres allowing review of retrosternal extension, tracheal deviation and tracheal compression.

▋ Differentiated thyroid carcinoma

Differentiated thyroid carcinoma includes the histological subtypes of papillary, follicular and follicular variant of papillary carcinoma. The imaging for these follows the fundamental principles of the BTA guidelines for nodule evaluation [8]. As well as primary lesion evaluation, ultrasound has the advantage of histological evaluation with fine needle aspiration. Further to this, ultrasound also allows assessment of nodal metastatic spread. This is essential for subsequent management plans discussed in the MDT meeting.

Cross-sectional imaging (either MR or CT) can help in assessing invasion of adjacent structures, particularly the trachea, and in assessing retrosternal extent. However, when performing CT it is important to perform a scan without iodinated contrast, as administration of this can potentially delay radioiodine treatment.

▉ Medullary carcinoma

Nodular evaluation follows BTA guidelines as for differentiated thyroid cancer. However, medullary carcinoma has the added angle of association with type 2 multiple endocrine neoplasia (MEN). This involves systemic imaging for assessments of MEN type 2, for example, diagnosing the presence of pheochromocytomas. Nuclear medicine such as octreotide scintigraphy can help with assessment of MEN type 2.

▉ Anaplastic carcinoma

Anaplastic carcinoma will clinically present as a rapidly growing thyroid mass. In the case of anaplastic subtype, cross-sectional imaging is useful. CT in particular will show extent of the tumour along with invasion of adjacent structures, particularly the trachea. Calcification is a common feature. CT findings demonstrate heterogeneous enhancement with hypoenhancing necrosis.

▉ Thyroid lymphoma

Thyroid lymphoma may clinically present similar to anaplastic but is prognostically much better. CT imaging will demonstrate a thyroid mass. However, the radiological difference between anaplastic and lymphoma is that the latter will be much more homogeneous in attenuation characteristics and enhancement. Calcification and necrosis are rare. In addition, lymphoma comparatively respects adjacent structures and rather than invading them will tend to circumnavigate them or surround them.

PARATHYROID

A dual approach is adopted in many centres. This involves an ultrasound test to identify a parathyroid adenoma in the peri-thyroid region. This is combined with a nuclear medicine test, which confirms the presence and potential location of the adenoma. The isotope most commonly used is Technetium (Tc) 99 m Sestamibi. This will allow a focused approach during surgery.

More recent techniques involve the use of so-called 4D-CT. This involves three scans being performed at the same sitting including the upper thorax. The first scan is non-contrast, then an arterial phase contrast scan is performed and finally a delayed phase is completed. The theory involves the relative rapid washout of parathyroid adenomas, thereby being highest attenuation on the arterial phase scan. This will allow differentiation from other structures such as lymph nodes [11].

Choline PET-CT uses choline-based radiotracers to localise parathyroid adenomas. It has demonstrated favourable outcomes with high sensitivity and detection rates [12]. In difficult-to-localise cases or patients requiring repeat operation, a combination of these modalities may be the best approach rather than considering one better than the other. It is preferable to have adjunctive approaches available for challenging cases [13].

In cases where parathyroid adenomas cannot be localised on nuclear medicine or cross-sectional imaging, then interventional radiology may have a role. This involves parathyroid venous sampling. This involves catheterising the femoral vein and sampling blood from veins closely associated with each parathyroid gland. The vein with the highest parathyroid hormone level is presumed to be draining the adenomatous gland [14]. However, since surgical intervention after equivocal investigations tends to involve four-gland parathyroid exploration, the use of venous sampling tends to be reserved for reoperation due to persistent post-surgical hyperparathyroidism.

REFERENCES

1 Harnsberger HR, Glastonbury CM, Michel MA, Koch BL. *Head and Neck.* 2nd ed. Lippincott Williams & Wilkins; 2010.

2 Adolphs AP, Boersma NA, Diemel BD et al. A systematic review of computed tomography detection of cartilage invasion in laryngeal carcinoma. *Laryngoscope.* 2015;125:1650–5.

3 Kuno H, Sakamaki K, Fujii S et al. Comparison of MR imaging and dual-energy CT for the evaluation of cartilage invasion by laryngeal and hypopharyngeal squamous cell carcinoma. *AJNR Am J Neuroradiol.* 2018;39:524–31.

4 Gregoire V, Ang K, Budach W et al. Delineation of the neck node levels for head and neck tumors: A 2013 update. DAHANCA, EORTC, HKNPCSG, NCIC CTG, NCRI, RTOG, TROG consensus guidelines. *Radiother Oncol.* 2014;110:172–81.

5 Mehanna H, Wong WL, McConkey CC et al. PET-CT surveillance versus neck dissection in advanced head and neck cancer. *N Engl J Med.* 2016;374:1444–54.

6 Slevin F, Subesinghe M, Ramasamy S, Sen M, Scarsbrook AF, Prestwich RJ. Assessment of outcomes with delayed (18)F-FDG PET-CT response assessment in head and neck squamous cell carcinoma. *Br J Radiol.* 2015;88:20140592.

7 Weiss MH, Harrison LB, Isaacs RS. Use of decision analysis in planning a management strategy for the stage N0 neck. *Arch Otolaryngol Head Neck Surg.* 1994;120: 699–702.

8 Perros P, Boelaert K, Colley S et al. Guidelines for the management of thyroid cancer. *Clin Endocrinol (Oxf).* 2014;81 (Suppl 1):1–122.

9 Chun AR, Jo HM, Lee SH et al. Risk of malignancy in thyroid incidentalomas identified by fluorodeoxyglucose-positron emission tomography. *Endocrinol Metab (Seoul).* 2015;30:71–7.

10 Bertagna F, Treglia G, Piccardo A, Giubbini R. Diagnostic and clinical significance of F-18-FDG-PET/CT thyroid incidentalomas. *J Clin Endocrinol Metab.* 2012;97:3866–75.

11 Chazen JL, Gupta A, Dunning A, Phillips CD. Diagnostic accuracy of 4D-CT for parathyroid adenomas and hyperplasia. *AJNR Am J Neuroradiol.* 2012;33:429–33.

12 Broos WAM, van der Zant FM, Knol RJJ, Wondergem M. Choline PET/CT in parathyroid imaging: A systematic review. *Nucl Med Commun.* 2019;40:96–105.

13 Amadou C, Bera G, Ezziane M et al. 18F-Fluorocholine PET/CT and parathyroid 4D computed tomography for primary hyperparathyroidism: The challenge of reoperative patients. *World J Surg.* 2019;43:1232–42.

14 Taslakian B, Trerotola SO, Sacks B, Oklu R, Deipolyi A. The essentials of parathyroid hormone venous sampling. *Cardiovasc Intervent Radiol.* 2017;40:9–21.

3 PERIOPERATIVE ISSUES

Gordon A. G. McKenzie and David J. H. Shipway

INTRODUCTION

The demographics of the surgical population are changing drastically. In 2050, triple the number of people are projected to be 80 years of age or over compared to 2015 [1]. Advanced *chronological* age closely correlates with adverse postoperative outcomes, and whilst age could be an independent risk factor, uncertainty exists whether it is the associated sequelae of ageing that are actually responsible. Recent interest has focused more closely on the features of adverse ageing. These include:

- Co-morbidity and multi-morbidity (three or more co-existing illnesses)
- Adverse functional status (degree of dependency)
- Frailty (discussed later) [2]

Older patients who lack these characteristics can be considered to have a lower *biological* age and therefore a lower risk profile.

Within the oncogeriatric population, where (radical) surgery offers an important curative modality for head, neck and thyroid cancer, decision-making and perioperative care particularly challenges the surgeon. It is increasingly recognised that many perioperative complications experienced by older surgical patients are in fact medical and not necessarily related to the specific surgical procedure. This observation has generated authoritative guidelines and successful models of geriatrician-led preoperative optimisation and proactive, embedded surgical liaison [3–5]. These models of care probably represent a future surgical model whereby issues with surgical training [6] can be overcome by greater collaboration between surgical and medical teams. For now, perioperative medicine remains the responsibility of the surgical team, with support from perioperative physicians, most of whom remain anaesthetists.

MANAGEMENT OF MEDICAL CO-MORBIDITY

Chronological age should not be a contraindication for otolaryngological surgery. For cancer surgery, age, medical background and biological behaviour of the tumour should be considered together with

the likely oncological, perioperative and long-term cosmetic, functional and quality-of-life outcomes. For example, the ability to provide tracheostomy and enteral feeding tube care needs to be considered [7].

Microvascular reconstructive options following radical oncological resection, such as total laryngectomy, have increased risk of complications in the older patient [7]. Furthermore, reduction of shoulder mobility after radical neck dissection has been associated with chronological age [8], exemplifying the need to consider the issue of compounding adverse functional outcomes in the older patient.

When considering a patient for surgery, the medical background provides the first insight into the patient's ability to survive, recover and ultimately benefit from surgery. An increased burden of co-morbidity, as measured by the Adult Comorbidity Evaluation–27, predicts worse survival, functional and quality of life outcomes in addition to higher risk of perioperative complications. Accurate co-morbidity data collection is therefore mandated for both risk counselling and future surgical oncological research [9]. The American Society of Anaesthesiologists (ASA) Grade 4–5 was independently associated with increased non-surgical complications following thyroid surgery, reaching 19% in one series. Length of stay increases linearly with chronological age in thyroid surgery, although mortality in specialist centres is favourable [10].

There are authoritative 2016 UK guidelines [9] on pre-treatment clinical assessment in head and neck cancer (HNC), although fast-paced medical research already outdates some elements [11]. Other guidelines referenced herein can be used track future validity.

▌ Cardiovascular

Decisions on preoperative cardiovascular investigation and intervention should ideally occur between the surgical multidisciplinary team (MDT), cardiologist, anaesthetist and, where available, perioperative geriatrician who may play a role in post-surgical inpatient management. A summary of definite recommendations from authoritative guidelines are made for clarity and brevity.

Preoperative risk assessment

The risk of perioperative myocardial infarction or cardiac arrest can be independently predicted by age,

Table 3.1 Type of surgery and cardiovascular risk.

Low risk (1%)	Intermediate risk (1%–5%)	High risk (>5%)
Superficial surgery	Head and neck surgery	Head and neck procedures involving oesophagectomy
Thyroid surgery		
Reconstructive		

Source: Modified from 2014 ESC/ESA guidelines, Kristensen SD et al. *Eur Heart J.* 2014;35(35): 2383–431.

type of surgery (see **Table 3.1**), functional status (i.e. degree of dependency), ASA grade and serum creatinine. This forms the Gupta Perioperative Cardiac Risk Calculator (http://www.surgicalriskcalculator.com/miorcardiacarrest) and may inform decisions relating to continuation of antiplatelet agents in the perioperative period, where routine practice may be to recommend temporary cessation [12].

Hypertension

Non-urgent surgery should be delayed until blood pressure is controlled below 160/100 mm Hg. However, moderate hypertension with target organ damage warrants counselling for the higher risk of perioperative major cardiovascular events. Preoperative optimisation of hypertension is recommended using established guidelines [13]; specialist medically *enhanced pre-assessment* services may achieve more rapid optimisation and prevent delays to surgery.

Structural heart disease

All patients undergoing head and neck surgery with known or suspected valvular heart disease should undergo preoperative resting echocardiography [12].

Ischaemic heart disease

All patients undergoing head and neck surgery with the following risk factors should undergo preoperative resting electrocardiogram (ECG):

- Age over 55 years
- Ischaemic heart disease (IHD)
- Heart failure, stroke
- Transient ischaemic attack (TIA)
- Serum creatinine >170 µmol/L (or creatinine clearance <60 mL/min/1.73 m²)
- Diabetes mellitus requiring insulin therapy

Only those patients undergoing high-risk (**Table 3.1**) procedures with poor functional capacity, as estimated by the inability to climb two flights of stairs (less than four metabolic equivalents), and three or more of these risk factors should undergo image stress testing [12].

The deployment of stents in the coronary vasculature requires antiplatelet cover to reduce the risk of stent thrombosis and myocardial infarction (MI) until the stent has undergone successful endothelialisation. The type of previous percutaneous coronary intervention (PCI) and stenting determines the minimum recommended duration of dual antiplatelet therapy (DAPT), and therefore may affect the timing of elective surgery. Cessation of DAPT prior to these timeframes represents an increased risk of perioperative in-stent thrombosis and acute MI, which is associated with greatly increased cardiovascular mortality:

a   Bare metal stent (30 days)
b   Drug-eluting stent (3–6 months, depending on product used; upper limit preferred)
c   Balloon angioplasty (2 weeks or more) [11]

Generally, indications for coronary angiography and preoperative coronary revascularisation mirror those in the non-surgical setting. Recent MI or coronary intervention requires discussion with cardiology, as rapid access to interventional cardiology or delay of surgery (even in the context of HNC) may outweigh the risk of perioperative ischaemia [12]. Current evidence indicates that prophylactic coronary intervention in asymptomatic IHD in the preoperative setting does not improve outcomes from surgery; it is therefore not advocated outside of a trial setting.

Arrhythmias

Existing anti-arrhythmic agents should be continued perioperatively, including on the morning of surgery, taken with a sip of water at least 2 hours before anaesthesia, even if nil by mouth (see Section 'Perioperative medication management and prescribing').

Intraoperative electrocautery use within 30 cm of pacing devices or leads can interfere with permanent pacemaker function, which requires battery and threshold checks to have been conducted within the last year before surgery. Pacemaker-patients should be referred to cardiac pacing services before surgery to determine if reprogramming is required to allow diathermy. Pacemaker-dependent patients may need their device rendered non-sensing by placing a magnet over the skin of the pacemaker during surgery. Implantable cardioverter defibrillator devices must be deactivated before surgery, continuously monitored intraoperatively and reactivated postoperatively by the cardiac pacing services [9,12].

Heart failure

The poor prognosis of advanced heart failure is under-recognised, although an important cause of perioperative morbidity. Fifty per cent of patients with severe heart failure or heart failure with untreatable aetiology will die within 1 or 4 years, respectively. Perioperative risk is higher than IHD alone. Preoperative optimisation is required in new or poorly controlled heart failure. Where not contraindicated, an angiotensin converting enzyme (ACE) inhibitor and beta blocker should be commenced or uptitrated before surgery. Right heart failure carries higher perioperative risk than left ventricular failure, as patients with pulmonary hypertension represent a significant anaesthetic challenge. Planned critical care admission may be advised [9].

▉ Respiratory

Smoking is an established risk factor for HNC and smoking cessation at any time preoperatively improves outcomes [14]. Combined extended cognitive behaviour therapy counselling with pharmacotherapy appears effective [15]. Concomitant and undiagnosed chronic obstructive pulmonary disease (COPD) is common in HNC and this should be optimised preoperatively (see **Box 3.1**). Suspected or unconfirmed COPD is one of a few indications for requesting preoperative spirometry [16,17].

> **Box 3.1 Preoperative optimisation of respiratory disease**
> - Smoking cessation and pre-operative pulmonary rehabilitation
> - Sputum sampling to tailor antibiotic regimens for postoperative pneumonia
> - Delaying surgery during or immediately following lower respiratory tract infection
> - Optimise bronchodilator therapy per established treatment algorithms and trial steroid responsiveness in moderate and severe disease
> - Optimise continuous positive pressure (CPAP) mask fitting and anticipate any postoperative anatomical changes
> - Plan to convert inhalers to nebulisers perioperatively
>
> *Source*: Adapted from Robson A et al. *J Laryngol Otol.* 2016;130(S2):S13–S22.

Guidelines [17] recommend that patients undergoing head and neck surgery require perioperative intervention to reduce postoperative pulmonary complications. Higher-risk patients (COPD, age >60 years, ASA 2 or more, functionally dependent or heart failure) may benefit from deep breathing exercises or incentive spirometry postoperatively.

Routine chest radiographs are not advocated by national guidelines, and many HNC surgical patients will have had staging imaging of the chest [18]. Patients with saturations less than 93% on air should have arterial blood gas sampling to quantify hypoxia and hypercarbia. As discussed earlier, identification of right heart disease and pulmonary hypertension is essential, therefore an echocardiogram may be required. The presence of hypoxia, hypercarbia or cor pulmonale together with a forced expiratory volume over one second (FEV_1) of less than 25% associates strongly with postoperative ventilatory failure and support [9].

Obstructive sleep apnoea (OSA) is an important co-morbidity, and obese patients should be screened for OSA using validated scores (e.g. Epworth Scale and STOP-BANG) [19]. Preoperative diagnostic sleep studies may influence anaesthetic technique, airway management, extubation protocols and postoperative ventilatory support [20].

Postoperative high dependency admission may be advised in known or suspected OSA or those with significant pulmonary hypertension, heart failure or significant diastolic dysfunction [9].

▌ Neurological and cognitive disorders

Cognitive impairment and dementia

The risk of postoperative delirium (POD) is markedly elevated in patients with pre-existing cognitive impairment, and preoperative cognitive screening should be considered in older patients, or in those with known or suspected diagnosis of cognitive impairment or dementia [5]. There is no consensus on screening tool, and individual centres must balance the test sensitivity with pragmatic factors such as time taken for completion of cognitive screening. Where cognitive impairment is clearly suspected, the Montreal Cognitive Assessment is commonly used to document severity of impairment [21]. Informed consent for surgery requires the patient to display mental capacity to make decisions regarding medical treatment (see **Box 3.2**). In English law, where capacity is absent and no attorney has been legally appointed to make decisions of behalf of the patient, a best-interests decision must be made by the MDT, in accordance with the Mental Capacity Act (2005) [22]. Dementia is a terminal condition with limited prognosis, and where capacity is absent, specialist perioperative geriatrician advice should be sought to ascertain prognosis and the absolute risks and benefits of surgical intervention.

Undiagnosed cognitive impairment or dementia identified in the preassessment clinic require preoperative investigation for reversible causes (see **Box 3.3**).

Stroke

Perioperative stroke approaches 5% following HNC surgery and is usually embolic carrying mortality of 26%. Risk factors largely mirror the general population and past cerebrovascular disease is a strong predictor [23]. Where possible, surgery should be delayed within 3 months of a stroke due to higher risk of a major adverse vascular event [24]. Carotid Doppler imaging should be arranged for stroke in the past year according to national HNC guidelines [9], although international guidelines recommend carotid artery and cerebral imaging for stroke or TIA in the preceding 6 months [12]. Where possible, head and neck surgery should be delayed in symptomatic carotid disease (stroke or TIA of the corresponding vascular territory in the past 6 months) [12]. The focus preoperatively is optimisation of modifiable risk factors such as hypertension and continuation of antithrombotic or antiplatelet therapy (see section 'Perioperative medication management and prescribing'). Where surgery must proceed, hypotension must be avoided and meticulous intraoperative care taken to protect the carotid vessels [9].

Parkinson's disease

Parkinson's disease is associated with increased perioperative complications and length of stay.

Imaging due to movement artefacts from dyskinesia and deep brain stimulators (potential magnetic resonance imaging [MRI] contraindication) pose additional challenges. To avoid perioperative complications such as rigidity and bradykinesia ('off' states), enteral or parenteral access must be available for antiparkinsonian drugs to be administered with strict dosing schedules. This should be achieved via nasogastric feeding tubes, or conversion of oral antiparkinsonian drugs to transdermal rotigotine when the gastrointestinal tract is inaccessible or non-functioning. Preoperative input with a specialist in Parkinson's disease is recommended. Planned preoperative substitution of monoamine oxidase B inhibitors (which can interact with anaesthetic agents) should occur [9,23].

Epilepsy

Epilepsy is associated with elevated risk of postoperative infection, acute kidney injury (AKI) and stroke. Perioperative seizure risk is proportional to baseline seizure frequency and preoperative optimisation is recommended wherever possible. Perioperative medication management is highlighted in the section 'Perioperative medication management and prescribing'. Other perioperative considerations are vagal nerve stimulators (an MRI contraindication) and those controlled on ketogenic diets (additional biochemical monitoring). Perioperative seizure frequency is quoted as 2%–6% and opioids tend to be pro-convulsive [23].

▮ Endocrine and metabolic

Diabetes mellitus

Suboptimal preoperative control of diabetes is associated with multiple adverse outcomes of surgery. Preoperative HbA_{1c} measures glycaemic control over the past 3 months. Perioperative dysglycaemia tends to occur where HbA_{1c} is over 69 mmol/mol and associates with increased surgical site infections, postoperative complications, critical care admission and inpatient mortality. Wherever possible, these patients and those with hypoglycaemic unawareness should have their medication optimised by a diabetologist preoperatively. However, the perioperative risks of suboptimal diabetic control must be carefully balanced against the risks of surgical delay, especially in the context of HNC [9].

In the perioperative period, glucose levels should ideally be maintained within 6–12 mmol/L. Guidelines [25] recommend that admission on the day of surgery remains appropriate although 'first-on-the-list' operating priority and availability of diabetes-specialist support should be provided. Caution is advised with anti-embolism stockings in the context of coexistent peripheral vascular disease and diabetic neuropathy. Management algorithms can be complex and local guidelines should be followed. **Figure 3.1** illustrates the management of perioperative hyperglycaemia [25].

Key considerations for perioperative management are the existing control (HbA_{1c}), type of diabetes, starvation period, timing of the surgery and predicted self-management capabilities postoperatively. The key points of a variable rate intravenous insulin infusion are listed in **Box 3.4**. Postoperative high dependency admission may need consideration in patients with poor glycaemic control and those with significant cardiac and renal diabetic complications [25].

Thyroid disease

Mild hypothyroidism is associated with postoperative delirium (POD) and ileus, although elective surgery is generally considered safe. More significant hypothyroidism may warrant postponement of non-urgent elective surgery for thyroid hormone replacement (see also **Table 3.3**). In circumstances where urgent or emergent surgery is required and severe hypothyroidism is present (e.g. myxoedema coma or heart failure), perioperative treatment with intravenous liothyronine sodium and corticosteroids will be required [26].

Thyroid storm is the most significant perioperative risk in the patient with hyperthyroidism. This rare complication is characterised by delirium and fever with potentially life-threatening haemodynamic instability. Preoperative beta blockade is used for prevention of perioperative thyroid storm. Elective surgery should be delayed until euthyroid status is obtained in moderate or severe hyperthyroidism. Where surgery is urgent or emergent, premedication is required with antithyroid drugs (e.g. propylthiouracil) and beta blockade. Corticosteroids may also be required [26].

Hypovitaminosis D

Vitamin D insufficiency and deficiency are very common in the general population. Hypovitaminosis D is seemingly associated with diverse adverse surgical outcomes and may affect post-surgical rehabilitation and fatigue in cancer patients [27,28]. Preoperative vitamin D correction has not yet been proven to improve perioperative outcomes, but has non-surgical benefits in the frail older adult and is therefore recommended [29].

Anaemia

Anaemia adversely influences surgical outcomes with effects proportional to severity. It may also indicate important underlying coexistent disease requiring evaluation. Basic evaluation of the anaemia may identify a specific deficiency (**Box 3.5**). Iron deficiency may indicate potential gastrointestinal malignancy, but is also common in benign disease (e.g. angiodysplasia) in the elderly. Intravenous iron (ideally given >2 weeks preoperatively) may optimise marrow function and reduce the need for perioperative blood

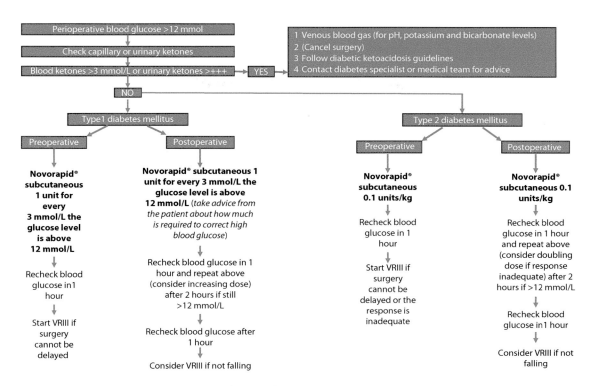

Figure 3.1 Perioperative management of hyperglycaemia.

Box 3.4 Key points relating to variable rate intravenous insulin infusion (VRIII)

- Previously termed 'sliding scale' (it is recommended to avoid this ambiguous term)
- Indications for VRII
  - Long starvation period anticipated (i.e. two or more missed meals)
  - Decompensated diabetes
- Recommended fluid prescription with VRIII
  - 5% glucose in 0.45% saline and 0.15% or 0.3% potassium
- Minimum investigations during VRIII
  - Hourly capillary blood glucose
  - Daily electrolytes
- Existing diabetes medications whilst VRIII running
  - Short-acting insulins (e.g. NovoMix): Stop until eating and drinking normally
  - Intermediate-acting insulins (e.g. Humulin I): Stop until eating and drinking normally
  - Long-acting insulins (e.g. Lantus, Levemir or Tresiba): Continue at 80% of the usual dose (reduces risk of rebound hyperglycaemia when VRIII discontinued)
  - Non-insulin medications: Stop all until eating and drinking normally
    - Except GLP-1 analogues (e.g. exenatide) – take as normal

transfusion. Where anaemia is severe, completion of blood transfusion should ideally occur 24–48 hours preoperatively. Other general strategies which may be important in individual circumstances include optimisation of erythropoiesis (e.g. preoperative erythropoietin-stimulating agents) and minimisation of perioperative iatrogenic blood loss [9,30].

◼ Chronic Kidney Disease

Chronic kidney disease is a risk factor for perioperative AKI. This risk can be mitigated (but not eliminated) by meticulous attention to fluid balance in the perioperative period to maintain euvolaemia, whilst avoiding nephrotoxic agents and hypotensive insults upon the kidneys. Patients with end-stage renal failure on renal replacement therapy, or those with solid organ transplants, require co-management with nephrology. Transplant patients will typically be continued on immunosuppression in the perioperative period, despite the moderate increased risks of perioperative infection or delayed wound healing.

◼ Chronic pain and musculoskeletal

Chronic pain is common in patients over 65 years old and is frequently caused by musculoskeletal complaints (e.g. osteoarthritis) and neuropathies (e.g. diabetes) [31]. Inadequately treated

preoperative pain increases the risk of uncontrolled postoperative pain. Moreover, long-term opiate use often necessitates postoperative doses 2–4 times higher than those required by opiate-naïve patients. Advanced interventions such as spinal cord stimulators and intrathecal drug delivery systems require specialist pain team referral for perioperative management [32].

All patients with rheumatoid arthritis should have flexion and extension views of the cervical spine interpreted by a senior radiologist, due to the risk of atlanto-axial subluxation and consequent spinal cord injury [9]. See the section 'Perioperative medication management and prescribing' for perioperative medication management.

◼ Chronic liver disease and alcohol dependence

Chronic liver disease

Patients with HNC have multiple risk factors (including alcohol abuse) for hepatic dysfunction, which itself increases the risk of perioperative morbidity and mortality very substantially. One large study [33] found that 6.8% of patients undergoing surgery for HNC demonstrated biochemical evidence of liver disease. Following major head and neck surgery, advanced liver disease was associated with a 14.6% 30-day perioperative mortality rate [33]. **Figure 3.2** is a guide to preoperative identification, risk stratification and perioperative management of chronic liver disease [34–36]. POD in a chronic liver disease patient should raise suspicion of hepatic encephalopathy and early correction of precipitants (e.g. drugs, infection, constipation) is necessary. Other considerations include monitoring for postoperative AKI, perioperative nutrition management and planned critical care admission. [37].

Alcohol dependence

A high prevalence of hazardous drinking exists within patients undergoing major HNC surgery, which is unsurprising given that alcohol is an established aetiological risk factor for HNC [38]. Alcohol dependency and the development of alcohol withdrawal symptoms has been associated with perioperative complications and increased length of stay [39]. Various screening

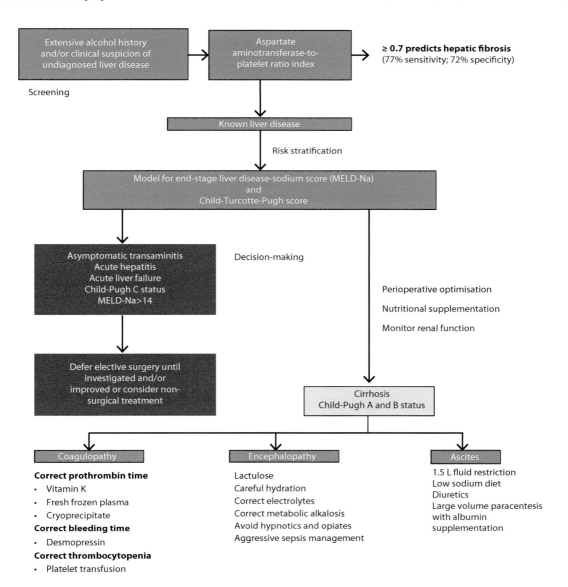

Figure 3.2 Preoperative identification, risk stratification and perioperative management of chronic liver disease.

tools (e.g. CAGE questionnaire) are available with attendant limitations. Screening enables referral to a cessation programme preoperatively, and reduction in alcohol consumption preoperatively has been shown to reduce postoperative complication rates [40]. Moreover, identification prompts the institution of perioperative nutrient supplementation to prevent Wernicke's encephalopathy and prophylactic pharmacological alcohol withdrawal protocols [5].

▮ Psychiatric

Depression, which frequently co-exists with anxiety, can be co-morbid or a symptom of the underlying endocrine disease (e.g. hypercalcaemia secondary to hyperparathyroidism). Depression is common in older patients and is associated with increased risk of postoperative infections, acute and chronic pain, delirium, and cancer mortality [41].

Screening for depression perioperatively is recommended [5]. Commonly used screening tools include the Patient Health Questionnaire-9 (**Figure 3.3**).

Scoring 10 or above indicates high depression risk, with sensitivity and specificity of 88% prompting appropriate referral [42]. It is currently unknown whether preoperative treatment of depression influences surgical outcomes [41]. Caution is advised regarding initiating selective serotonin uptake inhibitor antidepressants before surgery, as these have been associated with increased rates of perioperative haemorrhage. Where preoperative treatment of depression is indicated, our practice is to commence mirtazapine [43–45].

▮ Nutrition

Malnutrition is well recognised in HNC patients due to swallowing dysfunction, risk factors (e.g. alcohol abuse), cancer cachexia and treatments directly affecting the upper aerodigestive tract. In addition, benign disease of the upper aerodigestive tract may equally compromise nutritional state (e.g. pharyngeal pouches)[46,47]. Considerable perioperative morbidity (e.g. delayed wound healing and infective complications) and mortality are associated with malnutrition. Guidelines recommend dietetic input throughout the

---

Over the last two weeks, how often have you been bothered by any of the following problems?

- Little interest or pleasure in doing things?
- Feeling down, depressed, or hopeless?
- Trouble falling or staying asleep, or sleeping too much?
- Feeling tired or having little energy?
- Poor appetite or overeating?
- Feeling bad about yourself, that you are a failure, have let yourself or your family down?
- Trouble concentrating on things, such as reading the newspaper or watching television?
- Moving or speaking so slowly that other people could have noticed or being so fidgety or restless that you have been moving around a lot more than usual?
- Thoughts that you would be better off dead, or of hurting yourself in some way?

Scoring:
Not at all = 0
Several days = 1
More than half the days = 2
Nearly every day = 3

Total = __/27

Depression Severity:
0–4 none; 5–9 mild; 10–14 moderate; 15–19 moderately severe; 20–27 severe

Figure 3.3 Patient Health Questionnaire-9.

HNC care pathway. Nutritional screening at diagnosis is recommended using a tool such as the Subjective Global Assessment. Early referral enables preoperative optimisation of nutrition. If tube feeding is expected beyond 4 weeks, gastrostomy insertion is recommended. Patients with severe nutritional risk should have major surgery delayed to allow 10–14 days of of preoperative nutrition support where necessary. In accordance with the movement towards enhanced recovery programmes in head and neck surgery, preoperative carbohydrate loading should be considered [46].

▌ Geriatric syndromes

Frailty

Frailty is a clinical syndrome characterised by reduced physiological reserve across a range of organ systems. In surgical patients aged over 75 years, frailty strongly predicts perioperative complications, prolonged length of stay and postoperative mortality [48]. Whilst there is no current consensus on an optimal screening tool in the perioperative setting, evidence supports the use of either Edmonton Frail Scale or Clinical Frailty Scales in surgical populations [29]. In head and neck surgery, frailty measured using the modified frailty index retrospectively has been associated with increased Clavien-Dindo IV complications, especially following laryngectomy, and mortality [49,50].

Sarcopenia

Sarcopenia is an important component of the frailty syndrome, although it may exist in the absence of established frailty. *Sarcopenia* refers to reduced muscle mass, strength and overall performance; it is associated with poor oncological prognosis, increased perioperative complications, length of stay and postoperative mortality. The ability to assess sarcopenia using head and neck computed tomography may facilitate future risk stratification within the HNC population [51].

Falls

Preoperative falls predict postoperative falls, functional dependence and perioperative complications [52]. The Timed Up and Go Test can be used to assess falls risks. Difficulty in sit-to-stand (or where time to complete is over 15 seconds) associates with high risk for falls; preoperative referral to physiotherapy may be beneficial [5]. Postoperative falls may extend beyond the inpatient admission where patients suffer functional decline after surgery, and counselling frail older patients of this risk is advised [52,53].

Modification of geriatric syndromes

Preoperative identification of frailty is recommended for risk assessment and proactive planning of care. Though screening tools can play an important role in risk prediction, optimisation of the frailty syndrome is best achieved by comprehensive geriatric assessment (CGA) [29,49]. Frailty and sarcopenia are amenable to modification and frailty has been shown to be reversible in non-surgical cohorts. However, modification programmes typically involve multicomponent intervention which require considerable time and resources. Isolated parameters associated with frailty can be improved by exercise programmes and nutritional support, but evidence is limited that perioperative CGA-derived multicomponent interventions improves perioperative outcomes. [27].

▌ Preoperative testing

National guidelines grade procedures (see **Table 3.2**) to make specific rationalised recommendations about routine preoperative tests [18]. Most thyroid and major HNC surgery patients will require a resting electrocardiogram and basic blood panel (including full blood count and renal function tests). Cardiopulmonary exercise testing (CPEX) has demonstrated predictive capability for critical care admission, morbidity, length of stay and mortality in general surgery [54].

Table 3.2 Routine preoperative tests for elective surgery.

Minor	Intermediate	Major or complex
Excision of skin lesion	(Adeno) tonsillectomy	Thyroidectomy
		Radical neck dissection

Source: Adapted from NICE guidelines. Routine preoperative tests for elective surgery NICE guideline [NG45] (https://www.nice.org.uk/guidance/ng45; last accessed 14/02/2020)

PERIOPERATIVE MEDICATION MANAGEMENT AND PRESCRIBING

▨ Medication management

The physiological challenges and risk presented by anaesthesia and surgery mandate that a review of longstanding medication is conducted prior to surgery. Certain medications of long-term value may be hazardous in the perioperative period and require judicious management (e.g. anticoagulants, antiplatelet agents, diuretics, ACE inhibitors).

Second, older patients tend to accumulate medication with progressive multi-morbidity, rendering them vulnerable to polypharmacy (the co-prescription of five or more therapeutic agents) and its sequelae (e.g. drug interactions, falls, institutionalisation and mortality) [55]. There is some evidence polypharmacy may be associated with adverse postoperative outcomes, though whether this is an independent risk factor is uncertain [2,56].

Nonetheless, preoperative review of medication facilitates opportunity to optimise underlying chronic disease and rationalise growing medication lists. This can be challenging, and complex prescribing decisions are best made in a holistic physician-enhanced preassessment setting, where there is a surgical context to decision-making by perioperative physicians **Table 3.3** provides an evidence-based guide for reference. **Tables 3.4** and **3.5** cover antidiabetic drugs and insulins separately.

▨ Postoperative prescribing issues

Deliriogenic agents

Box 3.6 lists medications commonly prescribed during the perioperative setting, which may contribute to POD. Polypharmacy itself also increases the risk of POD, and regular review of

the drug chart should take place during inpatient admission to discontinue medications wherever no longer required [74].

▨ Analgesia

The surgical stress response augments pain, therefore intraoperative analgesia using local anaesthesia is advisable to improve postoperative pain and reduce opiate requirements and delirium [75]. A degree of adaptation to the World Health Organization (WHO) analgesia ladder is required in older surgical patients where fear of opiate toxicity is rightly a concern. However, it is important to reflect that uncontrolled pain is highly deliriogenic and also prevents mobilisation and rehabilitation. Management of severe post-operative pain can therefore be challenging, but must not be avoided (**Figure 3.4**) [75,76].

Box 3.6 Medications commonly prescribed prior to and during the perioperative setting, which may induce or contribute to POD

- Anticholingeric medications
  - Tricyclic antidepressants (e.g. amitriptyline)
  - Antihistamines (e.g. chlorphenamine)
  - Antimuscarinics (e.g. oxybutynin)
  - Antispasmodics (e.g. hyoscine butylbromide)
  - H2-receptor antagonists (e.g. ranitidine)
  - Antiemetics (e.g. cyclizine)
- Corticosteroids (e.g. prednisolone)
- Benzodiazepines (e.g. diazepam)
- Sedative-hypnotics (e.g. zopiclone)
- Opiate analgesics (e.g. morphine)

Table 3.3 Perioperative prescribing of common therapeutics.

Medication class (example agent)	Perioperative management	Alternative if enteral route unavailable	Rationale	Considerations	Reference
Alpha-2-agonists (e.g. clonidine)	CONTINUE including on morning of surgery	Transdermal clonidine	Omission may lead to rebound hypertension		[57]
Alpha blockers (e.g. tamsulosin)	CONTINUE including on morning of surgery	None required	May reduce risk of postoperative acute urinary retention and failed trial without catheter		[58]
Analgesic agents: chronic pain					
Anticonvulsants (e.g. gabapentin)	CONTINUE including on morning of surgery and restart when oral route available If must stop, slow dose tapering is required to avoid withdrawal syndrome	None required	Safe and have favourable associations with postoperative analgesia management	Arrange full blood count and electrolytes preoperatively as associated with derangement	[32]
Antidepressants: tricyclic antidepressants (e.g. amitriptyline), selective serotonin reuptake inhibitors (e.g. sertraline), selective noradrenaline reuptake inhibitors (e.g. venlafaxine)	CONTINUE including on morning of surgery and restart when oral route available	None required	Although concerns over bleeding risk elevated with SSRIs, discontinuation associated with increased postoperative cognitive and psychiatric symptoms	Watch out for serotonin syndrome, especially when co-prescribed with agents such as tramadol Also used for psychiatric conditions and can be continued	

(Continued)

Table 3.3 (*Continued*) Perioperative prescribing of common therapeutics.

Medication class (example agent)	Perioperative management	Alternative if enteral route unavailable	Rationale	Considerations	Reference
Opiates: modified release (e.g. 'MST')	CONTINUE including on morning of surgery and restart when oral route available	Use conversion tables as a guide to approximate total daily oral dose of opiates and convert this to a parenteral equivalent	Aim to maintain usual regimen as far as possible with supplementation and titration for acute postoperative pain	Recommended to start at 50% less when switching between opioids	
Transdermal patches (e.g. fentanyl)	CONTINUE perioperatively as per usual frequency and dose	None required		Titration for postoperative pain not recommended. Watch for side effects with fever (increased absorption)	
Angiotensin converting enzyme inhibitors (e.g. ramipril) and angiotensin receptor blockers (e.g. candesartan)	OMIT on morning of surgery generally (but see considerations)	IV enalaprilat is very rarely needed	Risk of intraoperative hypotension	Continuation in stable heart failure and LVSD	[12]
Anticoagulants – must weigh risk of life-threatening perioperative haemorrhage against thromboembolic risk					
New oral anticoagulants (e.g. dabigatran)	Average bleeding risk: discontinue 2–3 times their individual half-live. High bleeding risk: discontinue 4–5 times their individual half-live. Typically this will be 48–72 hours	See considerations	Short half-lives with well-defined 'on/off' action	Perioperative bridging therapy with unfractionated or low-molecular weight heparin generally not required	[59]

(*Continued*)

Table 3.3 (*Continued*) Perioperative prescribing of common therapeutics.

Medication class (example agent)	Perioperative management	Alternative if enteral route unavailable	Rationale	Considerations	Reference
Vitamin K antagonists (e.g. warfarin)	STOP 5 days before surgery and check international normalised ratio (INR) less than 1.5 preoperatively	Subcutaneous low molecular weight heparin if bridging therapy required	Balance between thromboembolic risk and bleeding risk needs to be carefully considered. If thromboembolic risk is significant (e.g. metallic valvular prosthesis), bridge with therapeutic low molecular weight heparin – last dose 24 hours preoperatively and continue until INR therapeutic	[9]
Antidiabetic drugs and insulins	Complex – see **Table 3.4** and **Table 3.5**	Variable rate intravenous insulin infusion	Maintain blood glucose between 6–12 mmol/L		[25]
Anti-epileptic drugs (e.g. valproate)	CONTINUE including on morning of surgery and restart as soon as able	IV alternatives available – discuss with neurology	Aim to minimise low serum levels – serum monitoring may be required		[23]
Antiplatelet agents					
Aspirin	Dependent on indication: Post-PCI (see below) – generally can be continued. Secondary cardiovascular prevention – consider continuation unless intraoperative bleeding risk too high	Intravenous and per rectum possible – use guided by cardiology	Perioperative aspirin withdrawal precedes up to around 10% of acute cardiovascular events. There is limited data on bleeding risk in head, neck and thyroid surgery: post-tonsillectomy bleeding is increased sevenfold; other (mainly retrospective) studies either show non-significant or significant increases in rate of bleeding versus severity	[11,60–62]
P2Y$_{12}$ inhibitors	See below. If outside PCI window: STOP: clopidogrel (5–7 days), pasugrel (7–10 days), ticagrelor (3–5 days) preoperatively	Not usually required	Clopidogrel may increase risk of postoperative haematoma in thyroid surgery		[61]

(Continued)

Table 3.3 (*Continued*) Perioperative prescribing of common therapeutics.

Medication class (example agent)	Perioperative management	Alternative if enteral route unavailable	Rationale	Considerations	Reference
Dual anti-platelet therapy (DAPT; aspirin and a P2Y$_{12}$ inhibitor)	DELAY NON-URGENT ELECTIVE SURGERY per timing of PCI (see text) Consensus required between patient, anaesthetist, surgeon and cardiologist in other circumstances	Available – use as guided by cardiology	Balance between bleeding risk and risk of stent thrombosis	If urgent or emergent, the risk of stent thrombosis is probably higher than risk of bleeding – consider operating on DAPT	[11,63]
Antipsychotics (e.g. olanzapine)	CONTINUE including on day of surgery	None required	Withdrawal may provoke recurrence of psychotic symptoms	Require careful monitoring and consideration of serotonin syndrome and neuroleptic malignant syndrome	[64,65]
Beta blockers (e.g. bisoprolol)	CONTINUE including on day of surgery	IV metoprolol, labetalol	Cardioprotective	Perioperative initiation may also be considered	[12]
Calcium-channel blockers (e.g. amlodipine)	CONTINUE including on day of surgery	None usually required – pause until oral route available	Little evidence of harm from continuation and may offer cardioprotective benefits		[66]
Digoxin	CONTINUE including on day of surgery	IV digoxin	May prevent tachyarrhythmias	Hypokalaemia can cause digoxin toxicity	[12]
Diuretics (e.g. furosemide)	Consider omission on morning of surgery	IV furosemide	Concern over intraoperative hypotension may not be as significant as previously thought		[67]

(*Continued*)

Table 3.3 (*Continued*) Perioperative prescribing of common therapeutics.

Medication class (example agent)	Perioperative management	Alternative if enteral route unavailable	Rationale	Considerations	Reference
Disease modifying anti-rheumatic drugs: non-biological (e.g. methotrexate) or biologics (e.g. etanercept)	Individualised decision – agreed between patient, specialist and surgeon Non-biologics can be continued if necessary STOP biologics according to their half-life	IV steroids (if required)	Balance of risk of disease flare versus risk of poor wound healing or infection	Consider need for stress dose steroid replacement (see steroids below) May also be used for inflammatory bowel disease, psoriasis, ankylosing spondylitis, systemic lupus erythematosus	[68]
H2 antagonists (e.g. ranitidine)	CONTINUE including on day of surgery	IV ranitidine	Reduces stress-related mucosal damage and aspiration chemical pneumonitis risk	Can be deliriogenic	[69]
Hormone replacement therapy	STOP 4–6 weeks prior to major surgery	None required	Increased VTE risk	Restart once fully mobile Graduated compression hosiery and unfractionated or low molecular weight heparin required if continued	[70]

(Continued)

Table 3.3 (*Continued*) Perioperative prescribing of common therapeutics.

Medication class (example agent)	Perioperative management	Alternative if enteral route unavailable	Rationale	Considerations	Reference
Inhaled bronchodilators: short-acting beta-2 agonists (e.g. salbutamol); long-acting beta-2 agonists (e.g. salmeterol); anticholinergic agents (e.g. ipratropium)	CONTINUE including on day of surgery	If using metered-dose inhalers is not suitable, change to nebulised alternatives	Reduced incidence of postoperative pulmonary complications in patients with asthma and chronic obstructive pulmonary disease		[71]
Inhaled corticosteroids (e.g. beclometasone)	CONTINUE including on day of surgery	Change to systemic routes if metered-dose inhaler not suitable	Maintain optimal lung function		
Leukotriene inhibitors (e.g. montelukast)	CONTINUE including on day of surgery	None – resume when oral route available	Beneficial effect on asthma control lasts up to 3 weeks after withdrawal		[72]
Levothyroxine	CONTINUE including on day of surgery	IV liothyronine sodium	Levothyroxine has a half-life of 5–9 days therefore omission for several days whilst nil by mouth is acceptable	IV treatment only required in severe hypothyroidism where undergoing urgent or emergent surgery	[26]
Lithium	STOP 72 hours before surgery	None required – resume once haemodynamically stable, oral route available and electrolytes are normal	Risk of perioperative lithium toxicity outweighs the risk of psychiatric recurrence	Discussion with psychiatry advisable to guide on perioperative symptom management	[64,65]

(*Continued*)

Table 3.3 (*Continued*) Perioperative prescribing of common therapeutics.

Medication class (example agent)	Perioperative management	Alternative if enteral route unavailable	Rationale	Considerations	Reference
Lipid modifying drugs (e.g. statins)	CONTINUE including on day of surgery	None available – restart once oral route available	May confer cardiovascular benefit		[12]
Oral contraceptive pill (oestrogen-containing)	STOP 4 weeks prior to surgery lasting longer than 30 minutes CONTINUE for minor surgery (e.g. <30 minutes)	None required	Risk of VTE must be weighed against risk of unwanted pregnancy	If stopping, advise on barrier method contraception preoperatively (and for 1 week after recommencing) and undertake pregnancy test prior to surgery	[73]
Proton pump inhibitors (e.g. omeprazole)	CONTINUE including on day of surgery	IV pantoprazole	See H2 antagonist above	Increased risk of Clostridium difficile infection	[69]
Selective serotonin reuptake inhibitors (e.g. fluoxetine)	CONTINUE including on day of surgery Consider stopping or changing to mirtazapine 2 weeks prior to high-bleeding risk surgery	None required	Perioperative safety concerns (including increased bleeding risk), but routine cessation linked to postoperative depression and delirium		[43–45]

(*Continued*)

Table 3.3 (Continued) Perioperative prescribing of common therapeutics.

Medication class (example agent)	Perioperative management	Alternative if enteral route unavailable	Rationale	Considerations	Reference
Steroids (e.g. prednisolone) and taking equivalent of more than 5 mg/day prednisolone	100 mg IM hydrocortisone at induction and 200 mg 4 hours later by IV infusion over 24 hours DOUBLE DOSE of oral steroids for 48 hours after major surgery	Continue IV hydrocortisone 50 mg QDS until oral steroids can be taken	Hypothalamic-pituitary-adrenal axis suppression possible	Consider testing for adrenal suppression Co-prescribe proton pump inhibitor if advanced cancer, older age, concomitant NSAIDs or anticoagulants, and previous peptic ulcer disease	[9,70]
Theophylline	OMIT evening before surgery	Utilise inhaled beta-2 agonists and anticholinergics	Narrow therapeutic range with potential for interactions		[71]

Table 3.4 Perioperative medication management of non-insulin antidiabetic agents.

Non-insulin medication group (examples)	Day prior to surgery/ admission	Day of surgery		Whilst on VRIII
		Scheduled for a.m. surgery	Scheduled for p.m. surgery	
Acarbose	Take as normal	Omit morning dose if NBM	Give morning dose if eating	Stop once VRIII commenced and *do not* recommence until eating and drinking normally
Meglitinide (repaglinide or nateglinide)				
Metformin (eGFR is greater than 60 mL/min/1.73 m^2 and procedure not requiring use of contrast media)		If taken *once or twice a day* – take as normal		
		If taken *three times per day*, omit lunchtime dose		
Sulphonylurea (e.g. glibenclamide, gliclazide, glipizide, glimeperide)		If taken *once daily in the morning* – omit the dose that day		
		If taken twice daily – *omit the morning dose that day*	If taken twice daily – *omit both doses that day*	
Pioglitazone	Take as normal			
DPP IV inhibitor (e.g. sitagliptin, vildagliptin, saxagliptin, alogliptin, linagliptin)				
GLP-1 analogue (e.g. exenatide, liraglutide, lixisenatide, dulaglutide)	Take as normal			
SGLT-2 inhibitors (e.g. dapagliflozin, canagliflozin, empagliflozin)	Take as normal	Omit on day of surgery		Omit until eating and drinking normally

Source: Adapted from Dhatariya K et al. *Management of adults with diabetes undergoing surgery and elective procedures: Improving standards,* Joint Diabetes Societies Inpatient Care Group, 2016.
Abbreviations: VRIII, variable rate intravenous insulin infusion; eGFR, estimated glomerular filtration rate; DPP IV, dipeptidyl peptidase-4 inhibitor; GLP-1, glucagon-like peptide-1; SGLT2, sodium-glucose co-transporter-2.

Table 3.5 Perioperative management of insulins.

Insulins	Day prior to admission	Day of surgery — Scheduled for a.m. surgery	Day of surgery — Scheduled for p.m. surgery	Whilst on VRIII
Once daily (evening) (e.g. Lantus®, Levemir®, Tresiba®, Insulatard®, Humulin I®, Insuman Basal®)	Reduce dose by 20%	Check blood glucose on admission	Check blood glucose on admission	Continue at 80% of the usual dose
Once daily (morning) (e.g. Lantus®, Levemir®, Tresiba®, Insulatard®, Humulin I®, Insuman Basal®)	Reduce dose by 20%	Reduce dose by 20% Check blood glucose on admission	Reduce dose by 20% Check blood glucose on admission	Continue at 80% of the usual dose
Twice daily (e.g. Novomix 30®, Humulin M3®, Humalog Mix 25®, Humalog Mix 50®, Insuman Comb 25®, Insuman Comb 50®, twice daily Levemir® or Lantus®)	No dose change	Halve the usual morning dose Check blood glucose on admission Leave the evening meal dose unchanged	Halve the usual morning dose Check blood glucose on admission Leave the evening meal dose unchanged	Stop until eating and drinking normally
Twice daily – separate injections of short acting (e.g. animal neutral, NovoRapid®, Humulin S®, Apidra®) and intermediate acting (e.g. animal isophane, Insulatard®, Humulin I® and Insuman®)	No dose change	Calculate the total dose of both morning insulins and give half intermediate acting only in the morning Check blood glucose on admission Leave the evening dose unchanged	Calculate the total dose of both morning insulins and give half intermediate acting only in the morning Check blood glucose on admission Leave the evening dose unchanged	Stop until eating and drinking normally
3, 4 or 5 injections daily (e.g. an injection of mixed insulin 3 times a day or 3 meal-time injections of short acting insulin and once or twice daily background)	No dose change	Basal bolus regimens: omit the morning and lunchtime short acting insulins If the dose of long acting basal insulin is usually taken in the morning then the dose should be reduced by 20% Premixed a.m. insulin: halve the morning dose and omit lunchtime dose Check blood glucose on admissions	Take the usual morning insulin (doses) Omit lunchtime dose Check blood glucose on admission	Stop until eating and drinking normally

Source: Adapted from Dhatariya K et al. *Management of adults with diabetes undergoing surgery and elective procedures: Improving standards*, Joint Diabetes Societies Inpatient Care Group, 2016.

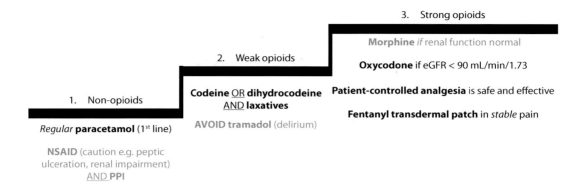

3. Strong opioids

Morphine *if* renal function normal

Oxycodone if eGFR < 90 mL/min/1.73

2. Weak opioids

Patient-controlled analgesia is safe and effective

Codeine <u>OR</u> **dihydrocodeine**
<u>AND</u> **laxatives**

Fentanyl transdermal patch in *stable* pain

1. Non-opioids

AVOID tramadol (delirium)

Regular **paracetamol** (1ˢᵗ line)

NSAID (caution e.g. peptic
ulceration, renal impairment)
<u>AND</u> **PPI**

Figure 3.4 Modified WHO analgesia ladder for elderly patients.

ANTICIPATING AND PLANNING DISCHARGE

Most young and straightforward patients are easy to discharge when surgically fit. However, older and multi-morbid patients may have social issues which require anticipation and planning to prevent unnecessary delays to discharge. Functional dependence and impaired mobility have been shown to predict perioperative complications and postoperative institutionalisation and mortality. **Box 3.7** demonstrates key points in the social assessment. Where any degree of dependence is identified, full screening of (instrumental) activities of daily living should be performed by nursing of therapy teams (e.g. Barthel scale) and optimisation explored [5].

> **Box 3.7 Short simple screening test for functional assessment**
>
> 1 Can you get out of bed or a chair yourself?
> 2 Can you wash and dress yourself?
> 3 Can you make your own meals?
> 4 Can you do your own shopping?
>
> *Source*: Modified from Mohanty S et al. *Optimal perioperative management of the geriatric patient: A best practices guideline from ACS NSQIP/American Geriatrics Society*. 2012.

SUMMARY AND CONCLUSIONS

Surgical patients frequently present with adverse features of ageing. These include co-morbidity, multi-morbidity and the geriatric syndromes. Head and neck oncogeriatric patients are particularly vulnerable, due to interactions between chronic medical conditions, risk factors and their primary disease process. Models of shared care between surgeon, anaesthetist and physician represent one solution to counter the challenge of the ageing surgical population. However, there can be no doubt surgeons of the future must engage with and maintain expertise in perioperative medicine. *Planning, patience* and *prioritisation* along with the concept of prehabilitation are the key strategies to successful preoperative surgical care.

REFERENCES

1 United Nations DoEaSA, Population Division. World Population Ageing. 2015. Contract No.: (ST/ESA/SER.A/390)s.

2 Huisman MG, Kok M, de Bock GH, van Leeuwen BL. Delivering tailored surgery to older cancer patients: Preoperative geriatric assessment domains and screening tools – A systematic review of systematic reviews. *Eur J Surg Oncol.* 2017;43(1):1–14.

3 Wilkinson K, Martin IC, Gough MJ et al. *An Age Old Problem: A review of the care received by elderly patients undergoing surgery.* National Confidential Enquiry into Patient Outcome and Death; 2010.

4 Shipway D, Koizia L, Winterkorn N et al. Embedded geriatric surgical liaison is associated with reduced inpatient length of stay in older patients admitted for gastrointestinal surgery. *Future Healthc J* Jun 2018, 5(2):108–116. DOI: 10.7861/futurehosp.5-2-108

5 Mohanty S, Rosenthal RA, Russell MM et al. *Optimal perioperative management of the geriatric patient: A best practices guideline from ACS NSQIP/American Geriatrics Society.* 2012.

6 Shipway DJ, Partridge JS, Foxton CR et al. Do surgical trainees believe they are adequately trained to manage the ageing population? A UK survey of knowledge and beliefs in surgical trainees. *J Surg Educ.* 2015;72(4):641–7.

7 Korc-Grodzicki B, Downey RJ, Shahrokni A, Kingham TP, Patel SG, Audisio RA. Surgical considerations in older adults with cancer. *J Clin Oncol.* 2014;32(24):2647–53.

8 Sheikh A, Shallwani H, Ghaffar S. Postoperative shoulder function after different types of neck dissection in head and neck cancer. *Ear Nose Throat J.* 2014;93(4-5):E21–6.

9 Robson A, Sturman J, Williamson P, Conboy P, Penney S, Wood H. Pre-treatment clinical assessment in head and neck cancer: United Kingdom National Multidisciplinary Guidelines. *J Laryngol Otol.* 2016;130(S2):S13–S22.

10 Ng SH, Wong KP, Lang BH. Thyroid surgery for elderly patients: Are they at increased operative risks? *J Thyroid Res.* 2012;2012:946276.

11 Levine GN, Bates ER, Bittl JA et al. 2016 ACC/AHA Guideline focused update on duration of dual antiplatelet therapy in patients with coronary artery disease: A report of the American College of Cardiology/American Heart Association Task Force on Clinical Practice Guidelines: An update of the 2011 ACCF/AHA/SCAI guideline for percutaneous coronary intervention, 2011 ACCF/AHA guideline for coronary artery bypass graft surgery, 2012 ACC/AHA/ACP/AATS/PCNA/SCAI/STS guideline for the diagnosis and management of patients with stable ischemic heart disease, 2013 ACCF/AHA guideline for the management of ST-elevation myocardial infarction, 2014 AHA/ACC guideline for the management of patients with non-st-elevation acute coronary syndromes, and 2014 ACC/AHA guideline on perioperative cardiovascular evaluation and management of patients undergoing noncardiac surgery. *Circulation.* 2016;134(10):e123–55.

12 Kristensen SD, Knuuti J, Saraste A et al. 2014 ESC/ESA Guidelines on non-cardiac surgery: Cardiovascular assessment and management: The Joint Task Force on non-cardiac surgery: Cardiovascular assessment and management of the European Society of Cardiology (ESC) and the European Society of Anaesthesiology (ESA). *Eur Heart J.* 2014;35(35):2383–431.

13 Hartle A, McCormack T, Carlisle J et al. The measurement of adult blood pressure and management of hypertension before elective surgery: Joint guidelines from the Association of Anaesthetists of Great Britain and Ireland and the British Hypertension Society. *Anaesthesia.* 2016;71(3):326–37.

14 Myers K, Hajek P, Hinds C, McRobbie H. Stopping smoking shortly before surgery and postoperative complications: A systematic review and meta-analysis. *Arch Intern Med.* 2011;171(11):983–9.

15 McCarter K, Martinez U, Britton B et al. Smoking cessation care among patients with head and neck cancer: A systematic review. *BMJ Open.* 2016;6(9):e012296.

16 Gottlieb M, Marsaa K, Godtfredsen NS, Mellemgaard A. Prevalence and management

of pulmonary comorbidity in patients with lung and head and neck cancer. *Acta Oncol.* 2015;54(5):767–71.

17 Qaseem A, Snow V, Fitterman N et al. Risk assessment for and strategies to reduce perioperative pulmonary complications for patients undergoing noncardiothoracic surgery: A guideline from the American College of Physicians. *Ann Intern Med.* 2006;144(8):575–80.

18 National Institute for Health and Care Excellence. Routine preoperative tests for elective surgery. NICE guideline [NG45]. 2016.

19 Chung F, Abdullah HR, Liao P. STOP-bang questionnaire: A practical approach to screen for obstructive sleep apnea. *Chest.* 2016;149(3):631–8.

20 Adesanya AO, Lee W, Greilich NB, Joshi GP. Perioperative management of obstructive sleep apnea. *Chest.* 2010;138(6):1489–98.

21 Axley MS, Schenning KJ. Preoperative cognitive and frailty screening in the geriatric surgical patient: A narrative review. *Clin Ther.* 2015;37(12):2666–75.

22 Nicholson TR, Cutter W, Hotopf M. Assessing mental capacity: The Mental Capacity Act. *BMJ.* 2008;336(7639):322–5.

23 Probasco J, Sahin B, Tran T et al. The preoperative neurological evaluation. *Neurohospitalist.* 2013;3(4):209–20.

24 Jorgensen ME, Torp-Pedersen C, Gislason GH et al. Time elapsed after ischemic stroke and risk of adverse cardiovascular events and mortality following elective noncardiac surgery. *JAMA.* 2014;312(3):269–77.

25 Dhatariya K, Flanagan D, Hilton L et al. *Management of adults with diabetes undergoing surgery and elective procedures: Improving standards.* Joint Diabetes Societies Inpatient Care Group. 2016.

26 Schiff RL, Welsh GA. Perioperative evaluation and management of the patient with endocrine dysfunction. *Med Clin North Am.* 2003;87(1):175–92.

27 Amrock LG, Deiner S. Perioperative frailty. *Int Anesthesiol Clin.* 2014;52(4):26–41.

28 Roy S, Sherman A, Monari-Sparks MJ, Schweiker O, Hunter K. Correction of low vitamin d improves fatigue: Effect of correction of low vitamin D in fatigue study (EViDiF Study). *N Am J Med Sci.* 2014;6(8):396–402.

29 British Geriatrics Society. *Fit for frailty: Care of older people living with frailty in community and outpatient settings.* British Geriatrics Society and the Royal College of Nursing; 2014.

30 Goodnough LT, Shander A. Patient blood management. *Anesthesiolog.* 2012;116(6):1367–76.

31 Reid MC, Eccleston C, Pillemer K. Management of chronic pain in older adults. *BMJ.* 2015;350:h532.

32 Farrell C, McConaghy P. Perioperative management of patients taking treatment for chronic pain. *BMJ.* 2012;345:e4148.

33 Cramer JD, Patel UA, Samant S, Yang A, Smith SS. Liver disease in patients undergoing head and neck surgery: Incidence and risk for postoperative complications. *Laryngoscope.* 2017;127(1):102–9.

34 Janssens F, de Suray N, Piessevaux H, Horsmans Y, de Timary P, Starkel P. Can transient elastography replace liver histology for determination of advanced fibrosis in alcoholic patients: A real-life study. *J Clin Gastroenterol.* 2010;44(8):575–82.

35 Pandey CK, Karna ST, Pandey VK, Tandon M, Singhal A, Mangla V. Perioperative risk factors in patients with liver disease undergoing non-hepatic surgery. *World J Gastrointest Surg.* 2012;4(12):267–74.

36 Rizvon MK, Chou CL. Surgery in the patient with liver disease. *Med Clin North Am.* 2003;87(1):211–27.

37 Suraweera D, Sundaram V, Saab S. Evaluation and management of hepatic encephalopathy: Current status and future directions. *Gut Liver.* 2016;10(4):509–19.

38 Shah S, Weed HG, He X, Agrawal A, Ozer E, Schuller DE. Alcohol-related predictors of delirium after major head and neck cancer surgery. *Arch Otolaryngol Head Neck Surg.* 2012;138(3):266–71.

39 Genther DJ, Gourin CG. The effect of alcohol abuse and alcohol withdrawal on short-term outcomes and cost of care after head and neck cancer surgery. *Laryngoscope.* 2012;122(8):1739–47.

40 Oppedal K, Moller AM, Pedersen B, Tonnesen H. Preoperative alcohol cessation prior to

elective surgery. *Cochrane Database Syst Rev.* 2012(7):Cd008343.

41 Ghoneim MM, O'Hara MW. Depression and postoperative complications: An overview. *BMC Surg.* 2016;16:5.

42 Kroenke K, Spitzer RL, Williams JBW. The PHQ-9: Validity of a brief depression severity measure. *J Gen Intern Med.* 2001;16(9):606–13.

43 Jeong BO, Kim SW, Kim SY, Kim JM, Shin IS, Yoon JS. Use of serotonergic antidepressants and bleeding risk in patients undergoing surgery. *Psychosomatics.* 2014;55(3):213–20.

44 Auerbach AD, Vittinghoff E, Maselli J, Pekow PS, Young JQ, Lindenauer PK. Perioperative use of selective serotonin reuptake inhibitors and risks for adverse outcomes of surgery. *JAMA Intern Med.* 2013;173(12):1075–81.

45 Kudoh A, Katagai H, Takazawa T. Antidepressant treatment for chronic depressed patients should not be discontinued prior to anesthesia. *Can J Anaesth.* 2002;49(2):132–6.

46 Talwar B, Donnelly R, Skelly R, Donaldson M. Nutritional management in head and neck cancer: United Kingdom National Multidisciplinary Guidelines. *J Laryngol Otol.* 2016;130(S2):S32–s40.

47 Boucher S, Breheret R, Laccourreye L. Importance of malnutrition and associated diseases in the management of Zenker's diverticulum. *Eur Ann Otorhinolaryngol Head Neck Dis.* 2015;132(3):125–8.

48 Huisingh-Scheetz M, Walston J. How should older adults with cancer be evaluated for frailty? *J Geriatr Oncol.* 2017;8(1):8–15.

49 Adams P, Ghanem T, Stachler R, Hall F, Velanovich V, Rubinfeld I. Frailty as a predictor of morbidity and mortality in inpatient head and neck surgery. *JAMA Otolaryngol Head Neck Surg.* 2013;139(8):783–9.

50 Abt NB, Richmon JD, Koch WM, Eisele DW, Agrawal N. Assessment of the predictive value of the modified Frailty Index for Clavien-Dindo Grade IV critical care complications in major head and neck cancer operations. *JAMA Otolaryngol Head Neck Surg.* 2016;142(7):658–64.

51 Swartz JE, Pothen AJ, Wegner I et al. Feasibility of using head and neck CT imaging to assess skeletal muscle mass in head and neck cancer patients. *Oral Oncol.* 2016;62:28–33.

52 Kronzer VL, Jerry MR, Ben Abdallah A et al. Preoperative falls predict postoperative falls, functional decline, and surgical complications. *EBioMedicine.* 2016;12:302–8.

53 Kronzer VL, Wildes TM, Stark SL, Avidan MS. Review of perioperative falls. *Br J Anaesth.* 2016;117(6):720–32.

54 Moran J, Wilson F, Guinan E, McCormick P, Hussey J, Moriarty J. Role of cardiopulmonary exercise testing as a risk-assessment method in patients undergoing intra-abdominal surgery: A systematic review. *Br J Anaesth.* 2016;116(2):177–91.

55 Harstedt M, Rogmark C, Sutton R, Melander O, Fedorowski A. Polypharmacy and adverse outcomes after hip fracture surgery. *J Orthop Surg Res.* 2016;11(1):151.

56 Gnjidic D, Hilmer SN, Blyth FM et al. Polypharmacy cutoff and outcomes: Five or more medicines were used to identify community-dwelling older men at risk of different adverse outcomes. *J Clin Epidemiol.* 2012;65(9):989–95.

57 Sanchez Munoz MC, De Kock M, Forget P. What is the place of clonidine in anesthesia? Systematic review and meta-analyses of randomized controlled trials. *J Clin Anesth.* 2017;38:140–53.

58 Madani AH, Aval HB, Mokhtari G et al. Effectiveness of tamsulosin in prevention of post-operative urinary retention: A randomized double-blind placebo-controlled study. *Int Braz J Urol.* 2014;40(1):30–6.

59 Kumar S, Moorthy R. New oral anticoagulants – A guide for ENT surgeons. *J Laryngol Otol.* 2016;130(4):324–8.

60 Dhiwakar M, Khan NA, McClymont LG. Surgical resection of cutaneous head and neck lesions: Does aspirin use increase hemorrhagic risk? *Arch Otolaryngol Head Neck Surg.* 2006;132(11):1237–41.

61 Oltmann SC, Alhefdhi AY, Rajaei MH, Schneider DF, Sippel RS, Chen H. Antiplatelet and anticoagulant medications significantly increase the risk of postoperative hematoma: Review of over 4500 thyroid and parathyroid procedures. *Ann Surg Oncol.* 2016;23(9):2874–82.

62 Francis DO, Dang JH, Fritz MA, Garrett CG. Antiplatelet and anticoagulation therapy in microlaryngeal surgery. *Laryngoscope*. 2014;124(4):928–34.

63 Song JW, Soh S, Shim JK. Dual antiplatelet therapy and non-cardiac surgery: Evolving issues and anesthetic implications. *Korean J Anesthesiol*. 2017;70(1):13–21.

64 Attri JP, Bala N, Chatrath V. Psychiatric patient and anaesthesia. *Indian J Anaesth*. 2012;56(1):8–13.

65 Huyse FJ, Touw DJ, van Schijndel RS, de Lange JJ, Slaets JP. Psychotropic drugs and the perioperative period: A proposal for a guideline in elective surgery. *Psychosomatics*. 2006;47(1):8–22.

66 Wijeysundera DN, Beattie WS. Calcium channel blockers for reducing cardiac morbidity after noncardiac surgery: A meta-analysis. *Anesth Analg*. 2003;97(3):634–41.

67 Khan NA, Campbell NR, Frost SD et al. Risk of intraoperative hypotension with loop diuretics: A randomized controlled trial. *Am J Med*. 2010;123(11):1059.e1–8.

68 Krause ML, Matteson EL. Perioperative management of the patient with rheumatoid arthritis. *World J Orthop*. 2014;5(3):283–91.

69 Nishina K, Mikawa K, Takao Y, Shiga M, Maekawa N, Obara H. A comparison of rabeprazole, lansoprazole, and ranitidine for improving preoperative gastric fluid property in adults undergoing elective surgery. *Anesth Analg*. 2000;90(3):717–21.

70 Joint Formulary Committee. British National Formulary (online). BMJ Group and Pharmaceutical Press. [Available from: http://www.medicinescomplete.com/.]

71 Licker M, Schweizer A, Ellenberger C, Tschopp JM, Diaper J, Clergue F. Perioperative medical management of patients with COPD. *Int J Chron Obstruct Pulmon Dis*. 2007;2:493–515.

72 Reiss TF, Chervinsky P, Dockhorn RJ, Shingo S, Seidenberg B, Edwards TB. Montelukast, a once-daily leukotriene receptor antagonist, in the treatment of chronic asthma: A multicenter, randomized, double-blind trial. Montelukast Clinical Research Study Group. *Arch Intern Med*. 1998;158(11):1213–20.

73 Faculty of Sexual and Reproductive Healthcare of the Royal College of Obstetricians and Gynaecologists. *UK medical eligibility criteria for contraceptive use (UKMEC)*. 2017.

74 American Geriatrics Society Expert Panel on Postoperative Delirium in Older Adults. Postoperative delirium in older adults: Best practice statement from the American Geriatrics Society. *J Am Coll Surg*. 2015;220(2):136–48.e1.

75 Aubrun F, Marmion F. The elderly patient and postoperative pain treatment. *Best Pract Res Clin Anaesthesiol*. 2007;21(1):109–27.

76 Falzone E, Hoffmann C, Keita H. Postoperative analgesia in elderly patients. *Drugs Aging*. 2013;30(2):81–90.

4

CONGENITAL NECK LUMPS

Jarrod J. Homer and Laura Warner

INTRODUCTION

The embryology of the head and neck region is complex. Defective embryological development can result in congenital neck lesions. Whilst some congenital neck masses are clinically evident at birth, others may present later in childhood or early adulthood. Congenital neck abnormalities include developmental anomalies of the branchial system, the thyroid gland, vascular and lymphatic systems, dermoid cysts, and teratomas.

THYROGLOSSAL DUCT CYSTS

Thyroglossal duct cysts are the commonest congenital neck mass. Although present at birth, most commonly become clinically apparent in childhood but may present in adulthood. Males and females are similarly affected.

▌ Aetiology

The thyroid gland develops at the foramen caecum (the junction between the anterior and posterior thirds of the tongue). Between 3 and 6 weeks gestation, the gland descends in the neck, passing through the middle of the developing hyoid bone, which has not yet fused in the midline. The descending tract usually obliterates; however, a persistent duct may remain, which gives rise to thyroglossal duct cysts. The cysts contain ectopic thyroid tissue, which very

occasionally may be the only functioning thyroid tissue.

▌ History

Usually a painless midline neck lump.

May have been noticed since birth or not.

Can present following infection as a midline neck abscess or, if this has discharged spontaneously, a fistula.

▌ Examination

A smooth, non-tender swelling in or near to the midline (left commoner than right).

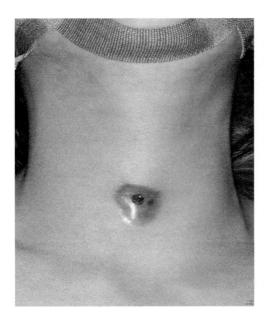

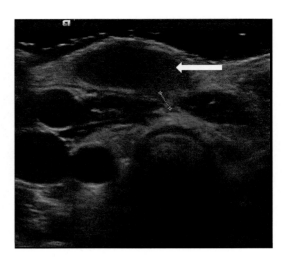

Figure 4.2 Ultrasound imaging of thyroglossal duct cyst (arrow). Measuring calipers indicate the thyroglossal duct.

Figure 4.1 Infected thyroglossal duct cyst.

They are commonly found between the hyoid and the normal position of the thyroid in the lower neck, but can occur at any location along the path of descent of the thyroid (see **Figure 4.1**).

Because of the attachment to both the larynx and base of tongue, these cysts move on swallowing and tongue protrusion.

▮ Investigation

The diagnosis of a thyroglossal duct cyst is usually made clinically; however, imaging is essential to ensure thyroid tissue is present in the normal location. Ultrasonography is commonly used and non-invasive (see **Figure 4.2**). Radionucleotide thyroid imaging was previously routinely advocated and may assist in cases of diagnostic uncertainty.

The commonest differential diagnosis is a dermoid cyst.

▮ Management

Whilst thyroglossal duct cysts can be managed conservatively, early surgery is advocated by most surgeons

to avoid complications such as repeated infection and fistula formation, and also for definitive histology.

Infections should be managed with broad spectrum antibiotics, and supplemented with needle aspiration if necessary. Infections are often polymicrobial, and antibiotic regimens should cover common oral pathogens due to the connection with the base of tongue.

Incision and drainage should be avoided where possible.

Surgical excision of the cyst alone leads to high recurrence rates. Sistrunk described excision of the cyst, tract and central portion of the hyoid bone in 1920 [1]. This approach reduces the recurrence rate when compared to excision of the cyst alone. The tract is often difficult to skeletonise and follow as well as often having microscopic tributaries which can be missed leading to recurrence. As such, a modified Sistrunk procedure has been described, advocating en bloc dissection of central neck tissues, incorporating a cuff of infrahyoid muscle tissue and resecting an area of the tongue base in addition to the central portion of the hyoid bone [2]. The recurrence rate when this technique is employed is approximately 3%; the wider extent of excision is considered necessary due to the potential for arborisation or multiple branching of the thyroglossal duct tract. Whilst a single transverse neck incision is usually sufficient, this can be extended to excise an ellipse of involved skin, and for cysts occurring low in the neck, a step-ladder incision may be required to facilitate adequate resection of the central hyoid bone and tongue base.

LINGUAL THYROID

▌ Aetiology

Complete failure of descent of the developing thyroid results in ectopic thyroid tissue in a mass at the base of tongue, known as a lingual thyroid. This thyroid tissue is typically the only functioning thyroid tissue. Whilst the mass may enlarge, causing compressive symptoms and swallowing difficulties, most patients are asymptomatic and this can be managed conservatively in the majority of cases.

Any ectopic thyroid tissue is susceptible to the disease processes that affect the thyroid, including thyroid malignancy, which is found in approximately 1% of thyroglossal duct cysts and lingual thyroid tissue [3,4].

▌ Dermoid cysts and teratomas

Aetiology

Teratomas are a form of germ cell tumour [5]. These uncommon masses are congenital neoplasms, arising from pluripotent cells, causing sequestration of skin cells along the line of embryonic fusion. They are defined histologically as containing tissues of all three germ cell layers (ectoderm, mesoderm and endoderm) [5]. They contain heterogeneous differentiated tissue, such as teeth, hair and bone. Dermoid cysts are cystic teratomas that are of ectodermal and mesodermal origin, lined by epidermis. Epidermoid cysts are simply lined with squamous epithelium (lacking adnexal structures), whereas true dermoid cysts may contain features of skin cells such as sebaceous glands and hair follicles. Teratomas may consist of mixed cystic and solid areas [6].

▌ History

Usually present at birth.

They are smooth, painless lumps.

▌ Examination

The cystic lesions typically arise along the lines of embryonic closure in the head and neck region (see **Figure 4.3**). They are found mostly in the midline of the neck, without movement on tongue protrusion, clinically differentiating from thyroglossal duct cysts. Dermoid cysts may also occur in the floor of the mouth or on the face affecting the lateral aspect of the orbit or as a midline nasal lesion, where a tuft of hair may be noted overlying the lesion. They less commonly affect the torso and genitalia.

Approximately 3% of congenital teratomas arise in the head and neck area [5]. These may present antenatally, detected on ultrasound imaging. Epiganthus is a large oropharyngeal teratoma, arising from the skull base, which is detected antenatally due to polyhydramnios and has the potential to cause neonatal airway compromise.

▌ Investigation

Ultrasonography may be useful in differentiating dermoid cysts from thyroglossal cysts, however, clinical correlation is essential.

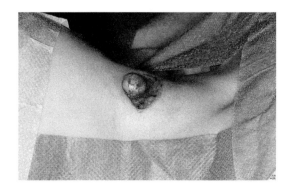

Figure 4.3 Intraoperative photograph of well encapsulated dermoid cyst.

Magnetic resonance imaging (MRI) is useful in surgical planning for teratomas and may be performed antenatally.

▌ Management

If asymptomatic, these may be managed conservatively, however, they have the propensity to grow, which needs to be explained to the patient.

Surgery is the mainstay of treatment for both dermoid cysts and teratomas. The exact procedure and extent of surgery depends upon the size and location of the lesion, and resection may need to be staged for larger cervical teratomas.

In cases of a large epiganthus causing airway compromise, ex utero intrapartum treatment (EXIT procedure) with tracheostomy may be required. Whilst teratomas carry a risk of malignancy, this is rare in cervical teratomas.

VASCULAR MALFORMATIONS

Congenital vascular abnormalities may be classified as vascular tumours or vascular malformations (see **Figure 4.4**).

▌ Haemangioma

Aetiology

Vascular tumours are benign endothelial neoplasms. The type most frequently encountered is infantile haemangioma; however, rarer vascular tumours in infancy such as angiosarcoma or kaposiform haemangioendothelioma may also arise in the head and neck region. Haemangiomas are the commonest benign tumours of infancy and commonly occur in the head and neck region, including the subglottis causing airway obstruction. Haemangiomata are characterised by a period of rapid proliferation of blood vessels and growth, followed by spontaneous involution. Growth is driven by vascular endothelial growth factor (VEGF). Involution may take years [7].

Clinical features

These will vary according to the location of the lesion.

Infantile haemangioma may be superficial cutaneous lesions or arise from deeper tissues. Cutaneous lesions appear as raised, dark red papules and can

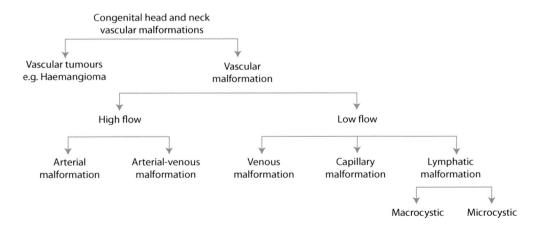

Figure 4.4 Flow chart to show the classification of congenital head and neck vascular malformations. (N.B.: Lymphatic malformations have historically been referred to as cystic hygromas.)

occur anywhere on the body but have a predilection for the head and neck.

Deeper lesions appear as soft, compressible, lobulated masses with a bluish discolouration and are commonly found in the parotid area or neck.

The oral cavity or subglottic airway may also be involved, resulting in airway compromise.

The typical history of infantile haemangioma is of initial rapid growth, followed by gradual involution, occurring within the first weeks of life.

Congenital haemangioma are lesions present at birth that display features of both vascular tumours and vascular malformations. After the initial phase of rapid growth, haemangioma begin to spontaneously involute, with complete resolution by 9 years of age in more than 90% of cases [7,8].

Investigation

Ultrasound imaging may assist in differentiation of haemangioma from other subcutaneous lesions, whereas MRI can delineate the exact location and extent of the lesion.

Management

Conservative management is sufficient in the majority of cases, as the lesion will eventually spontaneously regress.

For lesions in problematic anatomical locations, for example in approximation to the orbit or lesions of sufficient size to cause complications, medical or surgical intervention may be required.

Medical strategies include systemic corticosteroids, which may restrain growth if administered during the phase of rapid growth. Intralesional injection of triamcinolone may also be used. More recently treatment with propranolol, accidentally discovered in 2008, has revolutionised treatment of these lesions [9]. Patients must be monitored for hypoglycaemia and cardiac side effects such as bradycardia and hypotension. Surgery is reserved for cases resistant to medical therapies.

Vascular malformations

Vascular malformations are a result of defective development of vascular structures, resulting in an abnormal number of or abnormally sized vessels, which may be arterial, venous, lymphatic or a combination. Vascular malformations are classified into high- or low-flow malformations.

High-flow lesions are arterial or arteriovenous malformations.

Low-flow lesions include capillary malformations such as port-wine stains, venous malformations occurring in skin or subcutaneous tissues, and lymphatic or venolymphatic malformations [10].

Lymphatic and venolymphatic malformations

The head and neck area is the commonest sites for lymphatic malformations, which can also affect the trunk and limbs. Lymphatic malformations may affect the neck, commonly the posterior triangle but may also affect the oral cavity or facial tissues.

Aetiology

Lymphatic malformations are masses of dilated lymphatic channels or cysts filled with serous fluid. These may also be associated with venous anomalies, termed venolymphatic malformations. Lymphatic malformations are classified as macrocystic or microcystic but may exist together in a mixed lesion (see **Figure 4.5**).

Macrocystic lesions, also known as cystic hygroma, commonly arise in the infrahyoid neck. These are formed of multiple large, endothelium-lined, interconnected lymphatic cysts. Infrahyoid lesions may involve the laryngopharynx and may extend inferiorly into the mediastinum. Microcystic malformations arise above the hyoid and frequently involve the lips, floor of mouth and tongue (see **Figure 4.6**) [11].

History

Lymphatic malformations are usually present at birth, although some may become clinically apparent after enlarging following an upper respiratory tract infection or local trauma.

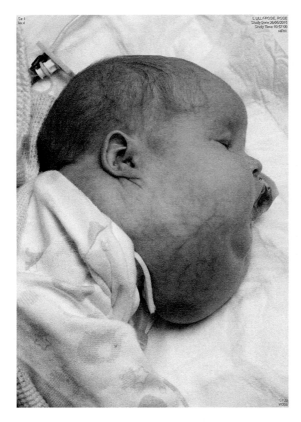

Figure 4.5 Infant with large micro- and macrocystic venolymphatic malformation, delivered by EXIT procedure with tracheostomy.

Large lesions may be detected antenatally on fetal ultrasound as early as 10 weeks' gestation.

Examination

Lymphatic malformations are soft, compressible, multiloculated lesions that transilluminate.

Whilst large lesions in the neck or mediastinum may cause airway compromise or swallowing difficulties, most lymphatic malformations cause no local symptoms.

Investigation

Magnetic resonance imaging provides accurate localisation of the lesion with identification of local

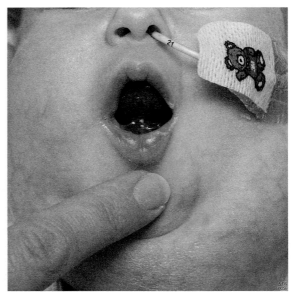

Figure 4.6 Microcystic venolymphatic malformation involving tongue and floor of mouth.

neurovascular structures which assist in surgical planning (see **Figure 4.7**).

Management

Treatment regimens for lymphatic malformations include clinical observation, sclerotherapy, medical treatment, laser and radiofrequency ablation, and surgery. A multimodal approach may be required for complex lesions. Airway compromise may necessitate tracheostomy and ex uterine intrapartum treatment may be required for large, antenatally diagnosed lymphatic malformations [11].

Smaller, non-disfiguring lesions may be managed with a period of 'watchful waiting', though only approximately 15%–20% will spontaneously regress. Whilst macrocystic lesions may be amenable to sclerotherapy, microcystic lesions do not typically respond. Agents such as doxycycline and OK432 may be inserted via a radiologically inserted pigtail catheter. Bleomycin has fallen out of favour as a sclerosing agent due to complications such as pulmonary fibrosis and risk of toxicity.

Medical therapies are not widely used but include treatment with sirolimus and sildenafil. Sirolimus,

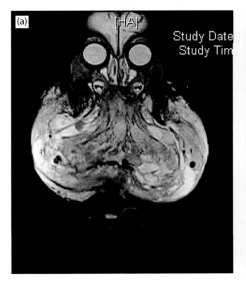
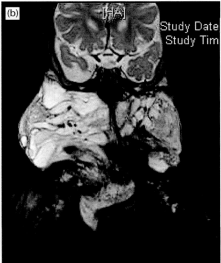
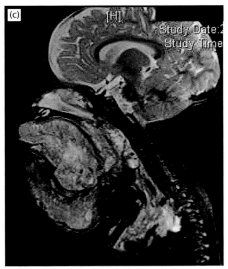

Figure 4.7 MRI imaging of large venolymphatic malformation demonstrating macrocystic neck disease (a), mediastinal involvement (b), and microcystic disease affecting the tongue and floor of the mouth (c).

a macrolide compound, has been reported in small case series and is well tolerated although high recurrences rates have been reported [12]. A phase 2 clinical trial is underway to investigate the efficacy of sildenafil (Viagra) in the treatment of lymphatic malformations [13].

Surgery is the mainstay of treatment for lymphatic malformations, with low recurrence rates

if complete excision is achieved. Surgery may be complicated by distorted anatomy and significant risks of intraoperative haemorrhage and injury to neurological structures. Multistage resections may be required for large, complex lymphatic malformations.

de Serres et al. proposed a staging system for lymphatic malformations (see **Table 4.1**). This has been

Table 4.1 de Serres staging classification for lymphatic malformations.

Stage	Position of lymphatic malformation	Unilateral or bilateral	Rates of complications
I	Infrahyoid	Unilateral	Increasing (↓)
II	Suprahyoid	Unilateral	
III	Suprahyoid and infrahyoid	Unilateral	
IV	Suprahyoid	Bilateral	
V	Suprahyoid and infrahyoid	Bilateral	

Source: de Serres LM, Sie KC, Richardson MA. *Arch Otolaryngol Head Neck Surg.* 1995;121(5):577–82.

shown to give prognostic information for risk of complications from treatment. In general, bilateral, suprahyoid lymphangiomas are more difficult to treat. This is because of the proximity to the pharynx, floor of mouth and tongue [14,15].

BRANCHIAL ANOMALIES

See **Table 4.2**.

■ Embryology

The branchial or pharyngeal arches first appear in the fourth week of gestation. The branchial system consists of arches, internal pouches and external grooves or clefts from which head and neck structures develop in utero (see **Table 4.2**). The branchial apparatus relates to a series of gill-like slits which are similar to those that develop into gills in fish, hence the name *branchial* meaning 'gills' in Greek [17].

Developmental abnormalities of the branchial system may give rise to cysts, fistulae and sinus tracts. Diagnoses rely upon sound knowledge of the branchial derivatives in order to determine the structures that may be involved. Fistulae and sinuses are epithelium-lined tracts. A branchial fistula represents persistence of both the external cleft and the internal pouch which are connected, whereas a sinus is persistence of the external cleft without an internal connection. The fistula tract is located caudal to the structures derived from the corresponding branchial arch. Branchial cysts are fluid-filled, epithelium-lined sacs which may derive from the internal pouch (endoderm) or external cleft (ectoderm) [17].

Branchial anomalies

First branchial cleft abnormalities are rare, representing approximately 5% of branchial disorders. These fistulae and sinuses are embryonic duplication abnormalities of the first branchial cleft (type I) or of the first cleft and arch (type II), as classified by Work in 1972 [18]:

- Type I represents duplication of the membranous external ear canal and is of ectodermal origin. Type I fistulae typically open anterior and inferior to the tragus, communicating with an opening in the external ear canal or middle ear. The fistula tract is closely related to the parotid gland and lies superficial to the facial nerve.
- The commoner type II fistulae arise as duplication of the membranous ear canal and pinna, consisting of both ectodermal and mesodermal tissues. An anterior opening is located close to the angle of the mandible with a posterior

Table 4.2 Branchial derivatives.

Arch	Nerve	Cartilage	Muscle	Artery	Internal pouch	External groove/cleft
1 Mandibular	Trigeminal	Meckel's: • Maxilla • Malleus • Incus	• Mylohyoid • Anterior digastric • Tensor tympani • Tensor veli palatini • Muscles of mastication	First aortic arch – maxillary artery	• Eustachian tube • Middle ear cleft • Tympanic membrane	• External auditory meatus • Tympanic membrane
2 Hyoid	Facial	Reichart's: • Lesser cornu and upper body of hyoid • Stapes superstructure • Styloid	• Muscles of facial expression • Posterior digastric • Stapedius	Second aortic arch – stapedial artery	• Palatine tonsil	• Overgrows remaining grooves
3	Glosso-pharyngeal	• Greater cornu and lower body of hyoid	• Stylopharyngeus • Superior and middle constrictor	Third aortic arch	• Inferior parathyroid glands • Thymic duct	• Obliterated
4	Vagus – Superior laryngeal nerve	• Thyroid lamina	• Cricothyroid	Fourth aortic arch – arch of aorta	• Superior parathyroid glands	• Obliterated
6	Vagus – Recurrent laryngeal nerve	• Cricoid • Arytenoid cartilages	• Inferior constrictor • Intrinsic muscles of larynx	Sixth aortic arch – ductus arteriosus	• Ultimobranchial body (forms parafollicular C-cells of thyroid)	• Obliterated

opening in the lateral portion of the external ear canal or conchal bowl, without middle ear involvement. Type II fistulae may lie either medial or lateral to the facial nerve. This inconstant relationship means that repair of a type II fistula carries greater risk of causing injury to the facial nerve than expected for a type I fistula repair.

First cleft fistulae are present at birth but often asymptomatic. They may present with recurrent skin infections or recurrent ear discharge.

Branchial anomalies

Second branchial abnormalities are the commonest encountered, representing approximately 90%–95% of all branchial abnormalities [19]. Second cleft fistulae or sinuses have an opening along the anterior border of the sternocleidomastoid muscle with a tract extending superiorly along the carotid sheath, and may pass between the internal and external carotid arteries at the carotid bifurcation. The tract can pass deep to the hypoglossal nerve to open in, or anterior to, the tonsillar fossa. Patients may present with recurrent discharge or recurrent skin infections, often triggered by an upper respiratory tract infection.

Third and fourth branchial anomalies

Third and fourth branchial arch and cleft abnormalities are rare and may be difficult to clinically differentiate from each other.

A third branchial fistula has a skin opening placed anterior to the sternocleidomastoid muscle in the lower neck. The tract courses superiorly, deep to the internal carotid artery and glossopharyngeal nerve and penetrates the posterolateral thyrohyoid membrane to open into the pyriform fossa, above the level of the superior laryngeal nerve.

Fourth branchial fistulae have a skin opening in a similar location, but the internal opening in the pyriform fossa apex is located inferior to the level of the superior laryngeal nerve.

Third branchial fistulae occur more commonly on the left side and present with recurrent skin infection or abscess in the lower anterior neck, or with recurrent thyroiditis.

Fourth branchial anomalies also present more commonly on the left side in a similar fashion with recurrent neck abscesses or thyroiditis, and a fistula opening may be visible in the apex of the pyriform fossa [20].

▌ Investigation

Fistulogram or sinogram imaging may be more useful in identifying the course of the tract and related anatomical structures.

In the case of second, third and fourth branchial anomalies, a contrast swallow can reveal the location of the internal opening.

Cross-sectional imaging with MRI or CT will delineate the anatomy and location of the aforementioned branchial abnormalities.

Fistulogram or sinogram imaging may be more useful in identifying the course of the tract and related anatomical structures.

▌ Management

Complete surgical excision of the sinus or fistula tract is the mainstay of management of symptomatic branchial cleft abnormalities. This is ideally performed at a time when infections are quiescent. Sound understanding of the related anatomy and local neurovascular structures is essential to avoid unnecessary complications.

When excising first branchial cleft abnormalities, an understanding of the proximity of the facial nerve is essential and intraoperative facial nerve monitoring should be considered.

With second branchial abnormalities, care must be taken to avoid vascular injury, as the tract may pass between the internal and external carotid arteries.

Third branchial abnormalities also lie in proximity to the carotid arteries and the hypoglossal and glossopharyngeal nerves.

The recurrent laryngeal nerve is at risk during open resection of fourth branchial abnormalities. These are approached from an incision that allows access to the ipsilateral thyroid (for removal) and inferior thyroid cartilage for excision of the tract. However, endoscopic diathermy obliteration of the pyriform fossae opening of fourth branchial fistulae has been described with excellent symptom control [21,22]. Recurrence occurs in at least 5% of cases after surgical excision of all branchial abnormality. A selective neck dissection is advocated by some for recurrent cases with good results [23].

BRANCHIAL CYSTS

▌ Aetiology

Branchial cysts are often described as the commonest congenital neck mass. There is considerable debate over the aetiology of branchial cysts and several theories as to their aetiology exist (see **Table 4.3**).

Lateral, cystic neck lumps above the hyoid presenting in children are likely to have developed from an embryological remnant, such as the branchial cleft. Those presenting in adults are thought to result from cystic degeneration of a lymph node originally proposed by Lucke and later supported by King [27,28]. This is based on the presence of lymphoid tissue in cyst walls on histological examination. Bhaskar and Bernier supported this theory and suggested that epithelium may become trapped within lymph nodes, known as 'epithelial inclusions', to explain the presence of epithelium within the wall of branchial cysts [29].

Genetic associations

First branchial cleft sinus or fistulae may be associated with first branchial arch abnormalities. Patients may have unilateral or bilateral facial palsy, hemifacial microsomia or first branchial arch syndromes such as Treacher Collins syndrome. Patients with first arch abnormalities have a higher propensity for concurrent otologic anomalies and hearing screening should be performed. In patients with any branchial abnormality, particularly if bilateral, the potential association with hearing loss, pinna abnormalities and renal malformations, known as branchio-oto-renal syndrome, should be considered with a low threshold for hearing assessment and renal ultrasound.

▌ History

- The lump usually presents in level II/III of the neck and may have become apparent acutely after an upper respiratory tract infection (URTI).
- Occasionally patients have noticed the cyst for an extended period and a size increase has prompted referral.
- Painless, unless infected, which can lead to acute presentation and confusion for an abscess.
- Smoking and alcohol history is essential.

Care must be taken to exclude metastatic squamous cell carcinoma (SCC) of unknown primary especially in patients over 40 and who smoke. Indeed it

Table 4.3 Theories for branchial cyst aetiology (see **Figure 4.8**).

Proposer	Theory
Ascherson [24]	Incomplete obliteration of branchial cleft
His [25]	Persistence of a cervical sinus
Wenglowski [26]	Incomplete obliteration of the thymopharyngeal duct
Lucke [27]	Cystic degeneration of the lymph node lying between the internal and external carotid arteries

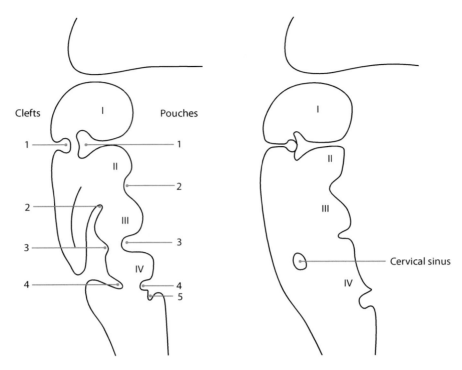

Figure 4.8 Caudal overgrowth of the second branchial cleft (left), trapping epithelium in the cervical sinus (right).

is said repeatedly that in these groups a suspected branchial cyst is a carcinoma until proven otherwise.

Examination

- Typically present under the junction of the upper and middle third of the sternomastoid muscle.
- It is solitary, mobile and non-tender unless infected.
- It is important to make a full assessment of the mucosal surfaces of the upper aerodigestive tract (UADT) and perform a skin survey. These examinations should all be clear if a presumption of a branchial cyst is to be made.
- It is worth examining the skin over the lower two-thirds of the sternocleidomastoid muscle (SCM) in detail to identify any sinus or fistula, which can be present as part of congenital branchial anomalies.

Investigation

Ultrasound scan (USS) imaging will reveal a thin-walled cystic lesion. The cyst can be aspirated under USS guidance, aiming to also capture cellular matter from the cyst wall for cytological diagnosis.

A low index of suspicion must be kept for the differential diagnosis of cystic lymph node metastasis from head and neck squamous cell carcinoma, particularly in patients over 40 years. This is discussed in detail in Chapter 5.

Management

Broad spectrum antibiotic treatment should be initiated for infection, with needle aspiration or incision and drainage in case of ongoing symptoms. The mainstay of treatment is surgical excision, performed once any infection has resolved.

The management of patients where the possibility of carcinoma of unknown primary is suspected is discussed in Chapter 5.

STERNOCLEIDOMASTOID TUMOUR OF INFANCY

▌ Aetiology

Sternocleidomastoid tumour of infancy (also known as fibromatosis colli of infancy) is the commonest neck mass diagnosed in the neonatal period. It is not a true mass, however, but rather an area of fibrosis within the sternocleidomastoid muscle causing congenital torticollis. Whilst the exact aetiology is unclear, it is widely accepted that the fibrosis occurs as a result of birth trauma [30].

▌ History

Usually presents at birth with a lateral, hard neck lump, which is generally quite alarming for parents and nursing staff.

The baby will often not be able to turn their head to the affected side (torticollis).

▌ Examination

A firm, non-tender fibrotic area or mass involving the mid to lower third of the sternocleidomastoid.

It may result in reduced head movement (torticollis).

▌ Investigation

Ultrasonography can confirm the diagnosis and will differentiate from other types of neck mass. In cases where resolution is incomplete, cross-sectional imaging and biopsy may be required.

▌ Management

Physiotherapy is the mainstay of treatment, aiming to promote a full range of motion. Symptoms can progress if untreated for up to 8 weeks, however, complete resolution typically occurs before 6 months of age.

Surgical excision is rarely required and is reserved for cases with severe symptoms that fail to resolve.

Long-term follow-up is recommended as the fibrosis may recur during periods of heightened growth [30].

REFERENCES

1 Sistrunk WE. The surgical treatment of cysts of the thyroglossal tract. *Ann Surg.* 1920;71(2):121–2.

2 Ahmed J, Leong A, Jonas N, Grainger J, Hartley B. The extended Sistrunk procedure for the management of thyroglossal duct cysts in children: How we do it. *Clin Otolaryngol.* 2011;36(3):271–5.

3 Sturniolo G, Vermiglio F, Moleti M. Thyroid cancer in lingual thyroid and thyroglossal duct cyst. *Endocrinol Diabetes Nutr.* 2017;64(1):40–3.

4 Sturniolo G, Violi MA, Galletti B et al. Differentiated thyroid carcinoma in lingual thyroid. *Endocrine.* 2016;51(1):189–98.

5 Peterson CM, Buckley C, Holley S, Menias CO. Teratomas: A multimodality review. *Curr Probl Diagn Radiol.* 2012;41(6):210–9.

6 Rothschild MA, Catalano P, Urken M et al. Evaluation and management of congenital cervical teratoma. Case report and review. *Arch Otolaryngol Head Neck Surg.* 1994;120(4): 444–8.

7 Eivazi B, Werner JA. Management of vascular malformations and hemangiomas of the head and neck – An update. *Curr Opin Otolaryngol Head Neck Surg.* 2013;21(2):157–63.

8 Cox JA, Bartlett E, Lee EI. Vascular malformations: A review. *Semin Plast Surg.* 2014;28(2):58–63.

9 Leaute-Labreze C, Dumas de la Roque E, Hubiche T, Boralevi F, Thambo JB, Taieb A. Propranolol for severe hemangiomas of infancy. *N Engl J Med.* 2008;358(24):2649–51.

10 Richter GT, Friedman AB. Hemangiomas and vascular malformations: Current theory and management. *Int J Pediatr.* 2012;2012:645–78.

11 Defnet AM, Bagrodia N, Hernandez SL, Gwilliam N, Kandel JJ. Pediatric lymphatic malformations: Evolving understanding and therapeutic options. *Pediatr Surg Int.* 2016;32(5):425–33.

12 Lackner H, Karastaneva A, Schwinger W et al. Sirolimus for the treatment of children with various complicated vascular anomalies. *Eur J Pediatr*. 2015;174(12):1579–84.

13 Swetman GL, Berk DR, Vasanawala SS, Feinstein JA, Lane AT, Bruckner AL. Sildenafil for severe lymphatic malformations. *N Engl J Med*. 2012;366(4):384–6.

14 Hamoir M, Plouin-Gaudon I, Rombaux P et al. Lymphatic malformations of the head and neck: A retrospective review and a support for staging. *Head Neck*. 2001;23(4):326–37.

15 Perkins JA, Manning SC, Tempero RM et al. Lymphatic malformations: Review of current treatment. *Otolaryngol Head Neck Surg*. 2010;142(6):795–803, e1.

16 de Serres LM, Sie KC, Richardson MA. Lymphatic malformations of the head and neck. A proposal for staging. *Arch Otolaryngol Head Neck Surg*. 1995;121(5):577–82.

17 Bajaj Y, Ifeacho S, Tweedie D, Jephson CG, Albert DM, Cochrane LA et al. Branchial anomalies in children. *Int J Pediatr Otorhinolaryngol*. 2011;75(8):1020–3.

18 Work WP. Newer concepts of first branchial cleft defects. *Laryngoscope*. 1972;82(9):1581–93.

19 Adams A, Mankad K, Offiah C, Childs L. Branchial cleft anomalies: A pictorial review of embryological development and spectrum of imaging findings. *Insights Imaging*. 2016;7(1):69–76.

20 Prasad SC, Azeez A, Thada ND, Rao P, Bacciu A, Prasad KC. Branchial anomalies: Diagnosis and management. *Int J Otolaryngol*. 2014;2014: 237015.

21 Rea PA, Hartley BE, Bailey CM. Third and fourth branchial pouch anomalies. *J Laryngol Otol*. 2004;118(1):19–24.

22 Derks LS, Veenstra HJ, Oomen KP, Speleman L, Stegeman I. Surgery versus endoscopic cauterization in patients with third or fourth branchial pouch sinuses: A systematic review. *Laryngoscope*. 2016;126(1):212–7.

23 Blackwell KE, Calcaterra TC. Functional neck dissection for treatment of recurrent branchial remnants. *Arch Otolaryngol Head Neck Surg*. 1994;120(4):417–21.

24 Ascherson GM. *Defistulis colli congenitis*. Berolini; 1832:1–21.

25 His W. Ueber der Sinus praecervicalis und uber die Thymusanlage. *Archiv fur Anatomic und Entwickelungsgeschichte*. 1886;9(421–33).

26 Wenglowski R. Ueber die Halsfisteln und Cysten. *Langenbeck Archivfur Klinische Chirurgie* 1912;98:151–208.

27 Lucke AI. Ueber atheromysten der Lymphdrusen. *Archiv fur Klinische Chirurgie*. 1861;1(356–365).

28 King ES. The lateral lympho-epithelial cyst of the neck; branchial cyst. *Aust N Z J Surg*. 1949;19(2):109–21, illust.

29 Bhaskar SN, Bernier JL. Histogenesis of branchial cysts; a report of 468 cases. *Am J Pathol*. 1959;35(2):407–43.

30 Krugman ME, Canalis R, Konrad HR. The sternomastoid 'tumor' of infancy. *J Otolaryngol*. 1976;5(6):523–9.

5

CERVICAL LYMPHADENOPATHY

Neil de Zoysa

INTRODUCTION

Cervical lymphadenopathy is relatively common but can encompass a large range of potential pathologies. The key goal of the clinician is to distinguish benign from malignant and identify those which are manifestations of systemic disease. The work-up of patients with pathology in the neck follows a logical sequence (see flow chart of **Figure 5.6**).

This chapter will discuss key points within patient demographics and presentation to help focus history taking and investigation. It will then go onto discuss important differentials and their management, including the important and controversial area of head and neck carcinoma of unknown primary.

ANATOMY

The location of a neck mass affects the differential diagnosis. Therefore, an understanding of the anatomy is key to assessment and subsequent communication.

There are two main ways to classify the location of cervical lymphadenopathy:

1 Triangles of the neck
2 Nodal levels

Differential diagnoses for palpable lymphadenopathy must include masses arising from solid organs such as the salivary glands, thyroid gland or even direct extension of the tumour from the upper aerodigestive tract (UADT).

▌ Triangles of the neck

For the purposes of teaching, particularly at the undergraduate level, triangles of the neck represent an easily understood and reproducible method of dividing the neck anatomically based on largely palpable landmarks.

The neck can be divided into anterior and posterior triangles using the sternocleidomastoid muscle, and further subdivided into smaller triangles using the digastric muscle and omohyoid muscle (see **Figure 5.1**). In general, masses in the posterior triangle of the neck are more likely to be neoplastic and malignant than the anterior triangle. The mandible, hyoid bone, clavicle and trapezius muscles make up the remaining boundaries.

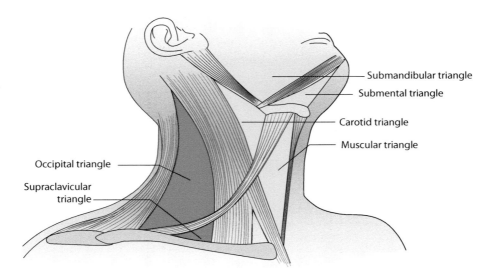

Figure 5.1 Triangles of the neck.

Submandibular triangle
Submental triangle
Carotid triangle
Muscular triangle
Occipital triangle
Supraclavicular triangle

▌ Nodal levels of the neck

For the purposes of documentation in specialist practice, nodal levels (see **Figure 5.2**) are considered the standard and should be used over triangles of the neck. Here the accuracy of documentation is crucial.

HISTORY

History is key to establishing a differential diagnosis and appropriately investigating the patient.

▌ Age

Aetiology of neck masses generally fall into three categories:

1 Congenital
2 Inflammatory
3 Neoplastic

The balance of these aetiologies varies by age, and this is demonstrated in the charts of **Figure 5.3**.

Sixty per cent of paediatric neck lumps are inflammatory, usually a form of cervical lymphadenitis. Only the minority are neoplastic. Clearly it is important to screen for and capture this small group of neoplastic lumps in this group. It is also important to recognise, however, that the majority of paediatric patients will see resolution of their lumps following observation or the commencement of appropriate antimicrobial therapy if indicated.

As a result, paediatric patients with neck masses, showing no other symptoms, signs or features of other disease can usually be reassured and conservatively managed in this way prior to performing imaging.

Congenital neck masses usually display characteristic features both on history and examination, have close ties with embryology, and make good exam cases! Congenital neck masses are discussed in detail in Chapter 4.

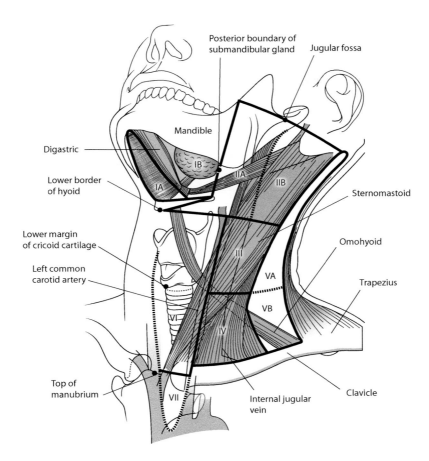

Figure 5.2 Levels of the neck.

In young adults, inflammatory masses still make up for the majority of presentations of neck masses, but neoplasia is now more common than the presentation of congenital neck lumps. Patients over 40 are far more likely to be demonstrating neoplasia, whether this is benign or malignant. These patients as a result require repeatable objective evidence to show the nature of their presentation before being reassured [1].

▮ Duration

Days: May suggest infective/inflammatory origin
Weeks/months: Chronic infections (e.g. TB), inflammatory diseases (e.g. sarcoid), neoplasia
Years: Less likely to represent malignancy unless there has been a recent change

▮ Growth pattern

Growth over 2 cm per month is clearly of concern and increases the likelihood of malignancy. Rapid growth over a week or a fortnight should raise concern of an infective/inflammatory origin, but be cognisant of the risk of high-grade lymphoma or poorly differentiated malignancy. Some neck lumps (often cystic ones) display rapid initial growth followed by a plateau in growth thereafter [2].

▮ Associated symptoms

These are very important to clarify.

Malignant neck lumps are often painless but can cause referred pain.

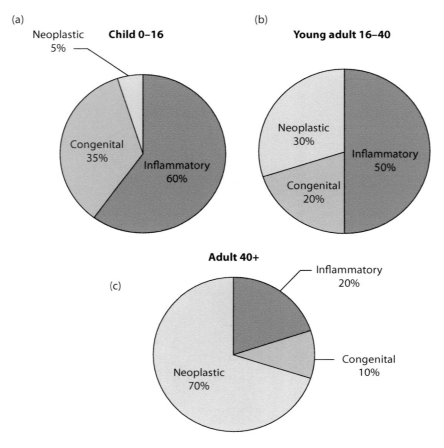

(a)

Neoplastic 5%

Child 0–16

Congenital 35%

Inflammatory 60%

(b)

Young adult 16–40

Neoplastic 30%

Inflammatory 50%

Congenital 20%

(c)

Adult 40+

Inflammatory 20%

Congenital 10%

Neoplastic 70%

Figure 5.3 Charts to demonstration distribution of neck lumps across different age groups.

Infective lymphadenopathy is often painful due to its rapid growth and inflammation.

It is important to screen the patient for UADT symptoms of malignancy.

Dysphagia

Suggests malignancy involving the pharynx (mainly hypopharynx).

Progressive dysphagia (i.e. initially to solids and later to solids and liquids) is a red flag symptom.

The onset is usually insidious over months and may predate the neck lump.

There may be weight loss and a change in the patients diet to a soft diet.

Odynophagia with and without sore throat

When acute, odynophagia may represent the original infection from which a reactive lymphadenitis has been triggered. In children in particular, a relatively mild upper respiratory tract infection can result in a marked lymphadenopathy and lymphadenitis of rapid onset and alarm.

May suggest malignancy involving the oral cavity and pharynx. Particularly if there is a persistently sore throat, regardless of swallowing, which does not remit and has been ongoing for >3 weeks.

In malignancy it is usually unilateral especially ipsilateral to the lump.

Otalgia

This usually represents referred pain from the neck pathology irritating the great auricular nerve or from a potential primary tumour in the UADT stimulating the glossopharyngeal or vagus nerves.

In the setting of a non-acute neck lump (i.e. one present for >2 weeks), it is a red flag symptom.

Remember that in otitis externa the intraparotid lymph node can become enlarged, as this is the echelon lymph node draining the ear.

Mouth ulcers

It is unusual for lymphadenopathy to occur in response to inflammatory/infective mouth ulcers.

Lymphadenopathy in the presence of a non-healing/enlarging ulcer should raise concern for oral carcinoma.

All non-healing/enlarging ulcers should be biopsied.

Dysphonia

Persistent hoarseness or a rough voice raises concern for malignancy involving the larynx.

Ask about aspiration, i.e. coughing and choking on ingestion.

In advanced cases there may be dyspnoea or stridor.

Weight loss

A well-known red flag symptom.

Unintentional loss of more than 5% of body weight over 6 months is a cause for concern.

Constitutional symptoms

Suggestive of systemic disease or lymphoma.

Fever, night sweats: So-called 'B symptoms' [3].

Flushing, palpitations, hypertension: In phaeochromocytoma associated with paragangliomas (glomus tumours).

Skin conditions

Of course it is important to ask about any suspicious moles/lesions that may have metastasised to the lymph nodes, but it is also important to ask about other skin conditions such as acne, dermatitis, eczema or rashes in the head and neck which may be the underlying cause of reactive lymphadenopathy. This is particularly common in submental, posterior chain and occipital lymph nodes, often in response to shaving.

▇ Risk factors

Clearly ask about the following risk factors for malignancy.

Smoking

Highly important.

Current status and pack-years are important for risk stratification.

Alcohol intake

Another important risk factor, particularly in oral and hypopharyngeal cancer, is alcohol intake. Units per week currently and any history of alcohol dependence should be recorded. High alcohol intake combined with smoking may have a synergistic effect on the risk of head and neck cancer.

Previous head and neck cancer

Patients in this group have a 10% chance of developing a second primary and also have a risk of recurrence of their original disease. Recurrent disease may present locally (in the UADT), regionally (in the cervical lymph nodes) or with distant metastases.

Other malignancy

Especially skin cancer: In countries with high rates of sun exposure, cutaneous rather than mucosal malignancy can make up a larger proportion of metastatic squamous cell carcinoma in the neck. In patients with previous skin malignancy, a detailed history of where and when any excisions were performed including margins is important.

Immunosuppression

Patients who are immunosuppressed especially post organ transplant and HIV-positive patients have an increased likelihood of developing virally associated tumours at most sites.

Family history

Fanconi anaemia is a rare inherited autosomal recessive condition. Sufferers are at increased risk of head and neck cancer (approximately 400- to 700-fold risk) at a younger age [4].

EXAMINATION

▉ Neck examination

Inspection of the neck is useful. Previous surgical scars as well as signs of sun damage and skin lesions are important to note. The location of the lump heavily influences the differential diagnosis (see **Figure 5.4**) [5].

A further factor of importance is the nodal draining basin for a given nodal level (see **Figure 5.5**). Primary tumours from different sites in the head and neck drain primarily to different nodal groups. The potential primary sites for each echelon region must be closely inspected.

Echelon node image

Skin changes over the lump are important. Signs of skin dimpling or darkening/breakdown can be seen in advanced nodal metastasis.

Congenital neck masses, such as branchial cleft anomalies, may have a skin pit or sinus which helps

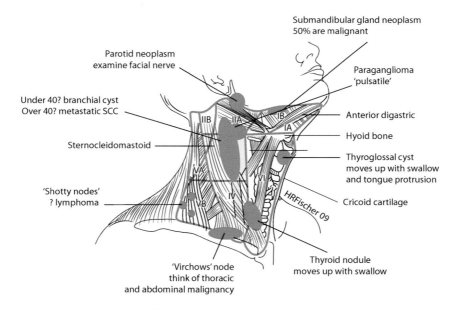

Figure 5.4 Diagram to demonstrate different underlying neck lumps according to location.

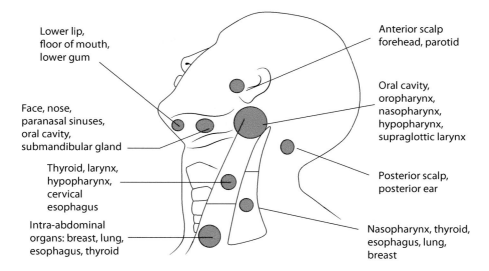

Lower lip,
floor of mouth,
lower gum

Anterior scalp
forehead, parotid

Oral cavity,
oropharynx,
nasopharynx,
hypopharynx,
supraglottic larynx

Face, nose,
paranasal sinuses,
oral cavity,
submandibular gland

Thyroid, larynx,
hypopharynx,
cervical
esophagus

Posterior scalp,
posterior ear

Intra-abdominal
organs: breast, lung,
esophagus, thyroid

Nasopharynx, thyroid,
esophagus, lung,
breast

Figure 5.5 Demonstration of the echelon node drainage for different potential primary tumour sites.

differentiate them between a cleft cyst, sinus or fistula (see Chapter 4).

Neck palpation must be comprehensive in covering all areas in a logical and repeatable fashion. Individual neck lumps can then be isolated and examined (see **Table 5.1**).

Movement on swallowing indicates fixation to the pre-tracheal fascia seen in the thyroid, thyroglossal duct and larynx.

Protrusion on tongue movement indicates attachment to the hyoid bone and is often associated the thyroglossal duct anomalies.

Low parotid and submandibular gland neoplasms also present as neck lumps. As a result, an appropriate cranial nerve examination is important in the assessment of neck lumps. Both thyroid, parotid and congenital masses are discussed in more detail in Chapters 6 and 14).

▌ UADT examination

A systematic examination of the head and neck should include headlight examination of the oral cavity and oropharynx.

Further examination of the UADT is mandatory and should begin with examination of the oral cavity and oropharynx including palpation of the tongue and bimanual palpation of the floor of the mouth.

In the specialist setting, full flexible nasoendoscopy has superseded the use of mirrors and has the added benefit of photo documentation and is a mandatory part of the routine examination of the neck lump.

Table 5.1 Features of neck lumps on examination that raise suspicion for malignancy.

Less suspicious	Suspicious
Small	Large
Soft/rubbery	Hard
Mobile	Fixed
Single	Multiple
No skin changes	Skin changes/breakdown
No neurology	Weak shoulder/face/voice/tongue

DIFFERENTIAL DIAGNOSIS

The differential diagnosis for enlarged cervical lymph nodes includes:

Infectious

- Lymphadenopathy/lymphadenitis
- Bacterial, viral, fungal, parasitic

Granulomatous

- *Infectious*
  - TB, atypical mycobacteria, cat scratch
  - Serology is useful but not always diagnostic
- *Non-infectious*
  - Sarcoidosis, Kawasaki, Castleman, Kikuchi, Kimura
  - Sialadenitis/sialolithiasis
  - Autoantibody titre including ANA, ENA, DsDNA, Anti Ro, Anti La and onward referral to rheumatology

Neoplastic

- *Benign*
  - Benign lymphoid hyperplasia, e.g. Castleman disease – very rare
  - Difficult to differentiate from a low-grade lymphoma
  - Requires excision biopsy for diagnosis

Malignant

- *Primary*
  - Lymphoma
- *Secondary*
  - Metastatic carcinoma, usually from lesion of mucosa of UADT or skin
  - Metastatic thyroid cancer or salivary gland cancer
  - Metastatic carcinoma from distant sites, e.g. Virchow's node from upper gastrointestinal malignancy

INVESTIGATION

Following history and examination, it may be apparent if the aetiology of the neck lump is infective. In paediatric and young adult patients with a short history, a trial or observation and appropriate antimicrobials may be the most appropriate initial step. Often however by the time patients are seen in secondary care this has already been done, and most palpable abnormalities require some form of imaging to further classify the mass. This is certainly the case for all patients over the age of 40. An outline of management is shown in **Figure 5.6**.

■ Ultrasound and fine needle aspiration cytology

Ultrasound scans (USS) have the advantage of no radiation exposure and are performable even in small children without anaesthesia in specialist hands.

- The main disadvantages of ultrasound are operator dependency and as a dynamic study, interpretation in retrospect is difficult making images poor for surgical planning.

However, USS in the appropriate hands can differentiate benign from malignant and assess local invasion and vascularity. The addition of ultrasound-guided fine-needle aspiration cytology (FNAC) makes USS the investigation of choice in neck lumps in the majority of cases.

FNAC has the advantage of offering negligible risk of tumour seeding and minimal trauma making vascular complications low. Palpable masses can undergo FNAC in clinic without the requirement of ultrasound and may expedite diagnosis whilst formal image-guided biopsy is awaited. Disadvantages include diagnostic yield, which can vary depending on the operator's technique, and whether a cytologist is present at the time of aspiration [6].

After diagnostic USS and/or FNAC, patients can be reassured, precede to surgery or be further worked up with appropriate cross-sectional imaging and discussion at the multidisciplinary team meeting if appropriate.

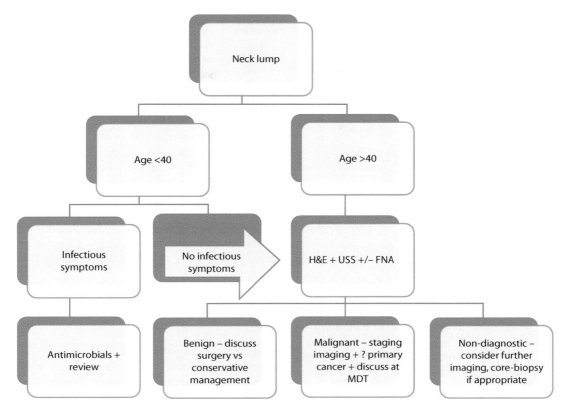

Figure 5.6 Flow chart to show initial work-up of patients with cervical lymphadenopathy.

▌ Core biopsy

The role of core biopsy (where a wide-bore needle obtains a slim tissue core) is controversial and can be judged on a case-by-case basis. Its main role is in the case of non-diagnostic FNAC. It also has the advantage of providing enough tissue for cell blocks and thus significant immunohistochemical information can be gleaned from the specimen, which is useful in identifying cell markers in the search for primary cancer if the tissue is metastatic cancer [7].

Core biopsy has a higher potential to cause tumour seeding and is on the whole used as a second choice after non-diagnostic FNAC. Another pathology where core biopsy can be useful is in the diagnosis of lymphoma, although certain centres may often prefer an excisional biopsy of a lymph node [8].

▌ Cross-sectional imaging

The role of cross-sectional imaging (CSI) is dependent on the clinical question being asked and often the local expertise in particular modalities of imaging. When requesting CSI it is important to bear these facts in mind rather than requesting thoughtless 'excludograms', which annoy the radiologists, your senior colleagues and the management!

Computed tomography (CT)

Advantages

- Images are very useful for operative planning and intraoperative guidance on localising pathology.
- Contrast enhances vessels and vascular tumours.
- It is widely available and local expertise is usually available.

- Excellent bony detail great for assessing bony involvement, e.g. mandibular or skull base, as well as thoracic extension of masses, e.g. retrosternal thyroid masses.
- No movement artefact on modern scanners.
- Can be reconstructed into 3D models.

Disadvantages

- Significant radiation dose.
- Contrast use is limited in those with renal impairment.
- Poor soft tissue differentiation.

MRI

Advantages

- T1-weighted 'anatomical' images have excellent soft tissue and spatial resolution.
- T2-weighted images preferentially highlight oedema and therefore associated pathology.
- Short tau inversion recovery (STIR) is a T2-weighted image which has fat signal suppression to further highlight abnormal tissue as a high signal.
- Has a much higher contrast resolution compared to CT and, in an appropriate patient, is the modality of choice to stage oral cavity and pharyngeal cancers as well as staging neck nodes (2016 consensus paper).
- Excellent for assessing soft tissue and organ invasion of tumours.
- Excellent for assessing large nerve peri-neural invasion (MRI neurograms can specifically be requested if patient displays neurological symptoms).

Disadvantages

- Longer scan times lead to movement artefact, which significantly reduces quality of scans. Therefore inherently poor for assessing the thorax and larynx.
- Contraindicated with some implantable pacemakers and defibrillators and implants, although newer scanners are able to overcome this drawback.

PET-CT

PET-CT is positron emission tomography combined with CT whole-body imaging using labelled tracers to fuse conventional, anatomical CT images with a functional 'map' of the disease process.

The commonest tracer is 18 fluorodeoxyglucose, which is preferentially transported and trapped into hypermetabolic cancerous or inflamed tissues.

Muscle activity causes artefact and potentially false positives. In the head and neck, these are commonly seen in the cricoarytenoid muscles when patients talk.

Main use in head and neck is for evaluating carcinoma of unknown primary where it can identify a primary in 33% of cases.

Another main role is in assessment of treatment response, detecting and restaging suspected recurrence of cancer, and staging certain cancers such as medullary thyroid cancer.

In the setting of cervical lymphadenopathy, a PET-CT cannot differentiate between an infective/inflammatory lymph node or a neoplastic lymph node, as both will be hypermetabolic.

PATHOLOGY

▥ Reactive lymphadenopathy

History

- Patients are usually young, from teenagers through to young adults, and of either sex.
- Typically solitary.
- Usually small nodal mass measuring 1–1.5 cm.
- May have come up after a URTI and simply not gone down afterward.
- Usually painless and persistent.
- Little in the way of other symptoms.

Examination

- Usually a single discreetly palpable node which is mobile, non-tender and has no skin changes.
- Common locations include levels I and II where the jugulodigastric node (high level II within the submandibular triangle) is the most common.
- Look out for skin conditions (see earlier)!

Investigation

Ultrasound is the modality of choice. Features include normal size, ovoid shape, fatty hilum and architecture The confident radiologist will not perform FNAC on such a node.

If performed, FNAC will yield a lymphoid cell population. Lymphoma is made less likely by a lack of monoclonal cell line on flow cytometry.

It is worth noting, however, that some cytologists will report that a low-grade lymphoproliferative disorder cannot be excluded regardless.

Management

Usually reassurance is all that is required in the otherwise asymptomatic low-risk patient (e.g. non-smokers <30 years old).

In any patient who is symptomatic or where there is a high index of clinical suspicion, the clinician should consider interval ultrasound over 6–12 months. Demonstration of no change is highly reassuring and patients can be discharged with appropriate safety netting.

▌ Branchial cyst

Several theories exist regarding the underlying aetiology, but most commonly these are thought to be due to cystic degeneration of a lymph node or a persistent embryologic cervical sinus [9].

Care must be taken to exclude metastatic squamous cell carcinoma (SCC) of unknown primary,

especially in patients over 40 and who smoke. Indeed it is said repeatedly that in these groups a suspected branchial cyst is carcinoma until proven otherwise.

History

- The lump usually presents in level II/III of the neck and may have become apparent acutely after an URTI.
- Occasionally patients have noticed the cyst for an extended period and a size increase has prompted referral.
- Painless, unless infected, which can lead to acute presentation and confusion for an abscess.
- Smoking and alcohol history is essential.

Examination

- Typically present under the junction of the upper and middle third of the sternomastoid muscle.
- It is solitary, mobile and non-tender unless infected.
- It is important to make a full assessment of the mucosal surfaces of the UADT and perform a skin survey. These examinations should all be clear if a presumption of a branchial cyst is to be made.
- It is worth examining the skin over the lower two-thirds of the sternocleidomastoid muscle (SCM) in detail to identify any sinus or fistula, which can be present as part of congenital branchial anomalies.

Investigation

Ultrasound will characterise a cystic structure.

FNAC should usually be performed. It often produces turbid or straw-coloured fluid with keratinised anuclear cells and squamous debris [10]. The presence of squamous cells makes squamous cell carcinoma impossible to exclude. Careful evaluation of the cyst wall is possible via ultrasound and may be targeted and more useful in ruling out carcinoma. Equivocal results combined with thick-walled cysts can be amenable to core biopsy dependent on local preference.

Cross-sectional imaging is useful for anatomical delineation and surgical planning. MRI will reveal attachment to the pharynx/tonsil as well as the relationship to the great vessels of the neck, accessory and hypoglossal nerve.

In patients where the index of suspicion is high despite equivocal FNAC or core biopsy, there may be a role for PET-CT. PET-CT has a high negative predictive value (96%) but a low positive predictive value (56%) in this setting [11]. A negative PET-CT scan is therefore reassuring allowing for the patient to proceed to surgical excision in most cases. It is worth noting, however, that FNAC or core biopsy can in itself create a false positive from the tissue trauma created by biopsy. Clearly the use of a valuable resource such as PET-CT in this context has to be balanced against the patient's perceived risk of malignancy. This author would therefore reserve the use of PET-CT to high-risk patients (i.e. smokers over 40 with no clinical sign of primary carcinoma) and request the scan to be performed before FNA or core biopsy takes place wherever possible.

Management

For the young, non-smoking patient with negative cytology and concordant imaging, the management is usually surgical excision. Patients who are either unfit for surgery or refuse surgery should be counselled appropriately and offered surveillance unless the aforementioned factors will not change in the future.

Incision and drainage should be avoided, where possible, if the cyst presents acutely infected. Aspiration under image guidance, if required, along with intravenous antibiotics is recommended with elective excision following the resolution of infection.

In a patient over 40, especially in smokers, a branchial cyst is said to be a carcinoma until proven otherwise. This may represent metastatic SCC of unknown primary or indeed true carcinoma within a branchial cyst, which is a debated entity.

In light of this, excision is best performed via a supraselective neck dissection of the involved levels. This allows for good access, identification of the internal jugular vein and carotid artery as well as cranial nerves X, XI and XII. A 'lumpectomy' is the more traditional approach and indeed is probably the most common approach worldwide. In the majority of cases this can be performed with good results. Conversion to a selective neck dissection should be strongly considered in cases where identification of anatomy is difficult and certainly in cases where the diagnosis is in doubt and carcinoma is suspected.

Oropharyngeal SCC related to human papillomavirus (HPV) is increasing in prevalence, which further complicates the issue, as this is seen in younger non-smokers. The majority of these carcinomas present with cystic nodal metastases and 5% have sub-clinical primaries in sites such as the base of the tongue.

With a lack of high-quality data to support any specific practice, this is a debated topic in many MDTs throughout the world. The principles are to avoid performing a 'lumpectomy'-type procedure on what turns out to be metastatic carcinoma despite a benign radiological appearance. This could 'seed' the neck and increase local treatment failure rates by threefold, which is significant, as the resection is not considered oncological [12].

It is this author's opinion that any cystic mass in the lateral neck should be treated with a high index of suspicion in patients over 40 and management should involve the multidisciplinary team (MDT).

If a branchial cyst is excised after equivocal cytology and carcinoma is found, centres should offer the patient a completion neck dissection and/or postoperative radiotherapy after the patient has been worked-up for carcinoma of unknown primary (see later).

A safe option in cases of doubt is to counsel the patient about possible malignancy, perform a supraselective neck dissection under frozen section control and proceed to comprehensive neck dissection if malignancy is confirmed.

Depending on the results of the PET-CT, a panendoscopy with blind or targeted biopsies can take place, including tonsillectomy with or without tongue base mucosectomy. If negative, the patient's procedure is complete. If carcinoma is confirmed, a complete comprehensive neck dissection is performed (usually levels II–IV) as well as bilateral tonsillectomy. Adjuvant treatment can then be dictated based on histological analysis and risk factors and/or presence of an index lesion.

▌ Lymphoma

History

Lymphoma should always be on the differential of patients presenting with neck masses.

- Single or multiple persistent nodes in groups within a nodal level.
- Can be painful
- May show a rapid increase in size in high-grade lymphomas.
- Systemic symptoms, i.e. 'B' symptoms of night sweats and weight loss, imply systemic disease and traditionally are a poor prognostic indicator.
- Risk factors include immunocompromise, previous lymphoma, viral infection with HIV, Epstein–Barr virus, HTLV, rheumatoid arthritis, Hashimoto's disease and coeliac disease.

Examination

- Findings usually range from multiple small 'shotty', rubbery nodes clustered in nodal levels within the neck to a large, rapidly growing nodal mass with smaller nodes palpable within the nodal level.
- It is important to fully assess the UADT with examination and flexible endoscopy, as lymphoma may present with extranodal disease particularly within mucosal-associated lymphoid tissue such as Waldeyer's ring (i.e. the Palatine tonsils, adenoids and the base of the tongue, lingual tonsils).
- If lymphoma is suspected, the patient's axillae and inguinal regions should be palpated for lymphadenopathy.

Investigation

FNAC is not diagnostic but has a crucial role in excluding metastatic carcinoma. Modern flow cytometry techniques are possible on FNAC specimens and allow for the identification of monoclonal B or T cells, which greatly raise the index of suspicion.

In order for accurate diagnosis and treatment planning, enough tissue to demonstrate cell architecture is required. This is traditionally optimally obtained via open biopsy. Excisional biopsy (i.e. complete excision) of a lymph node is preferable over incisional biopsy (cutting out a section of a node) as more tissue is obtained and less scarring is present in the neck. It is important to remember that once carcinoma has been excluded, incisional biopsy will not seed or upstage the lymphoma. As a result, diagnosis should not come at the cost of any functional structure, and when excision would cause morbidity, a large representative incisional biopsy is usually adequate enough for the progression of management. An important point is that upon biopsy, material should be sent fresh (i.e. not fixed in formalin) so that pathologists can use and fix the tissue as they see fit as well as perform flow cytometry.

Upon diagnosis, PET-CT scanning is now considered the staging modality of choice.

Management

The in-depth management of lymphoma is beyond the scope of this book as they are the remit of the haemato-oncologist. Most lymphomas are managed by chemotherapy, radiotherapy or a combination of both in the context of a specialist MDT.

▌ Carcinoma of unknown primary

History

Up to 5% of patients with head and neck cancer have no detectable primary lesion – that is they present with metastatic disease usually in the neck.

- Usually painless, an enlarging lateral neck mass is usually otherwise asymptomatic.
- A full smoking history with pack-years is useful in the context of risk stratification, prognosis and inclusion criteria for clinical trials.

Patients follow the demographic balance of all head and neck cancer, i.e. there are two main groups: the traditional SCC patient who is usually over 50 and a smoker possibly with a history of moderate to heavy alcohol use, and the younger patient under 50 who often is in good health and may or may not smoke.

The younger group represents a clinical entity of increasing incidence owing to HPV type 16 and 18 infections leading to SCC, which is biologically different in its behaviour to traditional non-HPV-related SCC.

Examination

- Assess the neck lump itself noting size, fixation to the sternomastoid, and deeper structures such as the prevertebral fascia and skin.
- Special care must be taken to assess for other palpable adenopathy, as a single large node or cluster of nodes can make others difficult to feel in comparison.
- Examination can then be directed to identify a primary lesion. Full mucosal survey of the UADT should be carried out.
- The tonsils and base of tongue require special attention, as even a small primary carcinoma at these sites can provide disproportionately large metastatic neck nodes.
- The skin should also be inspected for any changes and ulcerations, and a skin survey should be preformed noting any scars (which my indicate an old excised cutaneous malignancy) or suspicious skin lesions.

Investigation

Imaging

Ultrasound and FNAC are crucial in planning further work-up of patients. FNAC will usually be diagnostic but can show a spectrum from atypical squamous cells to frank clusters of squamous cell carcinoma. P16 immunohistochemistry is a useful surrogate biomarker for HPV overexpression and can be performed on a cytology sample if of high enough yield.

Core biopsy may be necessary if FNAC is non-diagnostic. This can produce sufficient tissue for additional immunostaining, which may help locate other primary tumour sites such as EBV (nasopharyngeal carcinoma), thyroglobulin (differentiated thyroid cancer) and calcitonin (medullary thyroid carcinoma).

Assuming no clinically apparent primary lesion has been identified, the patient is now a clinical unknown primary and further imaging is required to help locate the possible index lesion.

PET-CT has now overtaken both contrast CT and MRI scanning as the investigation of choice for locating an unknown primary and is now regarded as the standard of care in the UK [13]. Some MDTs may insist on cross-sectional imaging prior to PET-CT and only perform PET-CT if the MRI does not reveal a primary site. Meta-analysis has shown that PET-CT can identify a primary in up to 44% of cases. PET-CT has a high negative predictive value but is also sensitive and has a significant false positive rate. It can also miss mucosal primaries under 1 cm in maximal diameter.

Its main role therefore is to help target biopsies and to stage the patient. Biopsies will register on PET-CT as false positives, hence patients should be discussed at MDT meetings in light of their PET-CT before panendoscopy (see **Figure 5.7**).

Panendoscopy and biopsy

Patients must undergo panendoscopy under general anaesthesia. If imaging has been useful, targeted biopsies are performed. If the patient still has a carcinoma of unknown primary, a full mucosal survey of the UADT must take place.

Sites should include the nasal cavity, nasopharynx, oral cavity, hard and soft palates, tongue base, tonsil, posterior pharyngeal wall, vallecula, supraglottis, glottis, subglottis, pyriform fossa, post-cricoid region, and proximal oesophagus. Palpation of the oral cavity and tongue base should also be carried out.

If imaging (including PET-CT) has not revealed a primary site, then 'blind biopsies' are still performed in some units. More recently there is more evidence to support the resection of oropharyngeal lymphoid tissue, i.e. bilateral tonsillectomy and base of tongue

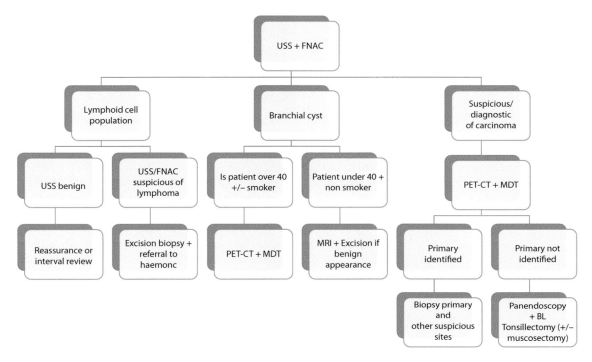

Figure 5.7 An algorithm for investigating cervical lymph nodes.

mucosectomy. It is now recommended that bilateral tonsillectomy is carried out in patients with carcinoma of unknown primary [14].

Base of tongue mucosectomy, which can be regarded as a mucosal stripping of the lingual tonsil, has shown promising results identifying between 80% and 90% of otherwise unknown primaries. This is commonly performed using a surgical robot so it is therefore limited to centres with appropriate facility [15].

P16 immunohistochemistry can be performed on FNAC. If positive this supports the presence of a microscopic oropharyngeal primary tumour, even if none can be found after full investigation. As such the vast majority of head and neck carcinoma of unknown primary is now thought to be an occult oropharyngeal carcinoma.

Management

If a primary is found, then the patient is managed according to the primary site with nodal metastasis.

A true unknown primary can be classified as T0. Nodal staging is as per other nodal staging in the neck (see **Table 5.2**).

The primary aim of treatment in all patients with SCC unknown primary is locoregional control. The rate of emergence of a primary in these patents is approximately 3% per year, which is in line with the rate of all other mucosal head and neck cancers demonstrating a second primary.

Table 5.2 Staging classification for carcinoma of unknown primary.

T	N	M	Stage
0	1	0	III
0	2a	0	IVA
0	2b	0	IVA
0	2c	0	IVA
0	3	0	IVB
0	1–3	1	IVC

In general, treatment options in head and neck cancer include surgery, radiation therapy and chemotherapy.

Surgery

Resection of tumour with a margin of healthy tissue. In this case, a neck dissection. Neck dissections are fascial dissections excising the contents of the deep layer of the investing cervical fascia down to the pre-vertebral fascia. The aim is a comprehensive clearance of all lymph nodes by systematically clearing fascia on structures, which are being preserved.

Neck dissections are classified into

Radical (RND): Removal of all tissue in levels I–V above the pre-vertebral fascia, sparing only the carotid artery, the vagus and hypoglossal nerve.

Modified radical (MRND): Involves the removal of all tissue in levels I–V but requires preservation of one or more of the following three non-lymphatic structures: the spinal accessory nerve, the internal jugular vein and the sternomastoid muscle.

Selective neck dissection (SND): As per modified radical and sparing as many structures not macroscopically involved in nodal disease including the sternomastoid, internal jugular vein and accessory nerve, and variably the cervical plexus nerves and the ansa cervicalis. It can be adapted to encompass levels as the disease dictates. The three most common types are:

– SND I–III (supraomohyoid) usually in the context of an N0 neck for oral cavity tumours.
– SND II–IV (lateral) usually for laryngeal and hypopharyngeal tumours.
– SND II–VI (posterolateral) for skin, parotid and thyroid tumours.

Radiation therapy

Radiation therapy is usually external beam radiation where a total dose (in grays) is delivered by cyclical techniques given over multiple visits (fractions) (e.g. 70 Gy in 35 fractions). Despite modern intensity-modulated radiotherapy (IMRT) treatments, radiation therapy particularly to the pharynx is plagued with the limitation of long-term toxicities including mucositis, xerostomia and neuropathies, which can be functionally debilitating and difficult to manage. It can also usually only be given once at a radical dose to a given site due to significant side effects on the brain stem, spine and bone necrosis (osteoradionecrosis).

Total mucosal irradiation (TMI)

The rationale for TMI is to deliver radical treatment dose irradiation to all potential mucosal primary sites (i.e. all of the UADT). The evidence to support this practice, however, is limited and as such it remains an area of controversy, although it is still popular in the UK. Patients undergoing TMI show significant acute and chronic toxicity as well as poor quality of life. This has improved using IMRTs but it is still an area where morbidity can be potentially reduced. Strategies to identify microscopic primary cancers such as base of tongue mucosectomy or lingual tonsillectomy could play a significant role in the future.

Chemotherapy

Platinum-based agents such as cisplatin (or carboplatin in those with reduced creatinine clearance) are not usually considered a radical modality of treatment on their own. They are used as adjuvant or concurrent therapy with radiation. Neoadjuvant chemotherapy has limited evidence for its use.

N1

See **Figure 5.8**.

This can usually be managed with a single modality (surgery or radiotherapy). There is debate within the literature about which is the best initial modality of treatment. Surgery allows the neck to be definitively staged and identification of pathological extracapsular spread, which is not reliably identified on preoperative imaging. In p16 negative head and neck cancer, extracapsular spread (spread of carcinoma beyond the capsule of the lymph node) is the most important negative prognosticator and indicates the need for adjuvant therapy [16]. In p16 positive oropharyngeal carcinoma, there is increasing evidence that this is not prognostic and may not require adjuvant therapy [17,18]. Most centres would advocate either a MRND or comprehensive SND (I–V) if this is being considered as a single modality treatment [19].

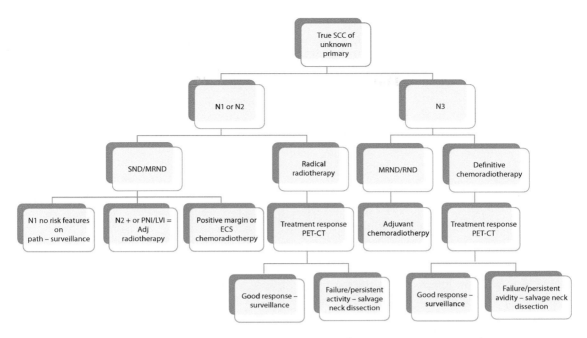

Figure 5.8 Algorithm for management of biopsy proven SCC of unknown primary in neck.

N2a/b/c

These patients will require adjuvant therapy (radiotherapy or chemoradiotherapy) if they undergo neck dissection. In light of this, it is often argued that they should be offered primary non-surgical management with surgery reserved for salvage. There is limited evidence to suggest outcomes between surgery and adjuvant therapy compared to radical radiotherapy alone is comparable [20]. Treatment options of upfront surgery versus non-surgical management should be offered to the patient after discussion at the MDT meeting [14].

N3

This represents stage IV disease and has a universally poor prognosis. Modified radical or a radical neck dissection has a role in both the curative and palliative setting. In the curative setting, postoperative chemoradiotherapy is usually necessary for a chance at local control. Upfront chemoradiotherapy is also a valid treatment strategy but, as with N2 disease, patients requiring salvage surgery suffer from higher rates of postoperative complications due to tissue damage from non-surgical treatment [21,22].

FOLLOW-UP

All patients should undergo at least 5 years of surveillance as per the recommendations on follow-up for other mucosal head and neck cancers. Review should include assessment of UADT and neck for recurrent disease or presentation of primary disease.

SPECIAL CONSIDERATIONS

Where thyroid tissue is identified in cervical nodes, this represents thyroid carcinoma until proven otherwise and should be investigated by ultrasound of the thyroid gland and FNAC or any nodules of suspicion (see Chapter 6). Where metastatic medullary carcinoma of the thyroid is identified on immunostaining, PET-CT in addition to ultrasound has a role in detecting a primary and other metastasis. Where PET-CT or immunostaining of nodal cytology suggest primaries outside the head and neck, referral should of course be made to the appropriate MDT for further management.

REFERENCES

1 Otto RA, Bowes AK. Neck masses: Benign or malignant? Sorting out the causes by age-group. *Postgrad Med*. 1990;88 (1):199–204.

2 Ruhl C. Evaluation of the neck mass. *Med Health R I*. 2004;87(10):307–10.

3 Weber AL, Rahemtullah A, Ferry JA. Hodgkin and non-Hodgkin lymphoma of the head and neck: Clinical, pathologic, and imaging evaluation. *Neuroimaging Clin N Am*. 2003;13(3):371–92.

4 Velleuer E, Dietrich R. Fanconi anemia: Young patients at high risk for squamous cell carcinoma. *Mol Cell Pediatr*. 2014;1(1):9.

5 Lopez F, Rodrigo JP, Silver CE, Haigentz M Jr., Bishop JA, Strojan P et al. Cervical lymph node metastases from remote primary tumor sites. *Head Neck*. 2016;38(Suppl 1):E2374–85.

6 Layfield LJ. Fine-needle aspiration in the diagnosis of head and neck lesions: A review and discussion of problems in differential diagnosis. *Diagn Cytopathol*. 2007;35(12):798–805.

7 Krane JF. Role of cytology in the diagnosis and management of HPV-associated head and neck carcinoma. *Acta Cytol*. 2013;57(2):117–26.

8 Amador-Ortiz C, Chen L, Hassan A et al. Combined core needle biopsy and fine-needle aspiration with ancillary studies correlate highly with traditional techniques in the diagnosis of nodal-based lymphoma. *Am J Clin Pathol*. 2011;135(4):516–24.

9 Golledge J, Ellis H. The aetiology of lateral cervical (branchial) cysts: Past and present theories. *J Laryngol Otol*. 1994;108 (8):653–9.

10 Valentino M, Quiligotti C, Carone L. Branchial cleft cyst. *J Ultrasound*. 2013;16(1):17–20.

11 Abadi P, Johansen A, Godballe C, Gerke O, Hoilund-Carlsen PF, Thomassen A. 18F-FDG PET/CT to differentiate malignant necrotic lymph node from benign cystic lesions in the neck. *Ann Nucl Med*. 2017;31(2):101–8.

12 Gleeson M, Herbert A, Richards A. Management of lateral neck masses in adults. *BMJ*. 2000;320(7248):1521–4.

13 Strojan P, Ferlito A, Medina JE et al. Contemporary management of lymph node metastases from an unknown primary to the neck: I. A review of diagnostic approaches. *Head Neck*. 2013;35(1):123–32.

14 Strojan P, Ferlito A, Langendijk JA et al. Contemporary management of lymph node metastases from an unknown primary to the neck: II. A review of therapeutic options. *Head Neck*. 2013;35(2):286–93.

15 Mehta V, Johnson P, Tassler A et al. A new paradigm for the diagnosis and management of unknown primary tumors of the head and neck: A role for transoral robotic surgery. *Laryngoscope*. 2013;123(1):146–51.

16 Jose J, Coatesworth AP, Johnston C, MacLennan K. Cervical node metastases in squamous cell carcinoma of the upper aerodigestive tract: The significance of extracapsular spread and soft tissue deposits. *Head Neck*. 2003;25 (6):451–6.

17 Sinha P, Kallogjeri D, Gay H et al. High metastatic node number, not extracapsular spread or N-classification is a node-related prognosticator in transorally-resected, neck-dissected p16-positive oropharynx cancer. *Oral Oncol*. 2015;51(5):514–20.

18 Sinha P, Lewis JS Jr., Piccirillo JF, Kallogjeri D, Haughey BH. Extracapsular spread and adjuvant therapy in human papillomavirus-related, p16-positive oropharyngeal carcinoma. *Cancer*. 2012;118(14):3519–30.

19 Dragan AD, Nixon IJ, Guerrero-Urbano MT, Oakley R, Jeannon JP, Simo R. Selective neck dissection as a therapeutic option in management of squamous cell carcinoma of unknown primary. *Eur Arch Otorhinolaryngol*. 2014;271(5):1249–56.

20 Demiroz C, Vainshtein JM, Koukourakis GV et al. Head and neck squamous cell carcinoma of unknown primary: Neck dissection and radiotherapy or definitive radiotherapy. *Head Neck*. 2014;36(11):1589–95.

21 Sanabria A, Kowalski LP, Shaha AR et al. Salvage surgery for head and neck cancer: A plea for better definitions. *Eur Arch Otorhinolaryngol*. 2014;271(6):1347–50.

22 Balaker AE, Abemayor E, Elashoff D, St John MA. Cancer of unknown primary: Does treatment modality make a difference? *Laryngoscope*. 2012;122(6):1279–82.

6
THYROID DISEASE

R. James A. England

The thyroid gland, being an endocrine gland, is susceptible to both disorders of structure and/or function and these may lead to local or systemic effects. The disease processes that may affect the thyroid gland include:

a Conditions of hypertrophy leading to direct pressure effects
b Malignant change
c Activity disorder

The disease processes may be inherited, and hence to some extent predictable, or due to environmental effects.

The aims of thyroid disease management include:

1 Exclusion or treatment of sinister disease
2 Exclusion or treatment of activity disorders to avoid systemic illness
3 Symptomatic amelioration including cosmesis

ANATOMY

The thyroid gland is composed of two lobes connected by a thin central isthmic portion. A third lobe ascending from the isthmus (usually not in the midline) called the pyramidal lobe is found in approximately 20% of patients [1]. The isthmus normally lies superficial to the third and fourth tracheal rings in the anterior neck directly below the sternothyroid muscles. The normal thyroid gland weighs just under 20 grams but the weight increases with age [2].

▌ Laryngeal innervation

This is discussed here due to the intimate relations of these nerves to the thyroid (see **Table 6.1**). A clear understanding of the location, course and function of these nerves is essential to the thyroid surgeon and the team caring for these patients pre- and post-operatively.

The superior laryngeal nerve is a branch of the vagus nerve. It descends on the lateral aspect of the pharynx deep to the internal carotid artery and divides into two branches. The external branch descends on the lateral aspect of the larynx deep to the sternothyroid to supply the cricothyroid muscle. It acts to increase vocal cord tension altering vocal pitch. It is seen when dissecting the medial aspect of the superior pole of the thyroid lobes.

The internal branch pierces the thyrohyoid membrane with the superior laryngeal artery. It supplies sensation to the supraglottis. The subglottis receives sensory innervation from the recurrent laryngeal

Table 6.1 Laryngeal innervation and effect of damage to each nerve.

Nerve	Supplies	Effect of damage	How this affects patient
Recurrent laryngeal nerve	*Motor*: All intrinsic laryngeal muscles except cricothyroid *Sensory*: Sensation below vocal cords	Paralysed vocal cord (N.B.: An inability to open the vocal cords due to the posterior cricoarytenoid muscle being paralysed)	*Unilateral*: Dysphonia (the precise character of voice depends on the position of the paralysed vocal cord) *Bilateral*: Potentially airway obstruction if the vocal cords are paralytic in the paramedian position
Superior laryngeal nerve			
External branch	*Motor*: Cricothyroid muscle	Loss of ability to change tension in vocal cord	Can affect vocal pitch
Internal branch	*Sensory*: Laryngeal mucosa above vocal cords	Loss of laryngeal irritation reflex cough	Can lead to aspiration

nerve. The glottis receives sensory innervation from both nerves. The recurrent laryngeal nerve (also a branch of the vagus) loops under the aortic arch on the left and the subclavian artery on the right. The left nerve travels in the tracheo-oesophageal groove lying deep to the superior parathyroid gland and enters the larynx at the cricothyroid joint. The right nerve travels at a more oblique angle, usually due to the effect of travelling under the subclavian artery, and also enters the larynx at the cricothyroid joint. It supplies all intrinsic muscles of the larynx. This nerve has to be identified and preserved during dissection of the thyroid lobes and parathyroid glands.

▌ Blood supply

The blood supply of the thyroid is symmetric bilaterally. The superior thyroid artery is a branch of the external carotid artery, whilst the inferior thyroid artery is a branch of the thyrocervical trunk (a branch from the first part of the subclavian artery).

A variable unique vessel is the thyroid ima artery. This is an embryonic remnant that is present in up to 10% of the population and usually arises from the brachiocephalic trunk but may also arise directly from the aortic arch.

The venous drainage is consistent. The superior and middle thyroid veins drain in the internal jugular, whilst the inferior thyroid veins drain into the brachiocephalic vein.

▌ Lymphatic drainage

The thyroid drains to the paratracheal lymph nodes. These are regarded as level VI. The boundaries of level VI are the hyoid superiorly, the suprasternal notch inferiorly and the carotid sheaths laterally.

▌ Innervation

The thyroid is innervated by the autonomic nervous system, the vagus and the sympathetic trunk providing the parasympathetic and sympathetic fibres, respectively.

PHYSIOLOGY

The basic functional unit of the thyroid gland is the follicle. This consists of a lumen filled with colloid surrounded by cuboidal epithelial cells. The principle component of colloid is the glycoprotein thyroglobulin. Thyroid hormone production involves the active uptake of inorganic iodide by thyrocytes and its subsequent oxidation and conversion to iodine. Iodine is combined with the tyrosine components of the thyroglobulin molecule to form mono- and diiodotyrosine. These molecules then combine to form the active metabolites tetraiodothyronine (T4) and triiodothyroonine (T3). All T4 is produced within the thyroid gland, but only 20% of the more active metabolite T3 is produced here. The remaining 80% is produced in the peripheral circulation from the conversion of T4.

The stroma of the thyroid contains parafollicular or C-cells, which are of neural crest origin. The C-cells comprise approximately 0.1% of the weight of the thyroid gland. They are predominantly situated in the mid and upper portions of the lateral thyroid. The C-cells produce calcitonin, a hormone that reduces serum calcium levels and therefore opposes the effect of parathyroid hormone. It does this mainly by inhibiting osteoclastic activity. Osteoblasts do not have calcitonin receptors and are therefore not affected by the hormone. A lesser action of calcitonin is the reduction in renal tubular resorption of calcium and phosphate.

PATHOLOGY

▮▮ The spectrum of thyroid disease

The thyroid gland, being an endocrine organ, may be affected by endocrine activity disorders. These comprise either under- or overproduction of thyroxine. In addition, the thyroid gland may develop an abnormal growth pattern leading to diffuse or localised enlargement of the gland, a condition known as goitre. Finally, thyroid tumours may develop, which may be benign or malignant. Each situation will be described in turn.

▮▮ Hypothyroidism

Hypothyroidism occurs when the thyroid gland produces insufficient thyroxine. It can be congenital or acquired.

Congenital hypothyroidism affects approximately 1 in 4000 births and is the most common treatable cause of congenital mental retardation [3].

The commonest acquired cause worldwide is iodine deficiency, but in iodine-replete areas the commonest cause is Hashimoto's thyroiditis or chronic autoimmune thyroiditis. First described in 1912 by Hakaru Hashimoto, it was not recognised as an autoimmune disorder until 1957. The condition is closely related to Graves' disease and is likely caused by both environmental and genetic factors. It is characterised by lymphocytic infiltration of the thyroid gland and associated high antibodies to thyroid peroxidase and thyroglobulin. The condition is far more common in women with a female preponderance of 7:1.

History

The common classical symptoms include:

a   *Constitutional*: Lethargy, weakness, cold sensitivity
b   *Gastrointestinal*: Constipation, weight gain
c   *Psychological*: Depression
d   *General*: Coarse hair, dry skin, thick tongue, deep voice, menstrual irregularity, myalgia, facial oedema

It is more common in women, iodine-deficient and middle-aged persons.

Drug history is also important, particularly amiodarone and lithium therapy.

A past medical history of autoimmune disorders, thyroiditis, Graves' disease, Turner/Down syndrome or radiation therapy are risk factors.

Examination

A goitre is uncommon in hypothyroidism.

Eyelid oedema and facial oedema is common. Bradycardia and diastolic hypertension is also often identified, as is delayed relaxation of tendon reflexes.

Flexible naso endoscopy (FNE) may identify oedematous vocal cords. A vocal cord palsy would be very rare and would generally be associated with a thyroid mass.

Investigation

Blood tests

Serum thyroid-stimulating hormone (TSH) test

Others – Serum T4, antithyroid peroxidase antibodies

Imaging

Ultrasound (US) is not part of a routine work-up for hypothyroidism in the absence of goitre or palpable nodule.

Management

This is treated with thyroid hormone replacement (thyroxine).

▌ Hyperthyroidism

Hyperthyroidism occurs when the thyroid gland overproduces thyroxine. This needs differentiation from thyrotoxicosis, which includes hyperthyroidism, but includes any situation leading to excess levels of circulating thyroxine, such as over-replacement with oral thyroxine.

The commonest cause of hyperthyroidism is Graves' disease, the cause in approximately 70% of cases. There is some evidence that the incidence of Graves' disease is increasing [4]. The cause of Graves' disease is thought to be multifactorial including a genetic predisposition leading to an increased risk of developing autoantibodies and non-genetic factors including stress, smoking and being female. Other common causes include toxic multinodular goitre, toxic solitary adenoma and thyroiditis, although many less common causes exist (**Table 6.2**).

Graves' disease

Graves' disease was first described in the 19th century as a condition comprising goitre with thyroid overactivity, tachycardia and ocular changes. It occurs in 20–50 per 100,000 of the population annually. It is 6 times more common in women than men and its peak age of incidence is between 30 and 50, although it may occur at any age. The lifetime risk is 3% for women and 0.5% for men.

Graves' disease is primarily a genetically mediated autoimmune disorder. Hypermethylation of several genes has been identified, including those encoding thyrotropin receptor and proteins involved in T-cell

Table 6.2 Less common causes of thyrotoxicosis.

Amiodarone treatment
De Quervain thyroiditis
Jod-Basedow thyrotoxicosis
Polyostotic fibrous dysplasia
Ovarian teratoma
Choriocarcinoma
Hydatidiform mole
Pituitary tumour
Post-partum thyroiditis
Struma ovarii
Testicular cancer
Thyroid cancer
Thyroxine overdose

signalling. Environmental factors such as dietary iodine, smoking, infections and stress have also been implicated. The condition involves the production by intrathyroidal B-cells of IgG subclass autoantibodies against the TSH receptor.

Clinical features

Graves' ophthalmopathy can be disfiguring and can threaten sight. It becomes clinically apparent in approximately one-third of Graves' patients. Its clinical course typically comprises an active phase lasting for up to 3 years involving increased tearing and ocular discomfort and proptosis, which may occasionally cause diplopia and even loss of vision. An inactive phase follows during which eye symptoms stabilise. More rarely, occurring in 1%–4% of Graves' patients, thyroid dermopathy involving characteristically non-pitting pretibial swelling is evident. In some with dermopathy, acropachy, which resembles finger clubbing, is also evident.

Investigation

If pathognomonic features such as ophthalmopathy or dermopathy are absent and a diffuse goitre is not detected, radionuclide scanning showing diffuse uptake can differentiate Graves' disease from thyroiditis and multinodular goitre.

Routine measurement of thyrotropin-receptor antibodies is not mandatory, but when such assays are performed, they have 99% sensitivity and specificity for Graves' disease.

Other common causes of hyperthyroidism

The other common causes comprise toxic multinodular goitre and toxic solitary adenoma. Thyroiditis may cause transient hyperthyroidism. Rarer causes are listed in **Table 6.2**.

Toxic multinodular goitre (TMNG)

This condition tends to occur in an older age group than Graves' disease. It is important to differentiate the two because TMNG will not respond to thionamide therapy as a curative treatment modality.

Toxic solitary adenoma

When a toxic patient has a dominant thyroid nodule, a toxic adenoma should always be considered. The diagnosis is confirmed by a radionuclide scan showing intense uptake within the nodule in a background of reduced uptake. The diagnosis is important, as the treatment of choice in most cases is a thyroid lobectomy, which optimises the chance of achieving cure without the need for post-treatment medication. Radioiodine treatment requires generally higher doses for success and normally results in permanent hypothyroidism. Most toxic adenomas are histopathologically follicular adenomas.

Thyroiditis

Thyroiditis comprises any thyroid disorder that causes inflammation of the thyroid. This group of conditions includes: Hashimoto's thyroiditis, postpartum thyroiditis, subacute thyroiditis, drug-induced thyroiditis and Riedel's thyroiditis.

Hashimoto's thyroiditis

This condition is covered in hypothyroidism, but it may initially present with hyperthyroidism. It is characterised by a swollen thyroid gland with initially elevated thyroid autoantibodies and either subclinical or overt thyrotoxicosis.

Postpartum thyroiditis

This classically occurs up to 6 months after giving birth and generally completely resolves, although the patient may ultimately become hypothyroid. It is important to differentiate the condition from Graves' disease by TSH receptor antibody testing or a radionuclide scan, the latter demonstrating reduced thyroid uptake in the case of thyroiditis.

Subacute or viral thyroiditis

Generally occurs after a viral illness. It is characterised by a swollen tender thyroid gland. Initially the patient will demonstrate symptoms of hyperthyroidism, but as the gland becomes depleted of thyroid substrate hypothyroid symptoms may be exhibited. Treatment is generally supportive with non-steroidal anti-inflammatory drugs and the majority of patients will completely resolve. However, 5% will become permanently hypothyroid. Once again a radionuclide scan will demonstrate reduced thyroid uptake.

Management

The American Thyroid Association consensus document for the management of thyrotoxicosis states that thionamide therapy, surgery and radioiodine treatment should all be considered as first-line therapies for the management of thyrotoxicosis [5]. For patients who currently smoke or formerly smoked tobacco, the efficacy of medical therapy is reduced and the importance of smoking cessation cannot be overstated.

In uncomplicated cases, antithyroid drugs remain the first-line treatment in Europe and are increasingly favoured over radioiodine in North America. Antithyroid drugs will control thyrotoxicosis in the short term and may induce euthyroidism in the long term after a 12–18 month course. However, this modality is only potentially effective in 40%–50% of patients. Whilst on thionamides patients must be made aware of the risk of neutropenia, so the development of a sore throat necessitates stopping medication and having a white cell count check prior to recommencing therapy. The recurrence rate is not further decreased by providing treatment for more than 18 months or by combining antithyroid drugs with levothyroxine (block and replace treatment).

Ablative therapy, either from radioactive iodine (RAI) or surgical thyroidectomy, necessitates lifelong thyroid hormone replacement post total thyroidectomy and in 90% of patients successfully treated with radioiodine. Thus, each treatment approach has advantages and drawbacks.

The patient's preference, after receiving adequate counselling, remains a critical factor in therapy decisions. According to a randomised study with 14–21 years of follow-up, quality of life was similar among the various treatment options, as was cost.

Surgery may be an attractive option for patients with large goitres, women with young children or women who are wishing to become pregnant shortly

after treatment, and patients who want to avoid exposure to antithyroid drugs or radioiodine. It is recommended that women who have undergone surgery wait until the serum thyrotropin level stabilises with levothyroxine therapy before attempting conception.

▌ Goitre

Aetiology

Goitre or thyromegaly is characterised by enlargement of the thyroid gland. The commonest worldwide cause is iodine deficiency, the cause in 90% of cases. Goitre affects 15.8% of the general population [6].

Goitre may be uninodular, multinodular or diffuse, and may be associated with hypothyroidism, euthyroidism, pituitary dysfunction, thyroid cancer or benign thyroid tumours.

The current World Health Organisation classification of goitre from 1994 involves a two-grade classification of goitre where the goitre is either palpable in the neutral neck position or visible in the neutral neck position [7]. This is a simple and useful classification for assessing goitre incidence but has little use otherwise.

In iodine-replete areas the aetiology of goitre is not fully understood, but primary factors include genetic propensity and female sex, and secondary factors include smoking, an elevated TSH and stress. In addition, dietary goitrogens including millet, selenium, cauliflower, sweet potato, cabbage, broccoli, kelp and turnip are recognised.

History

Goitre is commonly referred to as a neck lump. Compressive symptoms such as shortness of breath, noisy breathing or dysphagia should be excluded.

Patients should not be encouraged to blame goitres for vague symptoms such as globus pharyngeus, as in general there is little evidence to suggest thyroid surgery will resolve these symptoms [8].

Examination

Neck examination should assess any retrosternal extension and include FNE to assess vocal cord mobility. Vocal cord paralysis at presentation should raise immediate concern for malignant thyroid disease, though it is recognised to be a rare occurrence in benign thyroid disease [9].

Investigation

The likelihood of malignancy is first minimised by ultrasound evaluation with or without fine needle aspiration. The current British Thyroid Association (BTA) guidelines suggest adherence to the U classification when assessing thyroid nodules ultrasonographically (**Table 6.3**). Indeterminate nodules will often then be cytologically studied via fine needle aspiration cytology and graded using the 'Thy' classification (**Table 6.4**).

Management

Management depends on cause and symptoms. Thyroxine treatment has limited efficacy, but studies suggest a 15%–40% reduction can be achieved. If the thyroxine is withdrawn the gland returns to pretreatment size [10].

Radioiodine treatment can also result in volume decrease of up to 58% if recombinant human TSH is also used, although hypothyroidism may result in up to 65% of patients [10]. This option remains attractive for the older subgroup with comorbidities. Additionally, transient goitre swelling post-radioiodine administration may result in acute airway compromise.

Surgery represents the mainstay for the management of goitre in the UK. Although previously the standard surgical procedure was subtotal thyroidectomy, the move is towards total lobectomy or total thyroidectomy, as it is now recognised that the complication rates for this procedure are no higher, with a negligible recurrence rate. Additionally, the amount of thyroid tissue to leave in subtotal surgery cannot be accurately estimated and placing the patient on thyroxine post-subtotal surgery is generally advised anyway to keep serum TSH low and reduce the risk of recurrence.

▌ Thyroid cancer

Epidemiology

Thyroid cancer is the commonest endocrine malignancy comprising 3% of all cancers. It is the most rapidly increasing malignancy in the US in both men and women, with a 2.4-fold increase in differentiated thyroid cancer recorded between 1973 and 2002 [18]. Although some of the increase has been attributed to improved detection techniques, particularly via ultrasound, which has led to the increased discovery of incidental microcarcinomas (tumours less than 1 cm in maximum diameter), the incidence of tumours >5 cm in size has also increased 12% per year over the same period. However, the mortality rate has remained unchanged despite the increase.

Thyroid cancers comprise a spectrum of tumours arising from either the thyroid follicular cells or the parafollicular cells, or C-cells. The commonest types of thyroid cancers are the differentiated thyroid cancers divided into papillary thyroid cancers (accounting for 80% of thyroid malignancies) and follicular thyroid cancers (10%–20% of thyroid malignancies). These arise from the follicular cells. Medullary thyroid cancer, a neuroendocrine tumour, arises from the C-cells and comprises 6%–8% of thyroid cancers. Anaplastic thyroid cancer, which carries an appalling prognosis, is an aggressive tumour that is believed to develop either from a de-differentiating papillary tumour or de novo. This comprises 1% of thyroid cancers.

Aetiology

Known risk factors for the development of thyroid cancer include radiation exposure, genetic propensity, female sex and hypothyroidism.

The Chernobyl disaster in 1986 led to a large increase in the incidence of differentiated thyroid cancer among people who were young children and adolescents at the time of the accident and lived in the most contaminated areas of Belarus, the Russian Federation and Ukraine.

Patients with certain rare genetic disorders are more at risk of developing thyroid cancer.

Table 6.3 BTA classification for ultrasound assessment of thyroid nodules.

Classification	Findings	Risk of malignancy
U1	No thyroid nodules present on ultrasound examination	—
U2	Nodules benign on ultrasound examination Features may include: ● Hyperechoic or isoechoic nodule with a halo ● Cystic change with ring down artefact (colloid) ● Microcystic or spongiform appearance ● Peripheral eggshell calcification ● Peripheral vascularity	<3%
U3	Nodules indeterminate on ultrasound examination Features may include: ● Solid homogenous markedly hyperechoic nodule with halo (follicular lesions) ● Hypoechoic with equivocal echogenic foci or cystic change ● Mixed or central vascularity	5%–10%
U4	Nodules are suspicious on ultrasound examination Features may include: ● Solid hypoechoic (compared with thyroid) ● Solid very hypoechoic (compared with strap muscles) ● Hypoechoic with disrupted peripheral calcification ● Lobulated outline	10%–20%

U5	Nodules are malignant on ultrasound examination
	Features may include:
	
	● Solid hypoechoic with a lobulated or irregular outline and microcalcification
	● Papillary carcinoma
	  – Solid hypoechoic with a lobulated or irregular outline and globular calcification
	● Medullary carcinoma
	  – Intranodular vascularity
	  – Taller than wide axially (AP > TR)
	  – Characteristic-associated lymphadenopathy
		Up to 90%

Sources: Valderrabano P, McIver B, *Cancer Control*, 2017;24:doi:1073274817729231; Perros P et al. *Clin Endocrinol (Oxf)*. 2014;81(Suppl 1):1–122.

These include familial adenomatous polyposis of which Gardner syndrome is a subtype; Cowden disease with associated hamartomas and increased risk of breast and uterine carcinoma (PTEN gene) and Carney complex type 1 (PRKAR1A gene), which is also associated with a number of benign tumours.

Additionally, the BRAF and TERT mutations have been implicated with poorer prognosis in papillary thyroid carcinoma. Inherited mutations in the RET proto-oncogene are associated with the development of medullary thyroid cancer and account for approximately one out of four cases. This may or may not be part of the multiple endocrine neoplasia complex

Table 6.4 BTA classification for cytological grading of thyroid nodules.

Classification	Definition	Risk of malignancy
Thy1	Non-diagnostic	<10% 14% if cystic
Thy2	Benign	<3%
Thy3a	Atypical features present	5%–15%
Thy3f	Follicular neoplasm suspected	15%–30%
Thy4	Malignancy suspected	Up to 70%
Thy5	Diagnostic of malignancy	>90%

Sources: Perros P et al. *Clin Endocrinol (Oxf).* 2014;81(Suppl 1):1–122; Kwak JY et al. *Eur Radiol.* 2009;19:1923–31; Garcia-Pascual L et al. *Endocrine.* 2011;39:33–40; Orija IB et al. *Endocr Pract.* 2007;13:735–42; Trombetta S et al. *Int J Surg.* 2016;28(Suppl 1):S59–64; Wang CC et al. *Thyroid.* 2011;21:243–51.

(type 2). In addition, the risk of developing thyroid cancer is higher if previously diagnosed in a first-degree relative.

Three in every four thyroid cancer diagnoses are made in women. Obesity and previous diagnosis of other cancers, particularly breast cancer, are also believed to increase thyroid cancer risk.

Pathophysiology

Thyroid cancers are categorised by their histopathological characteristics.

Differentiated thyroid cancers (arising from thyroid follicular cells)

- Papillary thyroid cancer (80%)
- Follicular thyroid cancer (15%)
- Non-invasive follicular neoplasm with papillary-like nuclear features (NIFTP), a recently recognised subtype that may comprise up to 20% of differentiated thyroid cancer, characterised by no capsular or vascular invasion. *This is no longer considered malignant*

Poorly differentiated thyroid cancers

Comprise thyroid cancers arising from thyroid follicular cells with levels of differentiation that are intermediate between differentiated and undifferentiated tumours. They can be divided into solid, insular and trabecular subtypes.

Anaplastic thyroid cancers

A form of thyroid cancer comprising cells with poor differentiation, high mitotic rates and high levels of lymphovascular invasion. Comprising 1%–2% of thyroid cancers, prognosis is generally dismal with 5-year survival rates less than 5%. It tends to occur in patients over 65 years of age, those with previous radiation treatment and those with longstanding goitre.

C-cell–derived cancers

Medullary thyroid cancer (MTC) is a tumour arising from the parafollicular or C-cells and so behaves in a different way to other thyroid malignancies. Most cases, 75%, are sporadic, but 25% are genetically linked and caused by a mutation in the RET proto-oncogene. For this reason a new diagnosis in a potential proband mandates genetic testing.

When genetically predetermined, MTC has three forms: multiple endocrine neoplasia type 2A (MEN2A), type 2B (MEN2B) and familial MTC. All are inherited as autosomal dominant disorders. In MEN, the disease is associated with other endocrine disorders (see **Table 6.5**).

Table 6.5 Other disorders affecting MEN patients.

MEN type	Disorders associated	Incidence
MEN2A	MTC	100%
	Phaeochromocytoma	50%
	Hyperparathyroidism	10%–20%
MEN2B	MTC	100%
	Phaeochromocytoma	50%
	Mucosal neuromas	95%
	Marfanoid appearance	95%

History

The commonest mode of presentation of thyroid cancer is as a neck lump. Given that the majority of thyroid cancers demonstrate an indolent growth pattern and up to 20% of women have a goitre, the diagnosis may be delayed.

Paediatric thyroid nodules carry a 4 times greater malignancy rate than adult nodules.

Age less than 20 years or more than 60 years increases the risk of a malignant nodule.

Suspicions should be raised if patients demonstrate so-called red-flag symptoms which include [19]:

- Hoarseness
- Rapid growth of the mass
- Stridor
- Haemoptysis
- Other associated neck nodes

Other risk factors in the history include:

- Family history of thyroid disease, particularly thyroid cancer
- Symptoms to suggest thyroid activity disorders (an elevated TSH carries a higher malignancy risk)
- A previous history of radiation exposure

Examination

- A thorough examination includes: goitre assessment (uninodular, firmness of nodule to palpation, multinodular, fixity to surrounding structures)
- Examination for associated lymphadenopathy (particularly levels 2a, 3, 4, 5b)
- Laryngeal assessment – vocal cord palsy should raise suspicion for malignancy

Investigation

- Haematological – A serum TSH (a firm rapidly growing thyroid nodule may be a benign toxic nodule and FNA will always be misleading if the patient has thyrotoxicosis and may wrongly suggest sinister pathology so should therefore be avoided)
- An ultrasound scan (BTA guidelines, **Table 6.3**) – If a thyroid nodule is U2, then no further investigation is required unless other findings suggest a higher index of suspicion

Table 6.6 discusses how to react to different ultrasound scan (USS) FNAC results and their corresponding risk of malignancy.

Table 6.6 Options for managing different cytological and ultrasound findings in patients with thyroid nodules.

Classification	Action required
U1	No further action required
U2	No further action required unless there are risk factors for malignancy
U2 + Thy2	No further action unless there is strong clinical suspicion of malignancy
U2 + Thy3	Repeat USS-guided FNAC If Thy3 obtained again – diagnostic surgery
U3 + Thy1	Repeat USS-guided FNAC
U3 + Thy2	Repeat USS-guided FNAC
U3 + Thy3	Repeat USS-guided FNAC or Diagnostic surgery
AnyU + Thy4–5	Diagnostic or therapeutic surgery

If there is evidence of retrosternal extension, extrathyroidal extension or metastatic spread, three-dimensional imaging normally involving a computerized tomography (CT) scan including neck and chest is also appropriate.

All patients should be discussed in a thyroid-specific multidisciplinary team (MDT) and treatment modalities recorded. All tumours should be staged according to the tumour, node, metastasis (TNM) classification.

Staging

There are various risk stratification systems for differentiated thyroid cancer. Most use a combination of the size of the primary tumour, histological subtype, extrathyroidal and metastatic spread and age at diagnosis. They help to predict the risk of local recurrence and disease specific mortality. The TNM classification depends on the size of primary tumour, the number and location of metastatic lymph nodes and the presence of distant metastases (**Table 6.7**). The American Joint Committee on Cancer (AJCC) uses a combination of TNM classification and an age of more than 55 years at diagnosis as risk stratification tools (**Table 6.8**) [20].

Management

Surgery is the primary treatment modality in the management of all thyroid cancers. The extent of surgery is dictated by the tumour size and subtype, the tumour extent, the age at presentation and the extent of nodal involvement. MTC has a high propensity for lymph node metastases early, and therefore lymph node surgery at the time of thyroid resection is virtually mandatory.

Differentiated thyroid cancer (DTC)

Total thyroidectomy is indicated in patients with tumours >4 cm or in those whom post-operative RAI is felt to be appropriate (multifocal, bilateral, extrathyroidal spread or lymph node metastases).

Uninodular, intrathyroid disease with tumours <4 cm can be offered hemithyroidectomy with

Table 6.7 TNM classification for thyroid cancer.

Primary tumour (T)	
Categories may be subdivided as solitary tumour (s) or multifocal tumour (m); the largest determines the classification	
TX	Primary tumour cannot be assessed
T0	No evidence of primary tumour
T1	Limited to thyroid, 2 cm or less in greatest dimension
T1a T1b	Limited to thyroid, 1 cm or less Limited to thyroid, more than 1 cm but not more than 2 cm
T2	Limited to thyroid, greater than 2 cm but not more than 4 cm
T3	Limited to thyroid and >4 cm or gross tumour invasion of strap muscles
T3a T3b	Limited to thyroid Invasion of strap muscles
T4	Gross extrathyroid extension into major neck structures
T4a T4b	Extension into subcutaneous soft tissues, larynx, trachea, oesophagus or recurrent laryngeal nerves Tumour invades prevertebral fascia or encases carotid artery or mediastinal vessels
Anaplastic carcinoma – all are considered T4 tumours	
T4a	Intrathyroidal anaplastic carcinoma
T4b	Anaplastic with gross extrathyroid extension
Regional lymph nodes (N)	
NX	Regional lymph nodes cannot be assessed
N0	No regional lymph node metastasis
N1	Regional lymph node metastasis
N1a N1b	Metastasis to level VI (pretracheal, paratracheal and prelaryngeal/ Delphian lymph nodes) Metastasis to unilateral, bilateral or contralateral cervical (levels I, II, III, IV or V), or retropharyngeal or superior mediastinal lymph nodes (level VII)

Table 6.8 Stage grouping for differentiated thyroid cancer (AJCC 2017).

Stage	T	N	M
For differentiated thyroid cancer patients less than 55 years of age			
I	Any T	Any N	M0
II	Any T	Any N	M1
For differentiated thyroid cancer patients 55 years of age and over			
I	T1-2	N0	M0
II	T1-3b	N0-1	M0
(must be N1 for T1-2 tumours)			
III	T4a	Any N	M0
IVA	T4b	Any N	M0
IVB	Any T	Any N	M1

Source: Perros P et al. *Clin Endocrinol (Oxf).* 2014;81(Suppl 1):1–122.

Table 6.9 Post-operative risk stratification of differentiated thyroid carcinoma.

Risk category	Characteristics
Low	No local or distant metastases All macroscopic tumour resected No invasion of locoregional tissues/structures No aggressive histology (tall cell, columnar cell, diffuse sclerosing, poorly differentiated) No angioinvasion
Intermediate	Microscopic invasion of tumour into perithyroidal soft tissues (T3) at primary surgery Cervical lymph node metastases Aggressive histology (see aforementioned subtypes) Angioinvasion
High	Extrathyroidal invasion Incomplete macroscopic tumour resection (R2) Distant metastases

Source: Tuttle RM et al. *Thyroid.* 2010;20:1341–9.

completion offered to those who require or desire adjuvant RAI.

Total thyroidectomy may be offered to those with thy3 cytology if there are compressive symptoms or associated thyroid disorder such as Graves' disease.

Central (level VI) neck dissection should be performed in those with clinical, radiologic or cytologic evidence of nodal metastases. In patients at higher risk of metastases (e.g. T4 disease, multifocal disease) it may be performed prophylactically, but there is no definitive evidence that it improves survival or aids follow-up in the long term, and it increases the risk of permanent hypoparathyroidism and places the recurrent laryngeal nerves at greater risk.

Patients with DTC are stratified following surgery to aid recommendations for RAI (see **Table 6.9**) [12,21].

Adjuvant therapy

Radioactive iodine (Iodine-131) is the mainstay of adjuvant therapy in DTC. It can be used to ablate the remnant thyroidal activity in the thyroidal bed after

total thyroidectomy (radioiodine remnant ablation) or it can be used to treat known residual or recurrent local or metastatic disease.

Whilst it is known that post-operative radioiodine therapy is beneficial for some patients, there are many that the benefit is unclear. **Table 6.10** details those that may benefit from RAI [12,22].

Adjuvant therapies primarily involving radioiodine ablation but also involving external beam radiotherapy and tyrosine kinase inhibitors (TKIs) in poorer prognosis tumours are also used. Various chemotherapeutic regimens are employed mainly on a trial basis in patients with stage IV disease.

The use of radioiodine therapy is for intermediate tumours, and it is judged on stage and histopathological tumour characteristics. As tumours become more aggressive, they tend to lose iodine avidity and the effectiveness of radioiodine decreases; in such

Table 6.10 Recommendations for those who may benefit from RAI.

RAI not recommended	RAI recommended	May benefit from RAI
All criteria should be met	Any one of criteria may be met	One or more of criteria may benefit
Tumour <1 cm unifocal or multifocal Histology classical papillary or follicular variant of papillary carcinoma, or follicular carcinoma Minimally invasive without angioinvasion No invasion of thyroid capsule (extra thyroidal extension)	Tumour >4 cm Any tumour size with gross extra thyroidal extension Distant metastases present	Large tumour size Extrathyroidal extension Aggressive histology (tall cell, columnar or diffuse sclerosing papillary cancer, poorly differentiated elements) Widely invasive histology Multiple lymph node involvement, large size of involved lymph nodes, high ratio of positive to negative nodes, extracapsular nodal involvement

Sources: Orija IB et al. *Endocr Pract.* 2007;13:735–42; American Thyroid Association Guidelines Taskforce on Thyroid Nodules and Differentiated Thyroid Cancer et al. *Thyroid.* 2009;19:1167–214.

cases, the role of external beam radiotherapy and TKIs increases.

Medullary thyroid cancer

Once a diagnosis of MTC is made, a phaeochromocytoma diagnosis must be excluded prior to initial surgery to avoid the rare but potentially fatal complication of hypertensive crisis. In newly diagnosed MTC patients, subsequent familial screening may lead to prophylactic thyroidectomy in the paediatric patient. The timing of surgery is dictated by RET screening depending on the RET codon mutation. In MEN2B patients with codon 883 and 918 mutations, for example, thyroidectomy in the first year of life will cure MTC before it has developed. The American Thyroid Association has stratified the risk of each known mutation in MEN2A and B and accordingly provided guidance for the optimal timing of prophylactic surgery [23].

RAI has no role in the management of MTC.

Anaplastic thyroid cancer

Tumours that are small, intrathyroidal or easily excised completely macroscopically should be resected with total thyroidectomy, en bloc resection of adjacent involved structures, and where there is evidence of lymph node involvement, therapeutic lymph node dissection [12]. External beam radiotherapy can reduce morbidity often given with concurrent chemotherapy. EBRT can also be given in the palliative setting.

The 5-year survival rate for any anaplastic thyroid carcinoma is less than 10%.

Follow-up

Hypocalcaemia

The rates of hypocalcaemia following total thyroidectomy are up to 30% [24]. Serum calcium should be checked on the day after surgery. Hypocalcaemia should be treated with oral calcium supplementation. When the adjusted serum calcium is >2.1 mmol, the patient can be discharged. If hypocalcaemia persists beyond 72 hours on high dose calcium supplementation, then vitamin D (e.g. alfacalcidol or calcitriol) should be commenced. In severe symptomatic hypocalcaemia or biochemically <1.9 mmol intravenous calcium should be administered.

The majority of these patients will not need calcium replacement for life and they should be followed-up, monitored and the calcium weaned off gradually.

Differentiated thyroid cancer

Patients are followed-up using clinical examination, ultrasound and by monitoring serum tumour markers. These include thyroglobulin in DTC. Thyroglobulin can be measured as either unstimulated (in patients on thyroxine which is suppressing TSH) or stimulated (in patients who have had their thyroxine withdrawn for at least 4 weeks or who have received recombinant TSH prior to measurement). Stimulated thyroglobulin has been shown to be superior to unstimulated in detecting disease recurrence but can be more challenging, unpleasant for the patient (if suspending thyroxine treatment) and costly to obtain.

TSH suppression with supraphysiologic doses of levothyroxine is used to reduce the risk of cancer recurrence. However, long-term TSH suppression is associated with atrial fibrillation, cardiovascular disease and osteoporosis. As such patients are stratified into different responses to initial treatment for DTC and subsequently different levels of suppression (see **Tables 6.11** and **6.12**). All patients having undergone total thyroidectomy and radioiodine remnant ablation should be TSH suppressed <0.1 mU/L for 9–12 months before undergoing risk stratification according to **Table 6.11**. Following risk stratification patients' TSH suppression is categorised according to treatment response as shown in **Table 6.12**.

Patients regarded as low-risk (see **Table 6.9**) with tumours <1 cm do not require TSH suppression beyond that which is required to avoid clinical hypothyroidism.

Table 6.11 Classification of response to initial treatment for DTC.

Response category	Features
Excellent	All the following: ● Suppressed and stimulated Tg < 1 iU/L ● Neck US without evidence of disease ● Cross-sectional and/or nuclear medicine imaging negative (if performed)
Indeterminate	Any of the following: ● Suppressed Tg < 1 iU/L and stimulated Tg ≥ 1 and <10 iU/L ● Neck US with non-specific changes or stable subcentimetre lymph nodes ● Cross-sectional and/or nuclear medicine imaging with non-specific changes, although not completely normal
Incomplete	Any of the following: ● Suppressed Tg ≥ 1 iU/L or stimulated Tg ≥ 10 iU/L ● Rising Tg values ● Persistent or newly identified disease on cross-sectional and/or nuclear medicine imaging

Note: This should be assessed 9–12 months after completing treatment [21].

Table 6.12 Treatment response and TSH suppression recommendation.

Treatment response	Target TSH level	Time until restratification
Excellent	0.3–2.0 mU/L	9–12 months
Indeterminate	0.1–0.5 mU/L	5–10 years
Incomplete	<0.1 mU/L	Indefinite

Source: Perros P et al. *Clin Endocrinol (Oxf)*. 2014;81(Suppl 1):1–122.

Medullary thyroid cancer

Tumour markers used in follow-up are calcitonin and CEA levels in MTC. Rising calcitonin should trigger imaging to try to identify disease recurrence. This should begin with neck USS and CT of the neck and chest. If unremarkable in the presence of rising calcitonin, whole body imaging should be undertaken. This can be in the form of octreotide scanning, PET-CT or SPECT-CT using ^{123}I-MIBG.

Loco-regional recurrence should be resected wherever possible. Radiotherapy has a palliative role [12].

REFERENCES

1 Mortensen C, Lockyer H, Loveday E. The incidence and morphological features of pyramidal lobe on thyroid ultrasound. *Ultrasound.* 2014;22:192–8.

2 Pankow BG, Michalak J, McGee MK. Adult human thyroid weight. *Health Phys.* 1985;49:1097–103.

3 Gruters A, Krude H. Update on the management of congenital hypothyroidism. *Horm Res.* 2007;68(Suppl 5):107–11.

4 Nystrom HF, Jansson S, Berg G. Incidence rate and clinical features of hyperthyroidism in a long-term iodine sufficient area of Sweden (Gothenburg) 2003–2005. *Clin Endocrinol (Oxf).* 2013;78:768–76.

5 Ross DS, Burch HB, Cooper DS et al. 2016 American Thyroid Association guidelines for diagnosis and management of hyperthyroidism and other causes of thyrotoxicosis. *Thyroid.* 2016;26:1343–421.

6 Andersson M, Takkouche B, Egli I, Allen HE, de Benoist B. Current global iodine status and progress over the last decade towards the elimination of iodine deficiency. *Bull World Health Organ.* 2005;83:518–25.

7 World Health Organization, United Nations Children's Fund, and International Council for the Control of Iodine Deficiency Disorders. *Indicators for Assessing Iodine Deficiency Disorders and their Control through Salt Iodization.* World Health Organization; 1994.

8 Tomoda C, Sugino K, Tanaka T et al. Globus symptoms in patients undergoing thyroidectomy: Relationships with psychogenic factors, thyroid disease, and surgical procedure. *Thyroid.* 2018;28:104–9.

9 Collazo-Clavell ML, Gharib H, Maragos NE. Relationship between vocal cord paralysis and benign thyroid disease. *Head Neck.* 1995;17:24–30.

10 Cardia MS, Rubio IG, Medeiros-Neto G. Prolonged follow-up of multinodular goitre patients treated with radioiodine preceded or not by human recombinant TSH. *Clin Endocrinol (Oxf).* 2006;64:474.

11 Valderrabano P, McIver B. Evaluation and management of indeterminate thyroid nodules: The revolution of risk stratification beyond cytological diagnosis. *Cancer Control.* 2017;24:doi:1073274817729231.

12 Perros P, Boelaert K, Colley S et al. Guidelines for the management of thyroid cancer. *Clin Endocrinol (Oxf).* 2014;81(Suppl 1):1–122.

13 Kwak JY, Kim EK, Kim HJ, Kim MJ, Son EJ, Moon HJ. How to combine ultrasound and cytological information in decision making about thyroid nodules. *Eur Radiol.* 2009;19:1923–31.

14 Garcia-Pascual L, Barahona MJ, Balsells M et al. Complex thyroid nodules with nondiagnostic fine needle aspiration cytology: Histopathologic outcomes and comparison of the cytologic variants (cystic vs. acellular). *Endocrine.* 2011;39:33–40.

15 Orija IB, Pineyro M, Biscotti C, Reddy SS, Hamrahian AH. Value of repeating a nondiagnostic thyroid fine-needle aspiration biopsy. *Endocr Pract.* 2007;13:735–42.

16 Trombetta S, Attina GM, Ricci G, Ialongo P, Marini P. THY3 cytology: What surgical treatment? Retrospective study and literature review. *Int J Surg.* 2016;28(Suppl 1):S59–64.

17 Wang CC, Friedman L, Kennedy GC et al. A large multicenter correlation study of thyroid nodule cytopathology and histopathology. *Thyroid.* 2011;21:243–51.

18 Cramer JD, Fu P, Harth KC, Margevicius S, Wilhelm SM. Analysis of the rising incidence of thyroid cancer using the surveillance, epidemiology and end results national cancer data registry. *Surgery.* 2010;148:1147–52;discussion 52–3.

19 Kumar H, Daykin J, Holder R, Watkinson JC, Sheppard MC, Franklyn JA. Gender, clinical findings, and serum thyrotropin measurements in the prediction of thyroid neoplasia in 1005 patients presenting with thyroid enlargement and investigated by fine-needle aspiration cytology. *Thyroid*. 1999;9:1105–9.

20 Tuttle RM, Haugen B, Perrier ND. Updated American Joint Committee on Cancer/Tumor-Node-metastasis staging system for differentiated and anaplastic thyroid cancer (8th ed.): What changed and why? *Thyroid*. 2017;27:751–6.

21 Tuttle RM, Tala H, Shah J et al. Estimating risk of recurrence in differentiated thyroid cancer after total thyroidectomy and radioactive iodine remnant ablation: Using response to therapy variables to modify the initial risk estimates predicted by the new American Thyroid Association staging system. *Thyroid*. 2010;20:1341–9.

22 American Thyroid Association Guidelines Taskforce on Thyroid Nodules and Differentiated Thyroid Cancer, Cooper DS, Dougherty GM et al. Revised American Thyroid Association management guidelines for patients with thyroid nodules and differentiated thyroid cancer. *Thyroid*. 2009;19:1167–214.

23 American Thyroid Association Guidelines Task Force, Kloos RT, Eng C et al. Medullary thyroid cancer: Management guidelines of the American Thyroid Association. *Thyroid*. 2009;19:565–612.

24 Hannan FM, Thakker RV. Investigating hypocalcaemia. *BMJ*. 2013;346:f2213.

7

PARATHYROID DISEASE

R. James A. England

The parathyroid glands play a vital role in calcium homeostasis. They may be affected by various disease processes which alter their secretory function potentially giving rise to the symptoms of hyper- or hypocalcaemia and, in a more chronic scenario, end organ damage. Hypoparathyroidism is most commonly iatrogenic following thyroid surgery but may be secondary to autoimmune disease or other rare systemic disorders; it is not covered in great detail in this chapter. Hyperparathyroidism (HPT), of greater interest to the head and neck endocrine surgeon, may be due to the gland(s) themselves or due to a stimulus without the gland(s).

ANATOMY

The anatomy of the parathyroid glands is predicted partially by embryology and partially by the effect of increasing mass and deglutition. They arise from the endoderm of the third and fourth branchial pouches. There are normally four in number: two superior and two inferior. In a minority there may be as few as two glands or as many as six.

The superior glands arise from the fourth pouch and the inferior from the third pouch, which, due to a longer pathway of descent, have a broader range of ectopic positions and are more variable in where they lie in the neck. The fourth pouch also produces the ultimobranchial body which descends with the superior parathyroids. As the ultimobranchial body gives rise to the parafollicular C-cells of the thyroid gland, this means the superior parathyroid glands are always in close proximity to the posterior aspect of the thyroid gland.

The thymus is derived from the third pouch and migrates with the inferior parathyroid glands to the mediastinum. Though in the majority they separate, in some cases the inferior parathyroid gland may descend retrosternally with the thymus. A normal parathyroid gland weighs approximately 50–70 mg and is 5–7 mm in maximum dimension.

The superior parathyroid glands lie just deep to the recurrent laryngeal nerve (during surgery this relationship is often inversed as the thyroid is lifted out of the neck) and are closely related to the inferior thyroid artery. The inferior parathyroid glands tend to lie superficial to the recurrent laryngeal nerve and are usually located around the inferior pole of the thyroid gland, though their ectopic location can be anywhere from the angle of the mandible to the chest, including the retro-oesophagus.

Blood supply

The majority of the blood supply is provided by the inferior thyroid artery with some variable contribution from the superior thyroid artery. They drain into the superior, middle and thyroid veins.

Lymphatic drainage

The parathyroid gland lymphatics drain to the paratracheal nodes and deep cervical nodes.

Innervation

The thyroid branches of the cervical sympathetic chain provide sensory and some vasomotor supply.

PHYSIOLOGY

Calcium-sensing receptors exist on the cell surface of the parathyroid glands. A fall in serum calcium stimulates parathyroid hormone secretion. Parathyroid hormone (PTH) secretion mobilises calcium from the skeleton by promoting bone resorption (stimulating osteoclast activity and inhibiting osteoblasts). PTH increases renal resorption of calcium as well as phosphate excretion. It also initiates calcitriol (activated vitamin D_3) production in the kidneys, which stimulates increased intestinal absorption of calcium. These all lead to an increase in serum calcium. A negative feedback loop then inhibits further PTH production.

PATHOLOGY

Hyperparathyroidism

Parathyroid disease is divided into disease giving rise to underactivity of the parathyroid glands (hypoparathyroidism) and disease giving rise to overactivity (hyperparathyroidism).

Hyperparathyroidism (HPT) may be primary, secondary or tertiary.

Primary HPT is due to the development of a solitary adenoma in 85% of cases; hyperplasia affecting all glands in 12% of cases, which may be familial (such as in MEN1 or 2a) or non-familial; multiple adenomata in 2%; or parathyroid carcinoma in 1%.

Secondary HPT is due to external stimulation of the parathyroid glands and therefore removal of the external stimulus should result in return to euparathyroidism. Stimuli include low serum vitamin D levels, renal failure and lithium therapy.

Tertiary HPT exists when the secondary stimulus is removed but the HPT remains. The commonest example occurs in the post-renal transplant patient who still has HPT.

History

The symptoms of HPT can be initially vague and are related to the underlying pathology caused by pathologic hypercalcaemia.

a *Gastrointestinal*: Nausea, vomiting, constipation, peptic ulceration and pancreatitis
b *Renal*: Polyuria and polydipsia, renal calculi, nephrocalcinosis and renal failure
c *Musculoskeletal*: Muscle pain, joint pain, bone pain, pathological fractures and osteoporosis/penia
d *Cardiovascular*: Hypertension
e *Central nervous system*: Depression, confusion and lack of energy

It is imperative to ask in the past medical history specifically regarding these conditions.

Drug history is also important, particularly lithium therapy.

Examination

Specifically, no head and neck abnormal findings are expected to be found, as parathyroid glands rarely grow to a palpable size; if one is palpated in the setting of HPT, then parathyroid cancer should be suspected.

Though flexible naso endoscopy (FNE) is mandated to check vocal cord function, preoperative palsy due to parathyroid pathology invasion is extremely rare.

Investigation

Blood tests

Serum calcium: Nowadays, HPT is most frequently found incidentally due to the discovery of an elevated serum calcium on routine blood testing. When this is discovered, the test should be repeated with a simultaneous PTH assay.

Serum PTH: This will either be elevated or inappropriately normal. A suppressed PTH indicates the need for screening to exclude malignancy.

Others: Once HPT is suspected, potential causes of secondary HPT should be excluded, including renal failure, lithium therapy and hypovitaminosis D.

Urine

A 24-hour urine collection for calcium: creatinine clearance should be submitted and the ratio calculated. A ratio of >0.01 excludes the diagnosis of familial hypocalciuric hypercalcaemia (1:78,000 incidence), an autosomal dominant condition caused by an abnormal calcium-sensing receptor gene. This results in hypercalcaemia with a normal or mildly elevated PTH level, which will cause no end organ damage and requires no treatment.

Imaging

Imaging primarily aims to localise the pathologic parathyroid glands prior to surgical intervention.

This is important when trying to determine which parathyroid gland(s) are diseased and to try to predict ectopic locations. Different units use different protocols.

Ultrasound (US) has been reported to successfully identify single adenomas in 93% of cases [1]. This is highly operator dependent. The use of Doppler imaging to determine blood flow in different tissue is key to the success rate of US in this situation [2].

Nuclear scintigraphy utilises the radioisotope technetium-99 m (^{99m}Tc). This is absorbed faster by overactive parathyroid glands. Some centres have reported successful identification of up to 95% of solitary parathyroid adenomas and up to 80% of multigland disease (parathyroid hyperplasia) [3,4]. Many centres will use both US and scintigraphy as part of preoperative planning.

As secondary and tertiary HPT involve multigland disease, preoperative localisation may be of less use in primary surgery for these conditions. Some units will still employ preoperative localisation in inherited multigland disease to enable removal of the most active tissue only, minimising surgical trauma and scarring, due to the high likelihood of the requirement for multiple surgeries in this subgroup.

Other techniques being reported include 4D CT, C-methionine PET-CT, C-choline PET-CT and SPECT, although optimal imaging guidelines in primary surgery, multigland disease and revision surgery are still debated and these modalities are less readily available in most centres [5]. PET-MRI, a novel imaging modality in this field, has also shown promise in revision cases [6].

Management

In primary HPT, patients are classified as symptomatic or asymptomatic. Symptomatic patients should be offered surgery.

Asymptomatic patients may be offered surgery if they meet the requirements detailed in **Table 7.1**. Some argue that all asymptomatic patients should be offered surgery to avoid the need for long-term monitoring and prevent any long-term complications of HPT [7].

Table 7.1 Criteria for surgery for asymptomatic primary hyperparathyroidism.

Parameter	Measurement
Serum calcium	1.0 mg/dL (0.25 mmol/L) above upper limit of normal
Skeletal	• BMD by DXA: T-score <−2.5 at lumbar spine, total hip, femoral neck, or distal 1/3 radius • Vertebral fracture by x-ray, CT, MRI, or VFA
Renal	• Creatinine clearance <60 cc/min • 24-hour urine collection for calcium >400 mg/d (>10 mmol/d) and increased stone risk by biochemical stone risk analysis • Presence of nephrolithiasis or nephrocalcinosis by x-ray, ultrasound, or CT
Age	<50 years

Source: Bilezikian JP et al. *J Clin Endocrinol Metab.* 2014; 99:3561–9.

Asymptomatic patients who elect not to have surgery require long-term monitoring for the clinical features of HPT, as well as serum calcium and creatinine measurements.

Secondary HPT requires management of the underlying cause. This can involve the use of calcimimetic medications (e.g. cinacalcet). These negatively feed back on the parathyroid glands decreasing PTH and calcium levels [9]. Surgery is reserved for refractory cases.

Tertiary HPT most commonly occurs in patients with chronic kidney failure. Medical management is often commenced in these patients, but surgery remains the best option for refractory patients well enough to undergo surgery.

Surgical approaches

Single-gland versus multigland exploration

In patients where an adenomatous gland has been localised preoperatively, a minimally invasive approach can be taken to target this. This involves making a 1.5–2 cm incision over the suspected adenoma and directly dissecting down onto the abnormal gland [10]. Patients should be consented for the potential change in approach to the traditional thyroid-type incision and approach (involving mobilisation of the thyroid gland and identification of the recurrent laryngeal nerves) and exploration of all four glands in the event that the suspected adenomatous gland is found to be of normal size [11].

In patients with secondary or tertiary HPT, a four-gland exploration is advocated with three-and-a-half gland extirpation and reimplantation of half of a parathyroid gland into the sternocleidomastoid or forearm muscle [11,12].

Intraoperative monitoring

Successful parathyroidectomy can be predicted intraoperatively using intraoperative parathyroid hormone level monitoring. The half-life of parathyroid hormone is approximately 3–5 minutes and therefore the technology represents a realistic predictor of surgical success in real time [13]. A fall in parathyroid hormone levels of 50% or greater within 10 minutes of tumour resection indicates a successful operation [14].

Some units also utilise the gamma probe intraoperatively with a preoperative injection of technetium sestamibi as a localisation technique [15].

Surgical outcomes

Surgery for HPT has high success rates in most hands, although success rates in high-volume practices are greater. In primary HPT due to single-gland disease, success rates of >95% should be achievable. Surgical success in multigland disease will be lower, partly because of failure to recognise a multigland presentation, partly because the process may be surgically undertreated and partly because the process may have a genetic or external stimulatory drive that promotes recurrence.

Other than surgical failure, side effects include recurrent laryngeal nerve paralysis due to axonotmesis (permanent) or neurapraxia (temporary in most cases), haematoma and recurrence due to either metachronous adenoma formation or parathyromatosis due to disruption of adenomatous tissue resulting in remnant adenomatous tissue post-surgery. Overtreatment of HPT may also result in hypoparathyroidism in some instances.

In dialysis patients undergoing parathyroid surgery for tertiary HPT close post-operative monitoring of serum calcium levels is essential as hungry bone syndrome is expected with aggressive and prolonged calcium replacement therapy being required [16].

Recurrent hypercalcaemia in a patient having undergone surgery for HPT should prompt a systematic reevaluation of biochemical parameters including urine calcium and imaging to ensure familial hypercalcaemic hypercalciuria has not been previously mistaken for a surgically treatable disease.

Parathyroid cancer

Aetiology

Parathyroid cancer is rare, comprising approximately 1% of all presentations of HPT. Although not genetically predetermined, patients with MEN-1, HPT jaw tumour syndrome and isolated familial HPT have a higher incidence [17]. Only approximately 12% of cases are diagnosed preoperatively.

Clinical features

Parathyroid has been found to be associated with severe hypercalcaemia (>3.0 mmol/L) with a raised PTH level, and a neck lump should raise concern for this diagnosis [17].

Investigations

These patients should be investigated as per any patient with HPT.

Management

When suspected, the treatment of choice involves en bloc resection of the tumour and all immediately surrounding tissues including the ipsilateral thyroid lobe.

In terms of elective lymph node dissection, the ipsilateral and contralateral level VI are recommended to be excised, with other lymph node levels only to be

dissected if clinically (including radiologically) suspect of metastasis. There is some evidence to suggest tumours >3 cm in size are associated with lymph node metastasis [18].

Parathyroid cancer is relatively radioresistant.

As the disease has low metastatic potential, the 10-year disease specific survival is 49%–77% [17]. Medical management of inoperable parathyroid carcinoma includes calcimimetics and bisphosphonates. Death tends to occur as a result of uncontrolled hypercalcaemia.

Hypoparathyroidism

Hypoparathyroidism is most frequently iatrogenic as a result of thyroid surgery. However, it may also be autoimmune or due to other rare genetic causes (**Table 7.2**).

History

Symptoms of hypocalcaemia are present including paraesthesia, numbness and muscle spasm.

Examination

Neuromuscular hyperexcitability can be elicited by testing for Chvostek's sign (facial muscle spasms

Table 7.2 Causes of hypoparathyroidism.

Non-inherited	Iatrogenic post-thyroid/ parathyroid surgery (1%–5% of thyroid/parathyroid surgery) Haemochromatosis Wilson's disease Metastatic cancer
Inherited syndromic	Autoimmune polyglandular syndrome type 1 Di George type 1 CHARGE Hereditary deafness renal dysplasia syndrome Kenney-Caffey syndrome Dubowitz syndrome Bartter syndrome Kearns–Sayre syndrome
Inherited non-syndromic	Isolated hypoparathyroidism

caused by tapping the facial nerve in the preauricular region) and Trousseau's sign (carpal tetany secondary to inflating a blood pressure cuff around the arm).

Management

These patients require the input of an endocrinologist and are not managed surgically. They require calcium, vitamin D and magnesium replacement with replacement parathyroid hormone being a recent potential treatment option.

REFERENCES

1 Reeder SB, Desser TS, Weigel RJ, Jeffrey RB. Sonography in primary hyperparathyroidism: Review with emphasis on scanning technique. *J Ultrasound Med*. 2002;21:539–52; quiz 53–4.

2 Baskin HJ, Duick DD, Levine RA. *Thyroid Ultrasound and Ultrasound-Guided FNA*. 2nd ed. Springer; 2008.

3 Hindie E, Melliere D, Perlemuter L, Jeanguillaume C, Galle P. Primary hyperparathyroidism: Higher success rate of first surgery after preoperative Tc-99 m sestamibi-I-123 subtraction scanning. *Radiology*. 1997;204:221–8.

4 Thompson GB, Mullan BP, Grant CS et al. Parathyroid imaging with technetium-99m-sestamibi: An initial institutional experience. *Surgery*. 1994;116:966–72; discussion 72–3.

5 Lee GS, McKenzie TJ, Mullan BP, Farley DR, Thompson GB, Richards ML. A multimodal imaging protocol, (123)I/(99)Tc-Sestamibi, SPECT, and SPECT/CT, in primary hyperparathyroidism adds limited benefit for preoperative localization. *World J Surg*. 2016;40:589–94.

6 Purz S, Kluge R, Barthel H et al. Visualization of ectopic parathyroid adenomas. *N Engl J Med*. 2013;369:2067–9.

7 AACE/AAES Task Force on Primary Hyperparathyroidism. The American Association of Clinical Endocrinologists and the American Association of Endocrine Surgeons position statement on the diagnosis and management of primary hyperparathyroidism. *Endocr Pract*. 2005;11:49–54.

8 Bilezikian JP, Brandi ML, Eastell R et al. Guidelines for the management of asymptomatic primary hyperparathyroidism: Summary statement from the Fourth International Workshop. *J Clin Endocrinol Metab*. 2014;99: 3561–9.

9 Byrnes CA, Shepler BM. Cinacalcet: A new treatment for secondary hyperparathyroidism in patients receiving hemodialysis. *Pharmacotherapy*. 2005;25:709–16.

10 Desiato V, Melis M, Amato B, Bianco T, Rocca A, Amato M, Quarto G, Benassai G. Minimally invasive radioguided parathyroid surgery: A literature review. *Int J Surg*. 2016;28:S84–93.

11 Harari A, Allendorf J, Shifrin A, DiGorgi M, Inabnet WB. Negative preoperative localization leads to greater resource use in the era of minimally invasive parathyroidectomy. *Am J Surg*. 2009;197:769–73.

12 Pitt SC, Sippel RS, Chen H. Secondary and tertiary hyperparathyroidism, state of the art surgical management. *Surg Clin North Am*. 2009;89:1227–39.

13 Leiker AJ, Yen TW, Eastwood DC et al. Factors that influence parathyroid hormone half-life: Determining if new intraoperative criteria are needed. *JAMA Surg*. 2013;148:602–6.

14 Smith N, Magnuson JS, Vidrine DM, Kulbersh B, Peters GE. Minimally invasive parathyroidectomy: Use of intraoperative parathyroid hormone assays after 2 preoperative localization studies. *Arch Otolaryngol Head Neck Surg*. 2009;135:1108–11.

15 Friedman M, Gurpinar B, Schalch P, Joseph NJ. Guidelines for radioguided parathyroid surgery. *Arch Otolaryngol Head Neck Surg*. 2007;133:1235–9.

16 Ho LY, Wong PN, Sin HK et al. Risk factors and clinical course of hungry bone syndrome after total parathyroidectomy in dialysis patients with secondary hyperparathyroidism. *BMC Nephrol*. 2017;18:12.

17 Okamoto T, Iihara M, Obara T, Tsukada T. Parathyroid carcinoma: Etiology, diagnosis, and treatment. *World J Surg*. 2009;33:2343–54.

18 Hsu KT, Sippel RS, Chen H, Schneider DF. Is central lymph node dissection necessary for parathyroid carcinoma? *Surgery*. 2014;156:1336–41; discussion 41.

8

ORAL CAVITY

Jiten D. Parmar and Nick Brown

INTRODUCTION

The majority of oral head and neck cancer referrals for malignancy or potentially malignant lesions present via a neck lump referral or a referral based on the presence of a suspicious looking ulcer/white patch/red patch/lump in the oral cavity or neck. This chapter will focus on the management of oral cancers alone; however, the reader should be aware that approximately 5%–6% of head and neck malignancies are primarily salivary in nature [1]. There are many causes of neck lumps, of which head and neck metastasis could be considered as well as benign conditions, haematological malignancy, metastatic disease, infections and vascular anomalies to name a few, and these will test the diagnostic skills of any clinician to which the primary cause is not identifiable. This chapter will not deal with the separate entity and management of the 'Carcinoma with Unknown Primary' presentation, which will be discussed in another chapter.

ANATOMY

The oral cavity extends from the oral fissure to the oropharyngeal isthmus. The different anatomical subsites of the oral cavity include the mucosal lips (vermilion of the lips), upper and lower alveolar ridges (and teeth), hard palatal mucosa superiorly, floor of mouth inferiorly, buccal mucosae laterally retromolar trigone, and extends to the junction between the anterior two-thirds and posterior one-third of the tongue. The retromolar trigone is the triangular area of mucosa posterior to the final upper and lower molars. It extends from the level of the teeth to the hamulus of the medial pterygoid bone. The palatine tonsils, fauces, posterior two-thirds of the tongue and soft palate are part of the oropharynx.

The majority of the oral mucosa is lined by stratified squamous epithelium, interspersed with minor salivary glands, taste buds on the tongue and openings for the three major salivary glands (parotid, submandibular and sublingual glands).

The oral cavity is perhaps the easiest of areas to examine and diagnose directly without specialist equipment; however, the use of a dental mirror, gloved finger and a good light is highly advised.

Lymphatic drainage

The oral cavity drains to levels I, II, III and IV. The submandibular nodes in level Ib drain the buccal mucosa, lips, alveolar ridges, oral tongue and floor of mouth. The submental nodes in level Ia drain the anterior tongue, anterior floor of mouth, the incisors and central lower lip.

Innervation

The sensory innervation of the oral cavity is from the trigeminal nerve. The maxillary division (V2) supplies the greater palatine and nasopalatine nerves to the hard palate. It also supplies the superior alveolar nerve to the teeth. The mandibular division (V3) supplies the lingual nerve to the floor of mouth and tongue, inferior alveolar nerve to the teeth and buccal nerve to the buccal mucosa. Special taste sensation is also supplied to the anterior two-thirds of the tongue via the chorda tympani branch of the facial nerve.

Motor nerve supply primarily comes from the hypoglossal nerve to the intrinsic and extrinsic muscles of the tongue and the trigeminal nerve supplying the muscle of mastication.

PREMALIGNANT LESIONS/POTENTIALLY MALIGNANT LESIONS

The nomenclature for premalignant lesions has changed over the last few years to now call these lesions *potentially malignant lesions* [2]. Essentially, they fall into the definition of being any red, white or mixed red and white patch that cannot be otherwise diagnosed. Another subsection of this group includes the group diagnosed on biopsy as 'verrucous hyperplasia', which also has a higher malignant transformation rate.

History

Primarily these patients complain of an abnormal patch of mucosa in the oral cavity. This may be associated with itching, burning or pain. They may be asymptomatic and the lesion noticed by a dental or medical professional. A common pathway for the management can be found in **Figure 8.1**.

It is key to assess risk factors for malignancy, which remain traditionally tobacco and alcohol [3]. Other risk factors include:

- Use of betel nut [4]
- Genetic factors
  - Fanconi anaemia (especially after stem cell transplantation)
  - Ataxia telangiectasia
  - Bloom syndrome
  - Li-Fraumeni syndrome

- Arsenic exposure
- Previous cancer

Examination

As discussed in Anatomy section.

Investigation

A biopsy under local anaesthetic is performed if an obvious benign lesion cannot be diagnosed, or if the patient has high-risk factors which would steer the clinician towards a biopsy. This is easily achievable in the oral cavity due to ease of access.

Mehanna et al. looked at all red and white patches and concluded that these lesions were *dysplastic* in approximately 30% of cases, for which red patches were more likely to have dysplasia than white patches [5]. The overall conversion rate to malignancy has also been reported at 12% for the group as a whole. Ho et al. looked at the same cohort of patients from Liverpool and found the following risk factors for conversion to malignancy [6]:

- Female
- Non-smokers
- Lesions over 200 mm^2

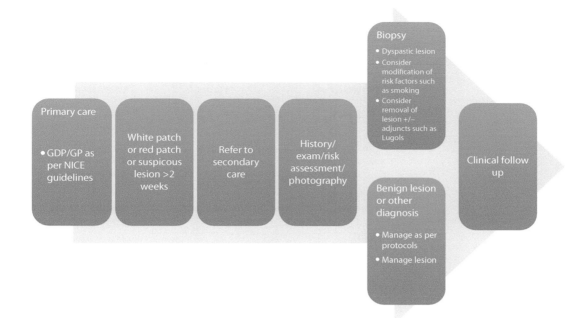

Figure 8.1 Flow chart to demonstrate work-up of potentially malignant oral cavity lesion.

- Present for over 2 years
- Age over 65

Management

Table 8.1 lists some common premalignant lesions and their management. The list is not exhaustive, and consideration must be given to the hundreds of completely benign lesions that are clinically diagnosable.

The management of patients with these 'potentially malignant lesions' has not changed. The identification of dysplastic tissue on biopsy would normally lead to its removal via a range of modalities, for which the most frequently used is the CO_2 laser.

Useful adjuncts

The LIHNCS trial used carbocysteine washes followed by *Lugol's iodine* to help identify the true extent of dysplastic tissue prior to removal via laser [10]. Data presented at the association of Clinical Oncology in 2017 showed using Lugol's iodine significantly reduced the need for reexcision of dysplastic margins [11].

Other adjuncts to help the clinician achieve improving outcomes in the management of the excision and clearance of potentially malignant lesions/dysplastic lesions include the use of fluorescence imaging techniques and the use of high-definition microscopic laser excision.

MALIGNANT LESIONS

History

In the majority of cases, oral cancers will present with an exophytic or endophytic ulcer which is growing in size and is often initially painless but becomes painful as the lesion grows, causing problems with eating and talking.

High-risk sites include the tongue and floor of mouth, which have traditionally always been thought to be

Table 8.1 Potentially malignant oral cavity lesions with symptomatology, risk of malignant transformation and management options.

Lesion	Presentation	Malignant transformation rate	Current management
Lichen planus	White, red or mixed (speckled)	<1% per annum [7]	Steroids; topical, intralesional, systemic
Oral submucous fibrosis	White, stiff mucosa, trismus, burning sensation Betel/areca chewing	Approximately 0.5% per annum [8]	Habit cessation. Surgery with caution – often exacerbates trismus
Chronic hyperplastic candidiasis	Variable; white or red patched or mixed Tongue, buccal muscosa, floor of mouth	Unknown Significant association [9]	Antifungals Consider laser excision if refractory
Actinic cheilitis	Ulcer/crust vermilion lower lip	Unknown	Lip shave, laser excision

due a gravitational 'pooling' effect of carcinogens. A common pathway for patients is seen in **Figure 8.2**.

▌ Examination

The oral cavity requires full examination as described earlier.

It is important to note that in the latest (8th) edition of the American Joint Committee on Cancer (AJCC) cancer staging manual, the anatomic specifics of the oral cavity have been adjusted to account for the differential in cause of lip and oral cancer. The vermilion border of the lip is staged according to skin cancer. The oral cavity is considered to begin at the border of the wet and dry mucosa [12].

Fibre-optic nasendoscopy and neck examination is also required to assess local extent, exclude synchronous primaries and clinically stage the neck for nodal metastases.

▌ Investigation

Imaging is essential, often in the form of a neck and chest computerized tomography (CT), to assess local extent and stage the neck and chest radiologically. Gadolinium contrast-enhanced MRI scans of the head, face and neck aid in assessing soft tissue extent. Lesions involving the bony structures of the mandible and maxilla will also benefit from CT scanning or cone beam CT (CBCT) scanning of these structures, as invasion into bone will upstage the tumour.

There are some lesions that are not obvious on clinical examination as to whether they are malignant; however, the clinician should be aware that the inflammatory process of a biopsy for confirmation of diagnosis may upstage the size of the lesion on MRI. This traditional misconception has been recently questioned and a recent study by Howe et al. has shown that there was no significant upstaging of the tumour on MRI and in fact showed that delays to biopsy when adopting a protocol for 'MRI first' investigation actually added delays to overall treatment (43 days vs 16 days) [11].

▌ Management

Once a tissue diagnosis is obtained the patient is discussed at the multidisciplinary team (MDT) meeting. The clinical, pathologic and radiologic information is collated to make definitive treatment recommendations. The patient is staged clinically (which includes radiologic evaluation) before definitive treatment, though the gold standard for staging disease is

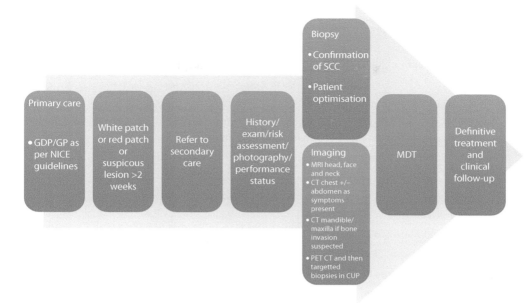

Figure 8.2 Flow chart for work-up of malignant oral cavity lesion.

considered to be following pathologic examination of the resected tumour and nodal compartments (see **Tables 8.2** and **8.3**).

Surgery still remains the mainstay of management of oral head and neck malignancy, with resection margins of 1 cm and an elective neck dissection (vital structures permitting) [15]. Up to 30% of clinically N0 necks have been found to have occult metastatic disease on histopathologic examination, upstaging them to N+ [16].

Neck dissection

The role of elective neck dissection has been the subject of much debate over the last 10 years. It was traditionally assumed that if a greater than 15%–20% risk of neck metastasis existed for identified oral squamous cell carcinoma (SCC) lesions, then an elective neck dissection should be undertaken [17]. Factors such as a tumour depth greater than 4 mm was thought to be an important threshold for metastasis; however, higher risk sites such as the floor of mouth, tongue and buccal mucosa have an increasing trend to metastasise at less invasive depths.

Verrucous carcinoma has traditionally been thought to have a lower risk of metastasis to the neck, but due to its location in the mouth (usually florid and associated with the alveolar tissues) bony reconstruction is usually required, commonly with a free flap and microvascular reconstruction, and therefore a neck dissection is often performed as part of the microvascular access procedure.

In the N0 neck, small T1 and T2 tumours can be resected and not reconstructed with a free flap, allowing for the possibility of a 'watch and wait' policy of the N0 neck. A landmark paper by D'Cruz et al. in 2016 showed that elective neck dissection in patients with early clinical and radiographic T1/T2 N0 head and neck cancer had an overall survival advantage (3-year survival 80%) over those who had watchful waiting and salvage neck dissection (3-year survival 67.5%) when originally diagnosed with a clinical/radiological N0 neck [16]. The paper also reported that the elective neck dissection group had an improved overall disease-free survival. A higher rate of metastatic disease in tumours over 4 mm in depth (3 mm [5.6%] vs 4 mm [16.9%]) was also found [16].

Table 8.2 TNM staging (8th ed.).

T stage	
T1	Size ≤2 cm or Depth of Invasion (DOI) ≤5 mm
T2	Size ≤2 cm but DOI >5 mm or tumour >2 cm and ≤4 cm with DOI ≤10 mm
T3	Size >4 cm or DOI >10 mm
T4a	Invasion of mandible, maxilla or skin (Note: Superficial erosion of bone/tooth socket (alone) by a gingival primary is not sufficient to classify a tumour as T4)
T4b	Invasion of masticator space, pterygoid plates, base of skull or encasement of internal carotid artery
N stage	
N0	No nodal involvement
N1	Single ipsilateral node ≤3 cm in size
N2a	Single ipsilateral node >3 cm but not greater than 6 cm
N2b	Multiple ipsilateral nodes, none greater than 6 cm
N2c	Any bilateral or contralateral nodes, none greater than 6 cm
N3a	Any node >6 cm
N3b	Any extranodal extension, clinical, radiologic or pathologic
M stage	
M0	No distant metastases
M1	Distant metastases

Sources: Brierley JD et al. *UICC TNM Classification of Malignant Tumours*, 8th ed. John Wiley & Sons Ltd, 2017; Amin MB et al. *CA Cancer J Clin.* 2017;67:93–9.
Note: DOI, depth of invasion not tumour thickness.

Lesions close to, or crossing, the midline will usually require bilateral neck dissection due to bilateral drainage of lymph. The majority of oral cancer patients (N0, N1, N2a) will undergo selective neck dissection of levels I–IV. Those with N2b–c or N3 (high volume) disease may undergo a modified radical (including levels I–V) neck dissection dependent on disease.

Trials investigating the use of sentinel lymph node biopsy (SLNB) and sampling to indicate the need for elective neck dissection have recently been published [18,19]. Despite promising trial data showing that SLNB can identify patients with metastatic disease, a review of the early literature reveals the issues of a steep learning curve and a higher than expected false negative rate (especially when used for areas such as the floor of mouth). Increased surgical experience with the technique and the use of improved tracers have been shown to reduce the false negative rate to approximately 2% [20]. Despite its accuracy and ability to spare the patient of a neck dissection, there has (to date) been a limited number of UK centres performing this diagnostic service, perhaps because of the steep learning curve, additional cost to the healthcare service and the additional man-hours required. Whether this saves overall patient morbidity and operating time is yet to be seen.

Reconstruction

As mentioned earlier, surgery for those patients who are fit enough still remains the mainstay of management, with reconstruction using well-established

Table 8.3 Stage grouping for oral cancer (8th ed.).

Stage I	T1	N0	M0
Stage II	T2	N0	M0
Stage III	T3	N0	M0
	T1	N1	M0
	T2	N1	M0
	T3	N1	M0
Stage IVA	T4a	N0	M0
	T4a	N1	M0
	T1	N2	M0
	T2	N2	M0
	T3	N2	M0
	T4a	N2	M0
Stage IVB	Any T	N3	M0
	T4b	Any N	M0
Stage IVC	Any T	Any N	M1

Sources: Brierley JD et al. *UICC TNM Classification of Malignant Tumours*, 8th ed. John Wiley & Sons Ltd, 2017; Amin MB et al. *CA Cancer J Clin.* 2017; 67:93–9.

options (from primary closure, local flaps, implants and obturators to microvascular hard and soft tissue reconstruction) available to the team. Advances in microvascular flap harvesting techniques have meant that increasing success rates of >95%–98% can be seen with flaps based on donor sites with reducing morbidity and functional deficit. The future of tissue engineering and transplant surgery is evolving, and may become increasingly more viable options for the reconstructive surgeon as the technology, techniques, biocompatibility and case selection improve. This is discussed in more detail in Chapter 16.

▮ Adjuvant therapy

At the primary site of resection

Indications for the use of adjuvant radiotherapy include close (generally defined as <5 mm in oral cancer) or involved margins where access to the site for further resection is not possible, perineural, perivascular spread and non-cohesive advancing front [15]. Apart from the situation of an involved margin, more than two other risk features in the primary resection site would normally be an indication

for adjuvant treatment as long as the patient was fit enough to complete up to 66 Gy in 33 fractions of intensity-modulated radiotherapy (IMRT).

It is, of course, essential that a dental assessment is carried out prior to commencing treatment, ideally by the restorative dentist as part of the MDT.

Radiotherapy to the neck

Radiotherapy to the neck would normally be indicated when more than one node is involved or if there is evidence of extracapsular spread.

Chemotherapy

Indications for chemotherapy in head and neck cancer include the presence of extracapsular spread from the nodes or evidence of an involved margin at the primary site. Cisplatin acts as a radiosensitiser in head and neck cancer treatment and confers some survival benefit (of the order of 6%–8%). It is not the mainstay of adjuvant therapy in this setting. Also, based on clinical data from the MACH-NC review, there is no evidence of improved survival over the age of 70 [21]. This is likely to be related to performance status rather than simply age itself. When indicated, chemotherapy is given concurrently with radiotherapy in the form of cisplatin (or carboplatin in those with impaired estimated glomerular filtration rate [eGFR]) to a dose of 100 mg/m^2. These are frequently given three weekly or in other equivalent regimes [22].

Neoadjuvant chemotherapy is not established as a routine treatment in oral cancer.

Biological treatments

In the head and neck, the agent most commonly used is the monoclonal antibody cetuximab, which is an anti-epidermal growth factor receptor (EGFR) antibody. EGFR overexpression is seen in 40%–95% of head and neck squamous cell carcinoma (HNSCC) and premalignant mucosa, and cetuximab prevents the attachment of growth factors to EGFR [23].

Cetuximab can be used instead of conventional chemotherapy when given in combination with radiotherapy [24]. It is also known to improve the activity of other chemotherapeutic agents, and Vermorken et al. showed that a combination of platinum, fluorouracil and cetuximab significantly improved survival as compared with platinum and fluorouracil alone [25]. It currently features heavily in clinical trials and has also been used in the palliative setting. Other biologics such as nivolumab have a role in the treatment of head and neck cancer that has progressed after having received chemotherapy, i.e. in the palliative setting as a potentially life extending treatment [26]. It is likely that biological treatments will become more prominent in the treatment of head and neck cancer in the future.

▐ Outcomes

Overall survival outcomes from oral cancer are approximately [27,28]:

- 86% for stage I
- 70% for stage II
- 50% for stage III
- 40% for stage IV

In the rehabilitation of the patient undergoing treatment for oral cancer, it is vital that there is early and ongoing regular input from dietetics, speech and language therapists, clinical psychologists and specialist cancer nurses. This is essential to get the best functional, psychological and survival outcomes for patients.

Osteoradionecrosis of the jaws

Osteoradionecrosis (ORN) of the jaws is one of the most severe chronic side effects of radiotherapy to the head and neck. It occurs in between 5%–10% of patients with oral or oropharyngeal cancer receiving radiotherapy [29,30]. ORN is radiation-induced fibrosis with disturbance of fibroblasts and the combination of osteoblastic death without replication of these cells. The mandible is susceptible to ORN due to the blood supply being limited to a single functional terminal artery (the inferior alveolar artery) [31].

The exposure of bone for greater than 8 weeks in a patient who has had previous radiotherapy to the jaws raises the suspicion of ORN. Many cases of ORN do resolve spontaneously after the dead bone breaks away as a sequestrum, but this can be a very a troublesome disease leading to chronically exposed bone which can progressively enlarge and lead to pathological fracture and fistula formation to the skin.

It can be prevented by removing any teeth of poor prognosis at least 2 weeks before the onset of surgery, meticulous oral hygiene after radiotherapy with high fluoride toothpastes and regular dental checkups. For this reason it is essential that a restorative dentist is a member of the MDT and assesses the patient's need for dental extractions before treatment commences. Some cases of ORN can be spontaneous; however, more often they are related to a dental extraction(s) or trauma from a denture. It is classified based on the Notani classification (see **Table 8.4**) [32].

ORN is unusual if areas that have been treated with less than 60 Gy, and the mandible is at much greater risk than the maxilla. Other risk factors include smoking, malnutrition, alcoholism, dose hypofractionation and brachytherapy. Bone resection during primary tumour surgery may also increase the risk of ORN [30].

Marx first proposed a theory of exposed bone based on the '3H' theory of *hypoxia, hypovascularity* and *hypocellularity* of irradiated bone predisposing to the condition, and he used hyperbaric oxygen to treat ORN [33]. He used varying protocols for prevention

Table 8.4 Notani classification of osteoradionecrosis of the jaws.

Class I	ORN confined to alveolar bone
Class II	ORN limited to alveolar bone and/or mandible above the level of inferior alveolar canal
Class III	ORN involving the mandible below the level of the inferior alveolar canal and ORN with a skin fistula and/or pathologic fracture

Source: Notani K et al. *Head Neck.* 2003;25:181–6.

of the disease prior to dental extraction and an altered protocol for patients that he was trying to treat with established disease. Unfortunately, none of his work has been reproduced in contemporary trials or research. Annane et al. published highly laudable and controversial results based on their experiments with hyperbaric oxygen therapy (they concluded that it was ineffective); however the study control groups were flawed and the inclusion study group were not correctly matched [34]. The HOPON trial (Hyperbaric Oxygen for the Prevention of Osteoradionecrosis) failed to show any benefit from having hyperbaric oxygen prior to dental extractions in patients who had previously had radiotherapy to the mandible [35].

Delanian et al. showed some promising results with treating ORN with pentoxifylline and vitamin E. This study was based on 18 patients and could not be reproduced by McLeod et al. in 2012 [36,37].

Follow-up

Follow-up is an area of controversy and variability. The most common time for loco-regional recurrence is within the first 2 years. Most cancer patients are followed-up for at least 5 years, with the frequency of follow up reducing as time goes on.

The oral cavity is easily examined as part of routine head and neck cancer follow-up. Neck examination is essential, as is monitoring weight at each visit. Most units will follow-up patients for 5 years, with a suggested dogmatic approach to follow-up as shown in **Table 8.5**.

Table 8.5 Example of common follow-up regime in oral cancer patients.

Year	Follow-up
1	Monthly
2	Every 2 months
3	Every 3 months
4	Every 4 months
5	Every 6 months

Signs of recurrence will include:

- New ulceration
- Nodal masses
- New onset weight loss

REFERENCES

1 Ferlay J, Colombet M, Soerjomataram I et al. Cancer incidence and mortality patterns in Europe: Estimates for 40 countries and 25 major cancers in 2018. *Eur J Cancer*. 2018; 103:356–87.

2 Warnakulasuriya S, Johnson NW, van der Waal I. Nomenclature and classification of potentially malignant disorders of the oral mucosa. *J Oral Pathol Med*. 2007; 36:575–80.

3 Blot WJ, McLaughlin JK, Winn DM et al. Smoking and drinking in relation to oral and pharyngeal cancer. *Cancer Res*. 1988;48:3282–7.

4 IARC Working Group on the Evaluation of Carcinogenic Risks to Humans. Personal habits and indoor combustions. Volume 100 E. A review of human carcinogens. *IARC Monogr Eval Carcinog Risks Hum*. 2012;100:1–538.

5 Mehanna HM, Rattay T, Smith J, McConkey CC. Treatment and follow-up of oral dysplasia: A systematic review and meta-analysis. *Head Neck*. 2009;31:1600–9.

6 Ho MW, Risk JM, Woolgar JA et al. The clinical determinants of malignant transformation in oral epithelial dysplasia. *Oral Oncol*. 2012;48:969–76.

7 Gandolfo S, Richiardi L, Carrozzo M et al. Risk of oral squamous cell carcinoma in 402 patients with oral lichen planus: A follow-up study in an Italian population. *Oral Oncol*. 2004;40:77–83.

8 Murti PR, Bhonsle RB, Pindborg JJ, Daftary DK, Gupta PC, Mehta FS. Malignant transformation rate in oral submucous fibrosis over a 17-year period. *Community Dent Oral Epidemiol*. 1985;13:340–1.

9 Alnuaimi AD, Wiesenfeld D, O'Brien-Simpson NM, Reynolds EC, McCullough MJ. Oral Candida colonization in oral cancer patients and its relationship with traditional risk factors of oral cancer: A matched case-control study. *Oral Oncol*. 2015; 51: 139–45.

10 McCaul JA, Cymerman JA, Hislop S et al. LIHNCS – Lugol's iodine in head and neck cancer surgery: A multicentre, randomised controlled trial assessing the effectiveness of Lugol's iodine to assist excision of moderate dysplasia, severe dysplasia and carcinoma *in situ* at mucosal resection margins of oral and oropharyngeal squamous cell carcinoma: Study protocol for a randomised controlled trial. *Trials*. 2013;14:310.

11 McCaul JA, McMahon JM, Quantrill J et al. LIHNCS: Lugol's Iodine in Head and Neck Cancer Surgery—A multi-centre, randomised, controlled trial assessing the effectiveness of Lugol's Iodine to assist excision of moderate dysplasia, severe dysplasia and carcinoma in-situ at mucosal resection margin of oral and oropharyngeal squamous cell carcinoma. *J Clin Oncol*. 2017;35:6065.

12 Lydiatt W, O'Sullivan B, Patel S. Major changes in head and neck staging for 2018. *Am Soc Clin Oncol Educ Book*. 2018:505–14.

13 Brierley JD, Gospodarowicz MK, Wittekind C et al. *UICC TNM Classification of Malignant Tumours*, 8th ed. John Wiley & Sons Ltd; 2017.

14 Amin MB, Greene FL, Edge SB et al. The 8th ed. AJCC Cancer Staging Manual: Continuing to build a bridge from a population-based to a more "personalized" approach to cancer staging. *CA Cancer J Clin*. 2017;67:93–9.

15 Kerawala C, Roques T, Jeannon JP, Bisase B. Oral cavity and lip cancer: United Kingdom National Multidisciplinary Guidelines. *J Laryngol Otol*. 2016;130:S83–9.

16 D'Cruz AK, Vaish R, Kapre N et al. Elective versus therapeutic neck dissection in node-negative oral cancer. *N Engl J Med*. 2015;373:521–9.

17 Weiss MH, Harrison LB, Isaacs RS. Use of decision analysis in planning a management strategy for the stage N0 neck. *Arch Otolaryngol Head Neck Surg*. 1994;120:699–702.

18 Alkureishi LW, Ross GL, Shoaib T et al. Sentinel node biopsy in head and neck squamous cell cancer: 5-year follow-up of a European multicenter trial. *Ann Surg Oncol*. 2010;17:2459–64.

19 Schilling C, Stoeckli SJ, Haerle SK et al. Sentinel European Node Trial (SENT): 3-year results of sentinel node biopsy in oral cancer. *Eur J Cancer*. 2015;51:2777–84.

20 Schilling C, Shaw R, Schache A et al. Sentinel lymph node biopsy for oral squamous cell carcinoma. Where are we now? *Br J Oral Maxillofac Surg*. 2017;55:757–62.

21 Pignon JP, le Maitre A, Maillard E, Bourhis J, MACH-NC Collaborative Group. Meta-analysis of chemotherapy in head and neck cancer (MACH-NC): An update on 93 randomised trials and 17,346 patients. *Radiother Oncol*. 2009;92:4–14.

22 Bernier J, Cooper JS, Pajak TF et al. Defining risk levels in locally advanced head and neck cancers: A comparative analysis of concurrent postoperative radiation plus chemotherapy trials of the EORTC (#22931) and RTOG (# 9501). *Head Neck*. 2005;27:843–50.

23 Specenier P, Vermorken JB. Cetuximab in the treatment of squamous cell carcinoma of the head and neck. *Expert Rev Anticancer Ther*. 2011;11:511–24.

24 Bonner JA, Harari PM, Giralt J et al. Radiotherapy plus cetuximab for squamous-cell carcinoma of the head and neck. *N Engl J Med*. 2006;354:567–78.

25 Vermorken JB, Mesia R, Rivera F et al. Platinum-based chemotherapy plus cetuximab in head and neck cancer. *N Engl J Med*. 2008; 359:1116–27.

26 Ferris RL, Blumenschein G, Jr., Fayette J et al. Nivolumab for recurrent squamous-cell carcinoma of the head and neck. *N Engl J Med*. 2016;375:1856–67.

27 Ganly I, Goldstein D, Carlson DL et al. Long-term regional control and survival in patients with "low-risk," early stage oral tongue cancer managed by partial glossectomy and neck dissection without postoperative radiation: The importance of tumor thickness. *Cancer*. 2013;119:1168–76.

28 Zhang H, Dziegielewski PT, Biron VL et al. Survival outcomes of patients with advanced oral cavity squamous cell carcinoma treated with multimodal therapy: A multi-institutional analysis. *J Otolaryngol Head Neck Surg*. 2013;42:30.

29 Moon DH, Moon SH, Wang K et al. Incidence of, and risk factors for, mandibular osteoradionecrosis in patients with oral cavity and oropharynx cancers. *Oral Oncol*. 2017;72:98–103.

30 Kuhnt T, Stang A, Wienke A, Vordermark D, Schweyen R, Hey J. Potential risk factors for jaw osteoradionecrosis after radiotherapy for head and neck cancer. *Radiat Oncol.* 2016;11:101.

31 Delanian S, Lefaix JL. The radiation-induced fibroatrophic process: Therapeutic perspective via the antioxidant pathway. *Radiother Oncol.* 2004;73:119–31.

32 Notani K, Yamazaki Y, Kitada H et al. Management of mandibular osteoradionecrosis corresponding to the severity of osteoradionecrosis and the method of radiotherapy. *Head Neck.* 2003;25:181–6.

33 Marx RE. Osteoradionecrosis: A new concept of its pathophysiology. *J Oral Maxillofac Surg.* 1983;41:283–8.

34 Annane D, Depondt J, Aubert P et al. Hyperbaric oxygen therapy for radionecrosis of the jaw: A randomized, placebo-controlled, double-blind trial from the ORN96 study group. *J Clin Oncol.* 2004;22:4893–900.

35 Shaw RJ, Butterworth CJ, Silcocks P et al. HOPON (Hyperbaric Oxygen for the Prevention of Osteoradionecrosis): A randomised controlled trial of hyperbaric oxygen to prevent osteoradionecrosis of the irradiated mandible after dentoalveolar surgery. *Int J Radiat Oncol Biol Phys.* 2019;104:530–9.

36 Delanian S, Depondt J, Lefaix JL. Major healing of refractory mandible osteoradionecrosis after treatment combining pentoxifylline and tocopherol: A phase II trial. *Head Neck.* 2005;27:114–23.

37 McLeod NM, Pratt CA, Mellor TK, Brennan PA. Pentoxifylline and tocopherol in the management of patients with osteoradionecrosis, the Portsmouth experience. *Br J Oral Maxillofac Surg.* 2012;50:41–4.

9

OROPHARYNX

Emma King and Neil de Zoysa

ANATOMY

An overview is provided in **Figure 9.1**.

The pharynx is subdivided into the nasopharynx, oropharynx and hypopharynx (cranially to caudally). It is lined by non-keratinised stratified squamous epithelium.

The oropharynx is dorsal to the oral cavity, extending cranially from the palate to the level of the hyoid bone (C2–C3). Its anterior boundaries include the tongue base, vallecula and lingual surface of the epiglottis. It opens anteriorly, through the isthmus faucium, into the oral cavity.

Superiorly it is bordered by the soft palate, which despite its external appearance is anatomically and functionally complex. On the lateral walls of the soft palate there are two muscular folds: anteriorly, the palatoglossus extends from the apponeurosis of the soft palate to the base of tongue. Posteriorly, the palatopharyngeus also arises from the soft palate apponeurosis and joins the stylopharyngeus muscle where it inserts into the posterior border of the thyroid cartilage. The palatopharyngeus is separated from the palatoglossus muscle by an angular interval or fossa, and within this the palatine tonsil is situated.

▌ Waldeyer's ring

Within the oropharynx are foci of mucosal associated lymphoid tissue. The main clusters are defined as tonsils and define Waldeyer's tonsillar ring (**Figure 9.2**). This refers to the collection of lymphatic tissue surrounding the pharynx. This lymphatic tissue responds to antigens either ingested or inhaled with priming of T- and B-cells and the secretion of antibodies into mucus and the blood stream.

▌ Pharyngeal spaces

There are two deep neck spaces which are intimately related to the oropharynx: the retropharyngeal space and the parapharyngeal space (**Figure 9.3**).

The retropharyngeal space

The retropharyngeal space runs from the base of the skull to the level of T6, posterior to the pharynx and oesophagus. Retropharyngeal lymph nodes are found in the portion of the retropharyngeal space superior to the hyoid bone. These lymph nodes drain the pharynx, nasal cavity, paranasal sinuses and the middle ear. Thus, infections in the pharynx can potentially lead to suppurative lymphadenopathy and

(a)

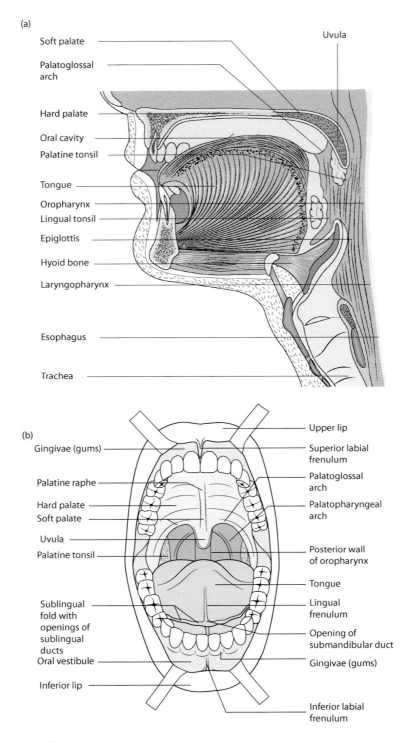

Soft palate

Palatoglossal arch

Hard palate

Oral cavity

Palatine tonsil

Tongue

Oropharynx

Lingual tonsil

Epiglottis

Hyoid bone

Laryngopharynx

Esophagus

Trachea

Uvula

(b)

Gingivae (gums)

Palatine raphe

Hard palate

Soft palate

Uvula

Palatine tonsil

Sublingual fold with openings of sublingual ducts

Oral vestibule

Inferior lip

Upper lip

Superior labial frenulum

Palatoglossal arch

Palatopharyngeal arch

Posterior wall of oropharynx

Tongue

Lingual frenulum

Opening of submandibular duct

Gingivae (gums)

Inferior labial frenulum

Figure 9.1 Anatomy of oropharynx.

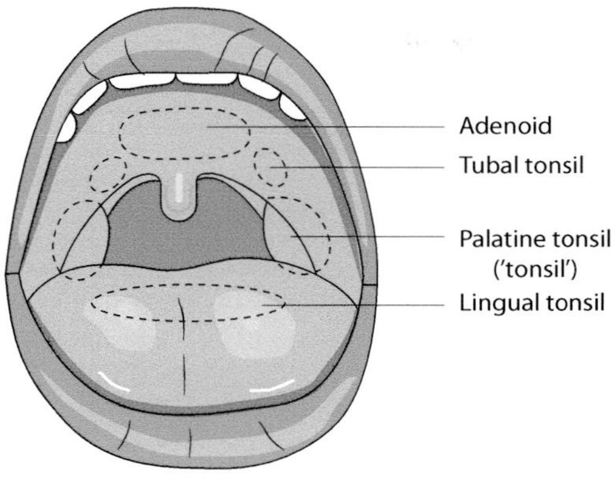

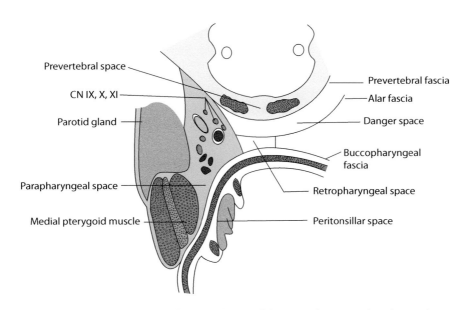

	Palatine tonsils	Located between the palatoglossal and palatopharyngeus folds. These are what are usually referred to as tonsils by patients and can be seen through the oral cavity.
	Lingual tonsil	Located on the superficial surface of the posterior third of the tongue and form the antero-inferior part of Waldeyers ring.
	Tubal tonsils	Located as the Eustachian tube opens into the nasopharynx, and form the lateral part of the ring.
	Pharyngeal tonsil	Also known as the adenoid, located on the posterior wall of the nasopharynx, forming the superior part of the ring.

Left side labels: Adenoid, Tubal tonsil, Palatine tonsil ('tonsil'), Lingual tonsil

Figure 9.2 Components of Waldeyer's ring.

Labels (left): Prevertebral space, CN IX, X, XI, Parotid gland, Parapharyngeal space, Medial pterygoid muscle

Labels (right): Prevertebral fascia, Alar fascia, Danger space, Buccopharyngeal fascia, Retropharyngeal space, Peritonsillar space

Figure 9.3 Diagrammatic representation of an axial view of the parapharyngeal and retropharyngeal spaces.

abscess formation in this space. These lymph nodes are more prominent in children, and largely atrophy by adulthood, explaining why retropharyngeal abscesses are more common in young children and adolescents. The contents include areolar fat, lymph nodes and small vessels.

Boundaries and relations of the oropharynx.

	Boundaries	Relations
Anterior	Middle layer of the deep cervical fascia	*Danger space* – also known as the alar space; extends freely from the base of the skull to the diaphragm, and spread of infection into this space can spread rapidly into the thorax leading to mediastinitis Carotid space
Posterior	Alar fascia, which separates the retropharyngeal space from the danger space	Pharyngeal mucosal space Parapharyngeal space
Lateral	Deep layer of the deep cervical fascia	
Superior	Clivus (skull base)	
Inferior	T4–6, the point of fascial fusion of the alar and middle layer of deep cervical fascia	

The parapharyngeal space

The parapharyngeal space consists largely of fatty areolar tissue and contains branches of the trigeminal nerve as well as the great vessels of the neck.

It is shaped like an inverted pyramid with its base at the skull base and apex inferiorly pointing to the greater cornu of the hyoid bone (**Figure 9.4**). It is split into two components (pre- and post-styloid) by the styloid process of the skull base (see **Tables 9.1** and **9.2**).

Abscesses and tumours are the main pathologies encountered in the parapharyngeal space. A detailed anatomical knowledge of this area is useful in the management of these entities, as well as a frequent topic of discussion in the intercollegiate examination!

■ Lymphatic drainage

The oropharynx drains to the deep cervical nodes in levels II–IV [1]. Anterior lesions, on the border of the oral cavity, can drain into level 1B [1,2]. Posterior lesions can in addition drain into the retropharyngeal lymph nodes, which as their name suggests lie posterior to the pharynx in the retropharyngeal space [3].

Lymph nodes of special note surgically

Retropharyngeal nodes are not usually resected in routine neck dissection. They are also not included in traditional staging systems for oropharyngeal cancer. Special dissection must be made to clear these if identified on preoperative imaging. With the advent of transoral robotic surgery, these nodes can be removed with the primary tumour if required, either due to preoperative identification on imaging or if identified during resection of the primary tumour. In addition, these nodes require removal as part of resection of advanced or recurrent pharyngeal cancers, with either transoral or open surgery [4].

■ Innervation

The pharyngeal plexus supplies most of the motor and sensory supply to the pharynx. The majority of the plexus is situated posterior to the middle constrictor muscle. It is composed of pharyngeal branches of the vagus (X), glossopharyngeal (XI) and trigeminal (V$_2$) nerves as well as sympathetic nerve fibres.

The motor neurons in the plexus arise mainly from the vagus and supply all the muscles of the pharynx

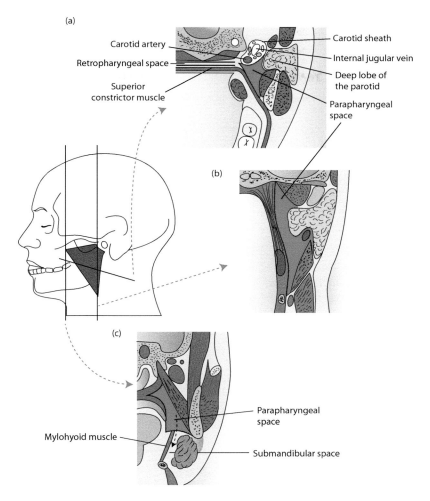

(a)

Carotid artery

Retropharyngeal space

Superior
constrictor muscle

Carotid sheath

Internal jugular vein

Deep lobe of
the parotid

Parapharyngeal
space

(b)

(c)

Parapharyngeal
space

Mylohyoid muscle

Submandibular space

Figure 9.4 Diagrammatic representation of the relations of the retropharyngeal and parapharyngeal spaces to the oropharynx. (a) axial (b) posterior coronal (c) anterior coronal.

Table 9.1 Contents of parapharyngeal space.

Contents	
Pre-styloid	**Post-styloid**
● Parapharyngeal fat ● Branches of the external carotid artery including the internal maxillary artery and ascending pharyngeal artery ● Pterygoid venous plexus and the retromandibular vein	● Internal carotid artery ● Internal jugular vein ● Glossopharyngeal nerve (IX) ● Vagus nerve (X) ● Accessory nerve (XI) ● Hypoglossal nerve (XII) ● Sympathetic trunk ● Lymph nodes

Table 9.2 Boundaries and relations of parapharyngeal space.

	Boundaries	**Relations**
Anterior	Fascia covering the medial pterygoid muscle (investing layer of the deep cervical fascia)	Prevertebral space
Posterior	Prevertebral fascia	Medial pterygoid
Lateral	Fascia covering the deep lobe of parotid (investing layer of the deep cervical fascia)	Pharyngeal mucosal space
Superior	Base of skull and styloid process	
Inferior	Greater cornu of the hyoid bone	
Medial	Middle (pretracheal) layer of the deep cervical fascia	Masticator space

and soft palate apart from the stylopharyngeus, which is supplied by the glossopharyngeal nerve, and tensor veli palatini, which is supplied by branches of the trigeminal nerve.

The sensory neurons to the plexus are conducted via the glossopharyngeal nerve, which supplies the greater portion of all three parts of the pharynx.

Clinical significance

High vagal neuropathy can be detected via palatal asymmetry both at rest (due to wasting) and during voluntary palatal elevation (saying 'ahh'). Isolated glossopharyngeal neuropathy is more subtle and usually only discernable via functional swallowing assessment (see Chapter 10).

Iatrogenic injury to the pharyngeal plexus is rare and is only usually seen in aggressive or salvage resections in the oropharynx, as a consequence of retrophayngeal nodal clearance or a late consequence of radiation therapy.

▌ Blood supply

The oropharynx receives blood supply from branches of the external carotid artery. These include the ascending pharyngeal, facial, maxillary and lingual arteries (**Figure 9.5**).

Surgical relevance during transoral surgery for oropharyngeal tumours

Of significance is the blood supply to the palatine tonsil, which is highly relevant during dissection and haemostasis of both benign and malignant lesions of the palatine tonsil. The palatine tonsil receives arterial supply via branches of the ascending pharyngeal (posterior tonsillar), facial (posterior tonsillar), lingual (anterior tonsillar) and maxillary (superior tonsillar) arteries. As a result, many surgeons ligate the linguofacial trunk, the ascending pharyngeal and linguofacial trunk, or indeed the entire external carotid artery to reduce the risk of haemorrhage after transoral resection of the lateral oropharynx.

SWALLOWING

The chief action in which the muscles of the pharynx combine is deglutition (swallowing); this is also discussed in detail in Chapter 10. Briefly, deglutition is a complicated, neuromuscular act whereby food is transferred from the oral cavity through the pharynx and into the oesophagus. The pharyngeal stage is the most rapid but also the most complex phase of deglutition. In the oropharyngeal phase of swallowing, the food bolus enters the base of the tongue triggering the phase.

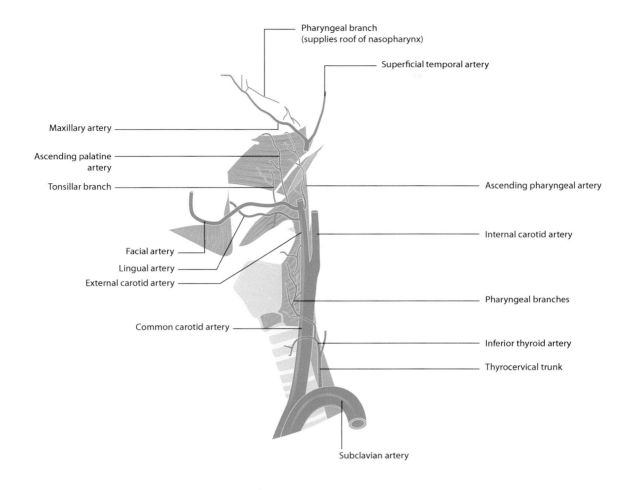

Pharyngeal branch
(supplies roof of nasopharynx)

Superficial temporal artery

Maxillary artery

Ascending palatine artery

Tonsillar branch

Ascending pharyngeal artery

Internal carotid artery

Facial artery

Lingual artery

External carotid artery

Pharyngeal branches

Common carotid artery

Inferior thyroid artery

Thyrocervical trunk

Subclavian artery

- Ascending pharyngeal artery, external carotid artery medial group
- Ascending palatine artery, from facial artery of external carotid artery
- Tonsillar artery
- Maxillary artery
- Lingual artery

Figure 9.5 Blood supply to the pharynx.

The soft palate (velum) elevates closing the oropharynx from the nasopharynx and preventing nasal regurgitation. When this fails to close completely, it is known as velopharyngeal insufficiency.

Palatal muscle contraction of the stylopharyngeus, salpingopharyngeus and palatopharyngeus assists the muscular peristaltic wave from the constrictor muscles (superior, middle and inferior) to propel the bolus into the oesophagus.

HISTORY

The main functions of the oropharynx include being a component of the airway and deglutition (assisting the transfer of food and liquid from the oral cavity to the hypopharynx). In addition, it acts as a valve to prevent nasopharyngeal (velopharyngeal) regurgitation and assists with speech articulation as a result of the nasopharyngeal valve.

Therefore, pathology usually encompasses one or more of the following symptoms:

- Stertor/stridor
- Dysphagia
- Odynophagia
- Referred pain (otalgia)
- Altered voice (muffling or dysarthria rather than hoarseness)
- Lateralising symptoms and the concomitant presence of a neck lump in association with the aforementioned symptoms are very concerning for malignancy

Important features in the history include details of:

- Sleeping habits (does the patient snore, have excessive somnolence, fatigue, delayed development in children)
- Lateralising odynophagia with otalgia: Both concerning features for malignancy
- Smoking and alcohol history: This is relevant for risk stratification especially in the context of malignancy
- Nasopharyngeal regurgitation/velopharyngeal insufficiency (does the patient regurgitate through the nose on swallowing: This is usually to liquids)
- Relevant medical history
  - Previous surgery/radiotherapy to head and neck; cardiac and pulmonary co-morbidities

ASSESSMENT OF PHARYNGEAL FUNCTION

See Chapter 10.

PATHOLOGY

▌ Tonsillitis

Between 50% and 80% of infective sore throats are virally induced, predominantly consisting of rhinovirus, coronavirus and parainfluenza viruses [5]. In addition, approximately 1%–10% of cases are caused by the Epstein–Barr virus (EBV; causing infectious mononucleosis or glandular fever). Bacterial tonsillitis can develop de novo or superimposed on an initially viral infection. The most common bacterial organism is group A beta-haemolytic streptococcus [6]. Other bacteria include *Chlamydia pneumoniae*, *Mycoplasma pneumoniae*, *Haemophilus influenzae*,

Candida, *Neisseria meningitidis* and *Neisseria gonorrhoeae* [6].

History

Specific points should include:

- Pain (sore throat)
- Odynophagia
- Dysphagia to liquids and solids
- Pyrexia and/or rigors
- Immunosuppression
- Known diabetic

Table 9.3 Symptoms of tonsillitis and peritonsillar abscess.

Symptom	Tonsillitis	Peritonsillar abscess
Sore throat	Bilateral	Unilateral
Odynophagia	Bilateral	Unilateral
Otalgia	Less common, bilateral	Common, unilateral
Trismus	Absent	Present
Length of time of symptoms	Longer (often several days)	Shorter (often 1 day or less)

Shortness of breath or noisy breathing (stertor) should be considered red flag symptoms that should mandate senior review. It is important to be able to differentiate swiftly on the basis of history between tonsillitis and peritonsillar abscess (see **Table 9.3**).

Examination

General patient overview:

● Temperature, blood pressure, respiratory rate, heart rate
● Ability to complete sentences

Specific examination includes:

● Cervical lymphadenopathy
● Oropharynx examination – size and symmetry of tonsils/palate
  – Presence of exudate
  – Trismus
● Fibre-optic examination to ensure safe airway and exclude supraglottitis – this is essential if there is any shortness of breath, stertor or if the patient is immunocompromised

Investigations

● Full blood count
● Urea and electrolytes
● C-reactive protein
● Monospot test

Management

If unable to maintain adequate oral intake the patient will require admission for i.v. fluids, analgesia, antibiotics (benzylpenicillin or clarithromycin if penicillin allergic) and steroids (i.v. dexamethasone). Steroids have been demonstrated to increase speed of resolution of pain [7].

When able to take oral medications and fluids and is haemodynamically stable, the patient can be discharged home on oral antibiotics and analgesia.

Complications

Complications include peritonsillar abscess, parapharyngeal space abscess and other deep space neck infection.

Obstructive sleep apnoea can occur secondary to reactive tonsillar hypertrophy during acute tonsillitis.

In the setting of untreated tonsillitis, scarlet fever, rheumatic fever and glomerulonephritis can occur. These are rare in developed countries due to the ease of access to antibiotics.

▌ Tonsilloliths

Tonsilloliths, or tonsil stones, are a soft collection of bacterial and cellular debris that form within the tonsillar crypts and are very common. They are most frequently associated with the palatine tonsils but can also be found within the lingual tonsils. Stoodley et al. demonstrated that tonsilloliths exhibit a biofilm structure and form chemical gradients through physiological activity [8]. There is oxygen respiration at the outer layer of the tonsillolith, denitrification toward the middle and acidification toward the bottom. The significance of this is not clearly understood yet.

History

Patients often notice tonsilloliths.

They are associated with halitosis but can more rarely present with unilateral pain and a feeling that 'something is stuck in the throat'.

As detailed later, tonsil tumours often present with unilateral symptoms and must not be mistaken for a benign tonsillolith.

Examination

Tonsilloliths are usually visible on oral inspection. If they have been recently removed, a large crypt can often be seen.

Investigation

Tonsilloliths are generally diagnosed clinically.

Management

Tonsillectomy is the definitive treatment for tonsilloliths. However, this is a benign condition and the absolute need for surgery can be debated. Patients often admit to using blunt instruments (e.g. cotton buds) to remove the debris from the crypt.

▉ Peritonsillar abscess (quinsy)

A peritonsillar abscess is a collection of pus between the tonsillar capsule and the pharyngeal constrictor muscles.

It is thought to occur either as a complication of acute tonsillitis or due to infection of a minor salivary gland (Weber's gland) which lies in the peritonsillar space. It is the most prevalent deep neck infection [9]. Teenagers and young adults are most commonly affected, and males are affected more frequently than females. Pathogens include group A streptococcus (cultured in approximately 20% of cases) and *Haemophilus influenzae*, though in many cases a mixed microbial growth of aerobes and anaerobes is obtained [9].

History

Peritonsillar abscesses have a similar but distinct presentation to tonsillitis (see **Table 9.3**). Usually a more severe spectrum of symptoms is seen, with a shorter history.

Examination

Usually trismus is present due to an inflammation-induced spasm of the medial pterygoid muscle. An asymmetrical soft palate in the acute setting with a septic patient is pathognomonic of a peritonsillar abscess. The ipsilateral tonsil is often not clearly seen due to the soft palate swelling. This differentiates quinsy from a parapharyngeal abscess where the tonsil is medialised.

Management

Management includes drainage of the collection of pus and treatment with intravenous antibiotics.

Drainage methods can include needle aspiration, incision and drainage, or a 'hot' tonsillectomy.

Following drainage, penicillin alone has been demonstrated to be sufficient. In cases where no pus has been drained yet or where it is yet to form metronidazole is a reasonable addition [10]. An alternative would be co-amoxiclav or clindamycin in those who are penicillin allergic.

Hot tonsillectomy is considered by some to be the gold standard of treatment for quinsy, but it is often only performed in cases refractory to drainage or in cases of airway compromise.

Complications

These are rare but significant if they arise. They include airway obstruction, parapharyngeal abscess, Lemierre's syndrome (infectious thrombophlebitis of the internal jugular vein), necrotising fasciitis, mediastinitis, erosion of the internal carotid artery and blowout, intracranial abscess and streptococcal toxic shock syndrome.

Adenotonsillar hypertrophy

Adenotonsillar hypertrophy is hypertrophy of the mucosally associated lymphoid tissue in Waldeyer's ring. The aetiology of this can be varied. It can be primary (unclear cause) or secondary (e.g. reactive to stimuli such as allergens or malignancy). Due to the complex relationship between adenotonsillar hypertrophy and facial shape and growth patterns as well as age and obesity, the clinical presentation of this can be varied.

Adenotonsillar hypertrophy results in nasal and Eustachian tube obstruction leading to mouth breathing, nasal congestion, hyponasal speech, snoring, obstructive sleep apnoea, chronic sinusitis and recurrent otitis media [11]. Adenotonsillar hypertrophy is the most important anatomical factor that has been associated with obstructive apnoea [12]. This syndrome is associated with several adverse outcomes, including cognitive impairment, metabolic and cardiovascular consequences, behavioural deficits and lower quality of life (QoL) [13]. Though not curative in all patients, the impact of adenotonsillectomy on these conditions can only be estimated prior to surgery and ascertained following surgery. With judicious patient selection, adenotonsillectomy results in improvement in most key outcomes [14].

In adenotonsillar hypertrophy there can be increased expression of inflammatory cytokines that respond well to anti-inflammatory agents such as corticosteroids. It has been shown that intranasal corticosteroids reduce cellular proliferation and the production of pro-inflammatory cytokines in a tonsil and adenoid mixed-cell culture system, and have been used clinically, decreasing rates of surgery for these patients [11].

Commonly, adenotonsillar hypertrophy affects all mucosally associated lymphoid tissue in the oropharynx (Waldeyer's ring). However, it can also be isolated to part of it, and then the question of managing an asymmetrical tonsil is raised. Patients regularly present with an asymmetric tonsil being the only symptom and examination finding. There are data sets that show a small percentage of cases representing underlying malignancy. Tonsillectomy

for histology is one option, but retrospective studies show an alternative is a watch-and-wait policy if the patients are otherwise clinically asymptomatic [15,16]. Patient choice is a significant factor in deciding treatment here.

Finally, incidental asymmetric tonsillar uptake on PET-CT scan is a regular referral to an ear, nose and throat clinic. Retrospective studies have suggested the risk of malignancy in the absence of clinical symptoms or if signs are low, and may be managed along the lines of an asymmetric palatine tonsil [17]. This of course excludes patients being investigated for carcinoma of unknown primary (CUP), in whom panendoscopy and bilateral tonsillectomy is recommended as first line.

Oropharyngeal tumours

Benign tumours

These can be divided into proliferative conditions of the epithelium including papilloma, and tumours of glandular structures including retention cysts and pleomorphic adenomas.

A tissue diagnosis is required to confirm the diagnosis. This may include excisional biopsy (with papillomas) and needle aspirations if a pleomorphic adenoma is suspected.

Malignant: Oropharyngeal carcinoma

Historically, oropharyngeal squamous cell carcinoma (OPSCC) was caused by exposure to cigarette smoke and/or alcohol. In a study by Hashibe et al. [18], the sum of the population attributed risk was 72%; tobacco causes 33% and alcohol 4%, however, synergistically the effect is 35%. More recently, a virally driven subset of cancers (human papillomavirus subtype 16 [HPV 16]) has emerged as the leading cause of squamous cell carcinoma (SCC) within the oropharynx. Though other subtypes (such as 18) have been identified in thee cancers, by far the most common in subtype 16. Today, up to 70% of oropharyngeal malignancies are thought to be driven by HPV 16 [19,20] This change in aetiology has been associated with a twofold increase in OPSCC in both the US and UK between 1990 and 2006 [21]. p16 is a tumour suppressor protein that can be detected using immunohistochemistry. It is used as a surrogate marker by pathologists to identify HPV positive (+) cases.

Although many HPV(+) patients present with lymph node involvement, in comparison to HPV negative (−) cases, their prognosis is generally better. At 5 years, disease-specific survival (DSS) is approximately 80% in HPV(+) disease versus 40% in HPV(−) cancers, irrespective of treatment [22].

There are several notable pathophysiological differences between HPV(+) and HPV(−) OPSCC. Whilst HPV(+) is poorly differentiated, often presents with large nodal metastases and frequently displays extracapsular spread, which are traditionally strong negative prognosticators, they do not have a strong influence in HPV(+) OPSCC. Additionally, patients who display a prominent immune response to the tumour (with higher levels of tumour infiltrating lymphocytes on pathological examination) have improved survival [23,24].

History

Benign tumours generally present with local symptoms:

- Asymmetric tonsil
- Altered voice
- Dysphagia
- Feeling of something in throat
- Referred pain (otalgia) is uncommon in benign disease

Malignant tumours often present with:

- A neck lump (metastatic neck node)
- Unilateral sore throat/odynophagia
- Referred pain (otalgia) is common
- Altered voice (late)
- Dysphagia (late)

Examination

In patients presenting with metastatic neck nodes, the primary tumour may be difficult to spot in clinic. Lateralising symptoms should guide the gaze.

Neck examination should be followed by oral cavity inspection and flexible naso endoscopy (FNE). Some attempt may be made to palpate the tonsils/ tongue base in clinic but this is generally poorly tolerated, and absence of firmness would not preclude examination under anaesthesia.

Investigation

Contrast-enhanced MRI is the modality of choice for staging the oropharynx and neck. A CT scan of the chest is currently recommended to complete staging.

PET-CT has an important role in investigating patients with metastatic carcinoma in cervical neck nodes with no identifiable primary in the UADT (CUP). If performed following biopsies, post-surgical inflammation may affect imaging.

Examination under anaesthesia is recommended to assess the involvement of local structures, as this is difficult to assess on imaging. In the era of availability of transoral surgery (either laser or robotic) for oropharyngeal carcinoma, it is important to recognise the role of tonsillectomy or tonsil biopsy. In patients where the tumour is clinically obvious it is enough to perform incisional biopsy to obtain diagnosis. In patients where the tonsils are clinically normal, then tonsillectomy should be performed to ensure the optimal chance of identifying the tumour. Standard tonsillectomy, in the setting of tonsil cancer, is not therapeutic or advantageous to the patient; however, it can make subsequent transoral surgery more challenging and therefore limit the therapeutic options available to the patient.

Staging of oropharyngeal cancer

Staging combines radiological, endoscopic and clinical findings according to the Union for International Cancer Control (UICC) tumour, node, metastasis (TNM) classification. The most recent edition of this classification in 2017 has seen a significant change in the staging of OPSCC [25]. The impact of p16 (HPV) status is major (see **Tables 9.4** and **9.5**).

Table 9.4 Comparison of TNM 8th edition T-staging system for p16 positive and negative oropharyngeal tumours.

	p16 positive	p16 negative
T1	≤2 cm	≤2 cm
T2	>2–4 cm	>2–4 cm
T3	>4 cm or extension to lingual surface of epiglottis	>4 cm or extension to lingual surface of epiglottis
T4	N.B. – No division into T4a or T4b; tumour invades any of the following: larynx, deep/extrinsic muscle of tongue, pterygoid muscles, hard palate, mandible, pterygoid plates, lateral nasopharynx, skull base or encases carotid artery	T4a – Tumour invades any of the following: larynx, deep/extrinsic muscle of tongue, medial pterygoid, hard palate, mandible T4b – Tumour invades any of the following: lateral pterygoid, pterygoid plates, lateral nasopharynx, skull base or encases carotid artery

Source: Amin MB et al. *CA Cancer J Clin.* 2017;67:93–9.

Table 9.5 Comparison of TNM 8th edition N-staging systems for p16 positive and negative oropharyngeal tumours.

	Clinical	Pathological
N0	No regional lymph node metastasis	No regional lymph node metastasis
N1	Unilateral metastasis, all 6 cm or less	Metastasis in 1–4 lymph nodes
N2	Contra/bilateral lymph node metastasis all ≤6 cm	Metastasis in ≥5 lymph nodes
N3	Metastasis in lymph node(s) >6 cm	N/A

Source: Amin MB et al. *CA Cancer J Clin.* 2017;67:93–9.

The TNM system can be used to stage the patient's cancer as shown in **Table 9.6**.

HPV-driven oropharyngeal tumours often present with local nodal metastases, but survival in this cohort is good. In order to reflect the improved survival, in the recent update of the American Joint Committee on Cancer (AJCC) and the UICC, HPV(+) disease has been re-staged. For example, a patient with a 1.5 cm (p16 positive) tonsil cancer and

Table 9.6 TNM 8th edition staging system for p16 positive oropharyngeal tumours [25].

Cancer stage	Clinical			Pathological		
I	T1–2	N0–1	M0	T1–2	N0–1	M0
II	T1–2 T3	N2 N0-2	M0 M0	T1–2 T3	N2 N0–1	M0 M0
III	T1–4 T4	N3 Any N	M0 M0	T3–4	N2	M0
IV	Any T	Any N	M1	Any T	Any N	M1

Source: Amin MB et al. *CA Cancer J Clin.* 2017;67:93–9.

two positive lymph nodes in the ipsilateral neck is stage IV in TNM 7 but will become a stage I in the TNM 8, to reflect the good outcome.

At the time of this writing, the Royal College of Pathologists have recommended that pathologists use TNM 8 in reporting these tumours. The effect on patient outcome is unknown, as TNM 8 has not been validated with large prospective patient groups. As a result, this has raised concerns within the clinical community, as there may be a risk that by changing the staging from TNM 7 to TNM 8 clinicians may change their treatment, due to the 'down staging' of tumours in TNM 8, de-intensifying their treatment plans.

▌ Management

All cases of diagnosed oropharyngeal cancer should be discussed in the setting of a head and neck multi-disciplinary team meeting.

Treatment options include:

- Radical treatment with the aim of cure and an acceptance of a degree of morbidity
- Palliative treatment where the main treatment aim is to control symptoms without adding morbidity
- Best supportive care where the patient's symptoms are managed without managing the disease at all

Early disease

Conventionally, early stage disease (stage I+II) is treated with single modality therapy, either surgery or radiotherapy. There is currently no high-quality data comparing the two treatment modalities. Survival data is equivalent and as such the decision on treatment modality is based on the likelihood of resecting the tumour with adequate margins in most centres with the facility to perform transoral surgery (using either laser or robot) [26–28].

Where possible, transoral approaches are favoured over traditional open procedures (requiring lip split and access mandibulotomy) due to lower morbidity.

Mistakenly, many believe transoral surgery for early oropharyngeal cancer is a recent development when it has been in regular use in international centres for over three decades [29]. Transoral laser, robotic and endoscopic procedures have been described [30].

Up to 30% of patients who are N0 will have occult nodal metastases [31]. Therefore all patients should undergo elective neck treatment to level II–IV in the form of a neck dissection for surgical patients and radiotherapy for patients undergoing non-surgical treatment.

Although the goal for T1–T2 N0 disease should be single modality treatment, adjuvant radiotherapy (RT) with or without chemotherapy may be required due to adverse pathological features for recurrence following surgery. Postoperative chemoradiotherapy is currently recommended in patients treated with surgery who have:

- Involved primary tumour resection margins.
- Nodal extracapsular spread. This is increasingly becoming recognised as a less influential negative prognosticator in p16 positive oropharyngeal carcinoma in stark contrast to the massive impact it has on survival in non-oropharyngeal subsites and p16 negative oropharyngeal cancer [32].

In the case of close margins or lymphovascular invasion, adjuvant radiation alone may be indicated.

Postoperative RT should be planned using the same principles as radical RT; a dose of 60 Gy in 30 fractions is typically recommended. Adjuvant treatment may affect functional outcomes following surgery.

The European trial 'BEST OF' [NCT02984410] is recruiting for Stage I and II patients and randomising into traditional intensity-modulated radiotherapy (IMRT) versus transoral surgery and neck dissection, and will be the first trial directly comparing the two modalities of treatment in early disease.

Advanced disease

Late stage disease (stage III + IV) is conventionally managed with combined modality treatment: either surgery and adjuvant radiotherapy or more commonly with concurrent chemoradiation (CCRT). Chemotherapy is usually platinum-based chemotherapy such as cisplatin or carboplatin. The main side effects of platinum-based agents include ototoxicity, neurotoxicity and nephron toxicity. The additional survival benefit in patients receiving chemotherapy is 6.5% [33]. This benefit is, however, not seen in patients over 70 years of age, and in this group targeted biological agents such as cetuximab are sometimes used instead. It should be noted that cetuximab can also cause significant toxicity and is not without risk. This lack of benefit is likely related to increasing performance status rather than a solely age-related threshold.

Conventional radiotherapy comprises of a dose 70 Gy in 35 fractions to the primary tumour and radiologically involved lymph nodes. At risk but radiologically negative sites receive a prophylactic dose of 50 Gy in 25 fractions.

Because of the excellent prognosis from lower-risk HPV-positive disease, De-ESCALaTE-HPV, a randomised clinical trial compared radiotherapy and cisplatin chemotherapy to radiotherapy and cetuximab in an effort to reduce toxicity of chemotherapy. This trial found no benefit in terms of reduced toxicity and worse tumour control rates with cetuximab [34]. In high-risk patients (HPV negative, smokers with more advanced disease) the ongoing CompARE trial looks at whether escalating treatment will improve survival.

As a consequence of the better outcome associated with HPV(+) HNSCC of the oropharynx, there is movement towards patient stratification to minimise treatment-associated toxicity in HPV(+) tumours, while maintaining good outcomes. In the UK the PATHOS trial seeks to answer this question and move away from single-modality treatment in favour of reducing morbidity in a group of patients who have a high rate of survival despite their treatment modality. Patients enrolled in PATHOS are treated surgically by transoral resection and neck dissection, then risk stratified according to their postoperative histology. They are then randomised into adjuvant treatment arms of conventional versus de-escalated treatment [35].

Follow-up

HPV status is a strong and independent indicator of survival. HPV-positive OPSCC has a 58% reduction in the risk of death compared with HPV-negative OPSCC [36].

A 3-year overall survival rate of 82.4% for HPV-positive disease compared with 57.1% (p < 0.001) for HPV-negative disease [36].

Factors such as smoking, particularly smoking at presentation, and number of involved nodes increase the risk status of HPV-positive OPSCC patients [36].

PET-CT is established as the standard of care in assessing response to non-surgical treatment. This should be performed no sooner than 3 months after completing treatment and has a high negative predictive value (i.e. if there is no fluorodeoxyglucose [FDG] uptake in the cervical lymph nodes then there is little chance of residual cancer) [37]. Following this, patients are currently generally followed-up clinically with intervals between appointments increasing as times from treatment increases up to 5 years.

Palliation

In patients who are unfit for or do not want radical treatment, palliative treatment can be offered to control symptoms without increasing morbidity through therapy itself. This is usually delivered in the form of chemotherapy for locally advanced disease although short courses of radiotherapy may be given to control pain or bleeding.

Options such as tracheostomy or gastrostomy tube insertion to relieve obstruction and aid the airway and nutrition need to be discussed in context with the patient's symptoms, survival time and wishes, as they can potentially prolong a patient's suffering.

Haematological malignancies

It is not uncommon for haematological malignancies to present in the oropharynx, specifically lymphoma and extramedullary plasmacytoma. Both tumours are clinically distinct from squamous lesions, often appearing to be more benign in nature. Lymphomas are treated with chemotherapy, and surgery is used to remove sufficient tumour to confirm the diagnosis. If lymphoma is suspected, after tissue removal from the patient, the sample should be divided and half sent in normal saline and half sent in formalin. Ideally, each tissue sample (node) should be at least 1 cm³ [38]. Extramedullary plasmacytomas are rare, but 80% occur within the head and neck [39]. Although the treatment of choice is radiotherapy, surgery may be required for radiation failure [40].

REFERENCES

1 Lindberg R. Distribution of cervical lymph node metastases from squamous cell carcinoma of the upper respiratory and digestive tracts. *Cancer.* 1972;29:1446–9.

2 Byers RM, Clayman GL, McGill D et al. Selective neck dissections for squamous carcinoma of the upper aerodigestive tract: Patterns of regional failure. *Head Neck.* 1999;21:499–505.

3 Werner JA, Dunne AA, Myers JN. Functional anatomy of the lymphatic drainage system of the upper aerodigestive tract and its role in metastasis of squamous cell carcinoma. *Head Neck.* 2003;25:322–32.

4 Troob S, Givi B, Hodgson M et al. Transoral robotic retropharyngeal node dissection in oropharyngeal squamous cell carcinoma: Patterns of metastasis and functional outcomes. *Head Neck.* 2017;39:1969–75.

5 Bird JH, Biggs TC, King EV. Controversies in the management of acute tonsillitis: An evidence-based review. *Clin Otolaryngol.* 2014;39:368–74.

6 Ebell MH, Smith MA, Barry HC, Ives K, Carey M. The rational clinical examination. Does this patient have strep throat? *JAMA.* 2000;284:2912–8.

7 Hayward G, Thompson MJ, Perera R, Glasziou PP, Del Mar CB, Heneghan CJ. Corticosteroids as standalone or add-on treatment for sore throat. *Cochrane Database Syst Rev.* 2012;10:CD008268.

8 Stoodley P, Debeer D, Longwell M et al. Tonsillolith: Not just a stone but a living biofilm. *Otolaryngol Head Neck Surg.* 2009;141:316–21.

9 Klug TE. Peritonsillar abscess: Clinical aspects of microbiology, risk factors, and the association with parapharyngeal abscess. *Dan Med J.* 2017;64.

10 Herzon FS, Meiklejohn DA, Hobbs EA. What antibiotic should be used in the management of an otherwise healthy adult with a peritonsillar abscess? *Laryngoscope.* 2018;128:783–4.

11 Sakarya EU, Bayar Muluk N, Sakalar EG et al. Use of intranasal corticosteroids in adenotonsillar hypertrophy. *J Laryngol Otol.* 2017;131:384–90.

12 Dayyat E, Kheirandish-Gozal L, Sans Capdevila O, Maarafeya MMA, Gozal D. Obstructive sleep apnea in children: Relative contributions of body mass index and adenotonsillar hypertrophy. *Chest.* 2009;136:137–44.

13 Tan HL, Gozal D, Kheirandish-Gozal L. Obstructive sleep apnea in children: A critical update. *Nat Sci Sleep.* 2013;5:109–23.

14 Marcus CL, Moore RH, Rosen CL et al. A randomized trial of adenotonsillectomy for childhood sleep apnea. *N Engl J Med.* 2013;368:2366–76.

15 Puttasiddaiah P, Kumar M, Gopalan P, Browning ST. Tonsillectomy and biopsy for asymptomatic asymmetric tonsillar enlargement: Are we right? *J Otolaryngol.* 2007;36:161–3.

16 Sunkaraneni VS, Jones SE, Prasai A, Fish BM. Is unilateral tonsillar enlargement alone an indication for tonsillectomy? *J Laryngol Otol.* 2006;120:E21.

17 Heusner TA, Hahn S, Hamami ME et al. Incidental head and neck (18)F-FDG uptake on PET/CT without corresponding morphological lesion: Early predictor of cancer development? *Eur J Nucl Med Mol Imaging.* 2009;36:1397–406.

18 Hashibe M, Brennan P, Chuang SC et al. Interaction between tobacco and alcohol use and the risk of head and neck cancer: Pooled analysis in the International Head and Neck Cancer Epidemiology Consortium. *Cancer Epidemiol Biomarkers Prev.* 2009;18:541–50.

19 Chaturvedi AK, Anderson WF, Lortet-Tieulent J et al. Worldwide trends in incidence rates for oral cavity and oropharyngeal cancers. *J Clin Oncol.* 2013;31:4550–9.

20 Steinau M, Saraiya M, Goodman MT et al. Human papillomavirus prevalence in oropharyngeal cancer before vaccine introduction, United States. *Emerg Infect Dis*. 2014;20:822–8.

21 Price PRM, Crowther R, Wight R. *Profile of Head and Neck Cancers in England: Incidence, Mortality and Survival*. In: Unit NCI (ed.). Solutions for Public Health; 2010.

22 Mellin H, Friesland S, Lewensohn R, Dalianis T, Munck-Wikland E. Human papillomavirus (HPV) DNA in tonsillar cancer: Clinical correlates, risk of relapse, and survival. *Int J Cancer*. 2000;89:300–4.

23 Ward MJ, Thirdborough SM, Mellows T et al. Tumour-infiltrating lymphocytes predict for outcome in HPV-positive oropharyngeal cancer. *Br J Cancer*. 2014;110:489–500.

24 Wood O, Woo J, Seumois G et al. Gene expression analysis of TIL rich HPV-driven head and neck tumors reveals a distinct B-cell signature when compared to HPV independent tumors. *Oncotarget*. 2016;7:56781–97.

25 Amin MB, Greene FL, Edge SB et al. The Eighth Edition AJCC Cancer Staging Manual: Continuing to build a bridge from a population-based to a more "personalized" approach to cancer staging. *CA Cancer J Clin*. 2017;67:93–9.

26 Dowthwaite SA, Franklin JH, Palma DA, Fung K, Yoo J, Nichols AC. The role of transoral robotic surgery in the management of oropharyngeal cancer: A review of the literature. *ISRN Oncol*. 2012;2012:945162.

27 White HN, Moore EJ, Rosenthal EL et al. Transoral robotic-assisted surgery for head and neck squamous cell carcinoma: One- and 2-year survival analysis. *Arch Otolaryngol Head Neck Surg*. 2010; 136: 1248–1252.

28 Weinstein GS, O'Malley BW, Jr., Magnuson JS et al. Transoral robotic surgery: A multicenter study to assess feasibility, safety, and surgical margins. *Laryngoscope*. 2012;122:1701–7.

29 Steiner W, Fierek O, Ambrosch P, Hommerich CP, Kron M. Transoral laser microsurgery for squamous cell carcinoma of the base of the tongue. *Arch Otolaryngol Head Neck Surg*. 2003;129:36–43.

30 Zoysa N, Sethi N, Jose J. Endoscopic video-assisted transoral resection of lateral oropharyngeal tumors. *Head Neck*. 2017;39:2127–31.

31 Lim YC, Koo BS, Lee JS, Lim JY, Choi EC. Distributions of cervical lymph node metastases in oropharyngeal carcinoma: Therapeutic implications for the N0 neck. *Laryngoscope*. 2006;116:1148–52.

32 Sinha P, Lewis JS, Jr., Piccirillo JF, Kallogjeri D, Haughey BH. Extracapsular spread and adjuvant therapy in human papillomavirus-related, p16-positive oropharyngeal carcinoma. *Cancer*. 2012;118:3519–30.

33 Pignon JP, le Maitre A, Maillard E, Bourhis J, MACH-NC Collaborative Group. Meta-analysis of chemotherapy in head and neck cancer (MACH-NC): An update on 93 randomised trials and 17,346 patients. *Radiother Oncol*. 2009;92:4–14.

34 Mehanna H, Robinson M, Hartley A et al. Radiotherapy plus cisplatin or cetuximab in low-risk human papillomavirus-positive oropharyngeal cancer (De-ESCALaTE HPV): An open-label randomised controlled phase 3 trial. *Lancet*. 2019;393:51–60.

35 Owadally W, Hurt C, Timmins H et al. PATHOS: A phase II/III trial of risk-stratified, reduced intensity adjuvant treatment in patients undergoing transoral surgery for Human papillomavirus (HPV) positive oropharyngeal cancer. *BMC Cancer*. 2015;15:602.

36 Ang KK, Harris J, Wheeler R et al. Human papillomavirus and survival of patients with oropharyngeal cancer. *N Engl J Med*. 2010; 363: 24–35.

37 Mehanna H, Wong WL, McConkey CC et al. PET-CT surveillance versus neck dissection in advanced head and neck cancer. *N Engl J Med*. 2016; 374: 1444–54.

38 Ramsay A et al. *Tissue Pathways for Lymph Node, Spleen and Bone Marrow Trephine Biopsy Specimens*. Royal College of Pathologists; 2008.

39 Galieni P, Cavo M, Pulsoni A et al. Clinical outcome of extramedullary plasmacytoma. *Haematologica*. 2000;85:47–51.

40 Bachar G, Goldstein D, Brown D et al. Solitary extramedullary plasmacytoma of the head and neck – Long-term outcome analysis of 68 cases. *Head Neck*. 2008;30:1012–9.

10

HYPOPHARYNX

Patrick J. Bradley and Neeraj Sethi

ANATOMY

The hypopharynx communicates superiorly with the oropharynx and inferiorly with the oesophagus, and is located posterior to the larynx. The superior border of the hypopharynx is an imaginary line from the superior level of the hyoid bone (or floor of the vallecula). The inferior boundary is anteriorly formed by the aryepiglottic folds that separate the hypopharynx from the larynx and posteriorly is the level of the inferior border of the cricoid cartilage and the apex of one piriform sinus to the other [1].

Specific subsites within the hypopharynx are the left and right piriform sinus, the posterior pharyngeal wall, and the post-cricoid region. The piriform sinuses are elongated, pear-shaped (Greek: *piri* meaning 'pear', *form* meaning 'like'; Latin: *pyri* meaning 'fire'), three-walled gutters that open medially into the pharyngeal lumen and extend anteriorly and laterally on either side of the larynx (thyroid cartilage). Inferiorly, the piriform sinus is in continuity with the post-cricoid region, a funnel-shaped area extending from the posterior surface of the arytenoid cartilage to the inferior border of the cricoid cartilage, which continues inferiorly as the oesophagus.

The wall of the hypopharynx is composed of four layers: a mucosal layer, a fibrous layer, a muscular layer and a loose connective tissue.

1 The mucosal layer is composed of stratified, non-keratinising epithelium. The submucosa contains glands that are composed of mucus and serous acini. There is an abundance of lymphatic vessels accounting for the frequent lymphadenopathy in inflammatory and neoplastic disease.

2 An intermediate fibrous layer (the pharyngobasilar fascia) is situated between the mucosa and the muscular layer in place of the submucosa. It is attached to the basilar region of the occipital bone. The fascial layer becomes strengthened posteriorly by a fibrous band (the midline pharyngeal raphe) providing attachment for the constrictor muscles.

3 The muscle layer is composed of the inferior constrictor. This is composed of two parts: the thyropharyngeus and cricopharyngeus. The thyropharyngeus muscle runs obliquely arising from the lamina of the thyroid cartilage and the lateral surface of the cricoid cartilage. The fibres pass backwards and insert into the pharyngeal raphe. The upper fibres overlap the middle constrictor muscle. The cricopharyngeus arises from the side of the cricoid cartilage, encircles the pharyngo-oesophageal junction and inserts on the opposite side of the cricoid cartilage. The cricopharyngeus is continuous with the circular fibres of the oesophagus and are believed to act as a sphincter.

4 The buccopharyngeal fascia is a thin fibrous layer continuous with the deep surface of the pharyngeal muscles and contains the pharyngeal plexus of nerves and veins. Posteriorly the buccopharyngeal fascia is attached to the prevertebral fascia and laterally it is connected to the styloid process and the carotid sheath [1].

▍ Lymphatic drainage

The hypopharynx drains primarily to levels IIa, III and IV.

Primary tumours of the piriform sinus and post-cricoid area may also drain to the retropharyngeal and the paratracheal nodes.

▍ Innervation

The pharynx receives its motor, sensory and autonomic supply through the pharyngeal plexus, which is located in the buccopharyngeal fascia, and is formed by the pharyngeal branches of the glossopharyngeal nerve (CN IX), the vagus nerve (CN X) and the sympathetic fibres from the superior cervical ganglion. All of the constrictor muscles are supplied by this plexus except the stylopharyngeus. The sensory fibres in the pharyngeal plexus are derived from the glossopharyngeal nerve. The superior laryngeal branch of the vagus nerve contributes to the sensory nerve supply of the hypopharynx.

SWALLOWING

Insight into swallowing requires an understanding of hypopharyngeal pathology and long-term management. Swallowing is divided into three phases: oral, pharyngeal and oesophageal [2]. The oral phase includes mastication and presentation of the food bolus to the faucial pillars where the pharyngeal phase begins. At this point, several events occur simultaneously:

1 Elevation of the soft palate to seal off the nasopharynx
2 Glottal adduction
3 Elevation of the hyoid/laryngeal complex
4 Constriction of the pharyngeal walls to drive the bolus caudal in the direction of the oesophagus

Movement of the bolus through the pharynx is initially accomplished by contraction of the semi-concentric superior constrictor. In the lower pharynx, contraction of the middle and inferior constrictors continues the peristaltic wave. The cricopharyngeus muscle acts as a muscular valve (aka upper oesophageal sphincter [UES], or the pharyngo-oesophageal segment). The UES remains closed under tonic contraction of the muscle unless stimulated. The anterior and superior displacement of the larynx via attachments of the cricoid cartilage results in opening of the cricopharyngeus.

CLASSIFICATION OF HYPOPHARYNGEAL LESIONS

See **Table 10.1**.

Table 10.1 Classification of hypopharyngeal lesions.

By location	By aetiology	
Intraluminal	Congenital	Acquired
Mural		Neuromuscular Diverticula Neoplastic Iatrogenic
Extramural		

SYMPTOMS OF HYPOPHARYNGEAL LESIONS

The primary function of the hypopharynx is the safe transfer of a bolus from the oral cavity/oropharynx into the oesophagus without any significant hold-up or delay, and to avoid overspill into the laryngeal airway [3]. Symptoms include:

- Dysphagia
- Odynophagia
- Sore throat
- Dysphonia
- Referred pain (otalgia)

Lateralising symptoms are more concerning for possible malignancy.

The presence of a neck lump in association with the aforementioned symptoms is also concerning for malignancy.

Important features in the history include details of:

- Feeding habits (diet, feeding methods, duration of meals, weight loss, coughing, choking during meals)
- History of persistent cough
- Heartburn
- Regurgitation
- Relevant medical history
- Surgery/radiotherapy to head and neck
  - Neurological/neuromuscular disorder
  - Aspiration pneumonia
  - History of gastro-oesophageal reflux)
  - Medications (e.g. antihistamines, antipsychotics, antidepressants and diuretics)
  - Other factors – tobacco and alcohol use

ASSESSMENT OF PHARYNGEAL FUNCTION

Assessment of the pharyngeal phase of swallowing evaluates [4–6]:

- Transport and clearance of the swallowed bolus
- Airway protection
- Palate–pharyngeal closure
- Pharyngeal contraction
- Hyoid/laryngeal elevation
- Function of the cricopharyngeus

▌ Pharyngeal squeeze manoeuvre

First described by Bastian [7], the pharyngeal squeeze manoeuvre can be performed in clinic using the flexible laryngoscope. The patient is asked to make a high-pitched, strained phonation, preferably with increasing effort. This will in a normal pharynx result in obvious recruitment of the pharyngeal constrictor musculature. This recruitment is reduced or absent in patients with swallowing problems. A good correlation between this manoeuvre and the pharyngeal constrictor ratio has been validated as a measure of pharyngeal strength.

▌ Self-assessment

Patient self-assessment has been shown to be helpful in determining functional health status and health-related quality of life. Validated available instruments include the Eating Assessment Tool (EAT-10), the MD Anderson Dysphagia Inventory and the Sydney Swallow Questionnaire.

▌ Flexible endoscopic evaluation of swallowing and sensory testing (FEES and FEESST)

FEES visualises the base of tongue, hypopharynx and larynx, and allows evaluation of the structure and function of the upper aerodigestive tract. After placement of the flexible nasendoscope and assessing the appearance of the laryngopharynx, pooling of secretions is assessed as is laryngeal movement on phonation, coughing, inhalation and coughing. Test swallows are then conducted using visible foods and liquids.

The principle advantages for FEES include:

1 Direct observation of the laryngopharyngeal anatomy
2 Ease of execution in outpatient or inpatient settings
3 No need for radiological intervention
4 No need for contrast administration
5 Observing pre-swallowing or premature spillage, penetration and aspiration into the larynx, as well as pooling of the valleculae or pyriform sinus, and visualising post-swallow residue
6 The impact of manoeuvres can also be assessed

Disadvantages include:

1 It does not allow for evaluation of the oral phase of swallowing
2 Evaluation of the pharyngeal phase of swallowing is limited owing to the 'white out' (hyoid/laryngeal elevation) that occurs during swallowing

FEESST is a test to assess airway protection, which involves the delivery of a discrete pulse of air to the epithelium innervated by the internal branch of the superior laryngeal nerve to elicit the laryngeal adductor reflex, a brainstem-mediated airway-protective reflex. It has been reported that there is a strong association between motor function deficits and hypopharyngeal sensory deficits. Patients with an absent laryngeal adductor reflex show significant aspiration with thin liquids and pureed foods.

▥ Contrast swallow

A contrast swallow involves swallowing of contrast medium followed by x-ray imaging of the pharynx, oesophagus and stomach. The contrast medium is usually barium unless there is a history of allergy or a known perforation (in which case gastrografin can be used, as this is water soluble and less irritant to tissues). It is still the gold standard approach to diagnose a pharyngeal pouch and can indicate the presence of oesophageal dysmotility or pharyngeal incompetence.

▥ Videofluoroscopic swallow study (VFSS)

VFSS is also known as the modified barium swallow (MBS). This test is the mainstay of radiological swallowing evaluation and allows for all four phases of swallowing to be observed (**Table 10.2**). The test:

1 Identifies existing oral and pharyngeal motility disorders
2 Ascertains the presence of penetration or aspiration during swallowing of any food consistency
3 Assesses the speed of the swallow
4 Evaluates the effect of therapeutic strategies such as postural changes and swallowing manoeuvres
5 Allows for an oesophagram to be performed during the same visit

▥ Transnasal oesophagoscopy (TNE or TNO)

With TNO the upper aerodigestive mucosal tract from the nasal vestibule to the gastric cardia can be visualised. It is easy to perform and is well tolerated, safe and rarely requires topical anaesthesia. It is growing in popularity for patients with globus sensation, laryngopharyngeal and gastro-oesophageal reflux, and for head and neck cancer screening [8].

Table 10.2 Comparison of measurements capable with videofluoroscopy and FEES/FEEST.

	Contrast swallow /FNL	FEES/FEEST
Complete swallowing evaluation	✓	
Visualises laryngopharyngeal anatomy		✓
Assesses vocal cord function		✓
Diagnoses a pharyngeal pouch	✓	
Requires nasal instrumentation		✓
Can be performed at the bedside		✓

Abbreviation: FNL, fibreoptic naso-laryngoscopy.

Pharyngeal and oesophageal manometry (upper oesophageal sphincter: UES)

The use of manometry allows for pharyngeal and cricopharyngeal muscles (UES) coordination and pressures to be evaluated objectively. Pharyngeal strength and contraction duration, the completeness of UES relaxation, and coordination between the pharynx and UES during swallowing can also be evaluated.

Oesophageal manometry is indicated in dysphagia not diagnosed by endoscopy (including full oesophago-gastro-duodenoscopy) or radiology. It is regarded as the most accurate method of diagnosing oesophageal dysmotility and for pH electrode placement.

Other available tests:

- 24 hour PH monitoring
- Computed tomography
- PET-CT scanning
- Endoscopy and biopsy

PATHOLOGY

Third and fourth branchial anomalies

See Chapter 4 for details.

Webs, strictures and stenosis

These can occur secondary to various aetiological factors including trauma (caustic, penetrating or iatrogenic), neoplasms (benign or malignant) or syndromes such as Plummer–Vinson syndrome [9]. Plummer–Vinson (aka Paterson-Brown-Kelly syndrome or sideropenic dysphagia) is a symptom complex caused by iron deficiency, mostly seen in women aged 30–50 years. It produces atrophic glossitis caused by the atrophy of the piriform papillae, angular chelitis, and occasionally hyperkeratotic lesions of the oral mucosa, koilonychias, pagophagia (eating ice), and webs that can become malignant. The web is initially anterior, located in the post-cricoid area, but later become circumferential. It is reported that because of the generalised chronic inflammation associated with the deficiency, fibrosis develops, causing webs and irreversible long strictures.

History

- High dysphagia which may be progressive or non-progressive dependent on the aetiological nature of the underlying pathology

Past medical history is key in these patients

- Iron deficiency anaemia
- Certain mucosal and skin diseases such as epidermolysis bullosa, pemphigoid, Behçet's disease
- Strictures may be associated with blunt trauma, pharyngeal surgery, caustic ingestion and more recently with non-surgical management of pharyngeal cancer with chemoradiotherapy

Examination

There may be nothing to find on clinical examination, though Plummer–Vinson syndrome produces atrophic glossitis with hyperkeratotic oral mucosal lesions and koilonychia.

Investigation

Contrast swallow is reported in up to 8% of patients investigated [10]. Most webs are located within 2 cm of the pharyngo-oesophageal junction. The typical web appears on fluoroscopy as a perpendicular linear filling defect arising from the anterior wall (see **Figure 10.1**). Its thickness is uniform and rarely exceeds 2 mm. Rarely, webs are circumferential. The relationship between webs to dysphagia and other diseases remains controversial.

Management

Any iron deficiency requires correction and autoimmune disease appropriate management.

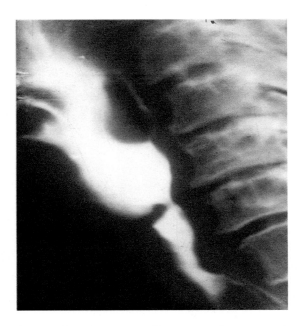

Figure 10.1 Contrast swallow image of an anteriorly based hypopharyngeal web.

These require direct visualisation, biopsy and dilatation. This can be performed using serial bougie instrumentation or balloon dilatation. The patient should be warned of the risk of perforation and dental/lip injury as well as recurrence of symptoms and the need for repeat procedures.

▌ Globus pharyngeus or globus syndrome

Globus pharyngeus is often described as the sensation of a lump in the throat associated with dry swallow, or the need to dry swallow, which disappears completely during eating or drinking and for which no organic cause can be established [11]. The symptom may be persistent or intermittent, but of major significance is there is no pain. The clinical symptom is usually long-lasting, difficult to treat and has a tendency to recur. The diagnosis of globus pharyngeus should be one of exclusion.

History

A feeling of something in the throat, catarrh or postnasal drip that will not clear.

This feeling is usually poorly localised.

There should be an absence of high-risk symptoms (dysphagia, odynophagia, throat pain, otalgia, weight loss, hoarseness).

Lateralising symptoms are of particular importance.

Common associated symptoms include:

- Reflux symptoms
- Psychological problems

Examination

Neck palpation, inspection and palpation of the oral cavity and oropharynx, and examination of the remaining mucosal surfaces of the upper aerodigestive tract by flexible nasendoscopy should be conducted.

Should TNO be available, then its use has been reported as efficient in reassuring patients that they do not have a serious diagnosis.

Investigation

Several reports emphasise that further investigations as a routine are usually uninformative, and sometimes with possible serious risk such as rigid endoscopy [12]. Almost all potential causes of globus can be excluded with a thorough history and examination.

Management

The aetiology of globus remains unknown but appears to be multifactorial (**Table 10.3**). Although data is limited, recent studies have focused on gastro-oesophageal reflux disease (GERD), abnormalities of the UES, psychological and psychiatric disorders, and stress as major factors contributing to the globus sensation. Since there is a paucity of controlled trials on the treatment of globus, evidence-based concepts are currently not available and thus treatment if indicated should be individualised for each patient. Given the benign nature of the condition, the likelihood of long-term symptom persistence and the absence of highly effective pharmacotherapy, the

Table 10.3 Causes of globus pharyngeus.

Gastro-oesophageal reflux
Abnormal upper oesophageal sphincter function
Oesophageal motor disorder
Pharyngeal inflammatory cause (pharyngitis primary/secondary)
Hypertrophy of tongue base
Retroverted epiglottis
Cervical heterotopic gastric mucosa
Forestier's disease (prominence of cervical vertebral bodies)
Psychological factors and stress
Thyroid disease
Upper aerodigestive malignancy

mainstays of treatment are explanation and reassurance [12]. A trial of anti-reflux medication (alginate) is a reasonable option but follow-up is likely to be of little use.

▌ Cricopharyngeal dysfunction

Cricopharyngeal dysfunction is a common cause of swallowing symptoms, which consists of a failure to appropriate relaxation of the cricopharyngeus muscle (UES) during the pharyngeal phase of swallowing. The possible aetiology is varied including anatomic, neuromuscular, iatrogenic, inflammatory, neoplastic and idiopathic. The opening of the UES necessitates three factors: neural inhibition of tonic intrinsic sphincter muscle contraction, anterior–superior laryngeal elevation that tends to the mechanical distraction of the UES, and passive stretching of the intrinsic sphincter muscles as the bolus passes through the lower pharynx. In a disease state, the UES compliance is altered or signalling impaired, leading to misdirection of the bolus into the laryngeal vestibule, triggering choking, cough or, failing that, aspiration (**Table 10.4**).

History

Typical symptoms include:

Table 10.4 Potential causes of cricopharyngeal dysfunction.

Central nervous system	Cerebellar infarct Brain stem infarct Parkinsonism Amyotrophic lateral sclerosis Base of skull neoplasm
Peripheral nervous system	Peripheral neuropathy Diabetic neuropathy Bulbar poliomyelitis Myasthenia gravis Neoplasm
Cricopharyngeus muscle	Polymyositis Oculo-pharyngeal muscular dystrophy Hyper/hypothyroidism
Cricopharyngeal disruption	Laryngectomy Supraglottic laryngectomy Neck irradiation Radical oropharyngeal resection Pulmonary resections
Cricopharyngeal spasm	Hiatus hernia Gastro-oesophageal reflux
Idiopathic cricopharyngeal achalasia	

- Dysphagia
- Globus sensation
- Coughing or choking episodes when eating

Examination

This will be largely unremarkable.

Pooling of secretions may be seen on flexible nasendoscopy.

Investigation

Contrast swallow shows a cricopharyngeal bar (though this can be present in normal subjects).

VFSS allows assessment of the dynamic actions of the muscle.

Manometry may add to confirming the diagnosis, though opinion varies as to its value.

Endoscopy may be indicated when there are clinical or radiological features suggestive of malignancy.

Electromyography has also been used by some researchers to diagnose swallowing disorders.

Management

Treatment of cricopharyngeal dysfunction depends on the underlying cause but in general involves:

- Enhancing the opening (dilatation, myotomy)
- Inducing relaxation (botulinum toxin injection)
- Enhancing current function (swallowing therapy and positional strategies)
- Diversion past the pharyngo-oesophageal segment (non-oral feeding)

The injections of botulinum toxin and cricopharyngeal dilatation are associated with a higher risk of recurrence, but are more suitable in the elderly and co-morbid patients. In patients requiring formal myotomy, the endoscopic approaches have been described and may be less morbid when compared with the classic transcervical surgical approach [13].

◼ Hypopharyngeal diverticula (pharyngeal pouches)

Hypopharyngeal diverticula (also referred to as pharyngeal or pharyngo-oesophageal pouch or

Table 10.5 Classification of diverticulae.

Classification system	Categories
By location	Hypopharyngeal Midthoracic Epiphrenic
By pathophysiology	Pulsion and traction diverticula
By composition	True and false diverticula

diverticula) have been described, with Zenker's diverticulum (ZD) being the most common with a reported annual incidence of about 2 per 100,000. The diagnosis is most frequent in elderly men with a peak incidence between ages 70–90 years [14]. Pharyngeal and oesophageal diverticulae can be classified in several ways (see **Table 10.5**).

Pulsion diverticula (see **Table 10.6**) herniate through a weakness in the outer muscular layer because increased intraluminal pressure are typically considered false diverticula (indicating the presence of only mucosa and submucosal in the wall of the pouch). Traction diverticula due to external tethering of the pharynx or oesophagus owing to some adjacent inflammatory process (e.g. resolution of a

Table 10.6 Types of pulsion hypopharyngeal diverticula.

Types of pulsion diverticula	Anatomy	Proportion of pulsion diverticula
Zenker's diverticulum (classical pharyngeal pouch)	Occur above the cricopharyngeus muscle, located at Killian's dehiscence (the triangular weakness between the oblique fibres of the thyropharyngeus muscle and the horizontal upper border of the cricopharyngeus muscle)	70%
Killian–Jamieson diverticulum	Protrudes through a weakness where the recurrent laryngeal nerve enters the larynx	25%
Laimer's diverticulum	Located between the divergent longitudinal muscle fibres of the proximal oesophagus where only the circular fibres of the oesophagus are present	<5%
Pharyngocele	Herniation of the pharyngeal mucosa through the thyrohyoid membrane	Rare

perforation, an inflamed lymph node or post-anterior approach cervical spine surgery) are considered true diverticula (indicating the presence of mucosa, submucosal and outer muscular layers).

History

Regardless of location or aetiology of a hypopharyngeal diverticulum, the clinical presentation and symptoms are similar. The primary presenting symptoms are:

- High dysphagia
- Regurgitation of undigested food (sometimes >24 hours later)

Additional symptoms may include:

- Halitosis
- Aspiration
- Cough
- Weight loss
- Hoarseness
- Gurgling in throat

Examination

Examination may be completely normal.

Rarely a neck swelling may be palpated, which may produce a gurgling on palpation (Boyce's sign).

Investigation

A contrast swallow is diagnostic (see **Figure 10.2**). Staging systems have been proposed but none is used universally (see **Table 10.7**). Most clinicians with

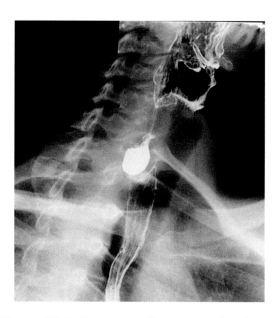

Figure 10.2 Contrast swallow image of a pharyngeal pouch.

experience consider such classifications to make little difference clinically and that ZD pouches are either small or large.

Endoscopic examination may be required to identify the more rare variants.

Management

Treatment is surgical. Of the more common Zenker's type of hypopharyngeal diverticula, the approach can be open or endoscopic (see **Table 10.8**). Much debate continues as to the advantages of each technique

Table 10.7 Three popular sizing systems for Zenker's diverticula; none is considered universal.

Stage	I	II	III	IV
Brombart (1973): Radiological measurement of pouch visible on UES	2–3 mm 'Rose thorn'	4–8 mm 'Club-like'	>9 mm	Compressing oesophagus
Morton and Bartley (1993): Based on barium length	<2 cm	2–4 cm	>4 mm	
Von Overbeek and Groote (1994): Based on vertebrae size	<1 vertebral body	>1 and <3	>3	

Table 10.8 Open and endoscopic approaches described to pharyngeal pouch surgery.

Open approach	Endoscopic approach
Excision of pouch and cricopharyngeal myotomy	'Stapling of pouch'; uses an endosurgical stapler that simultaneously divides the wall (cricopharyngeal bar) between the oesophagus and the pouch and staples the wound edges closed.
Cricopharyngeal myotomy alone	Dohlman's procedure (electrocautery of cricopharyngeal bar)
	CO_2 laser division of cricopharyngeal bar
	Transoral flexible endoscopic cricopharyngeal myotomy

(see below). What is common to both approaches is the cricopharyngeal myotomy. This is critical as the criocpharygeus muscle forms the bar behind which the pouch forms.

Endoscopic approach

The endoscopic approach can be performed on the majority of patients with a short duration of hospitalisation, with rapid initial improvement of symptoms. However, the pouch is not excised and myotomy is not as extensive as using an open approach. The recurrence rate of symptoms is higher (up to 20%) compared to the open approach, but the procedure can be repeated [15].

Relative and absolute contraindications to the rigid endoscopic approach include:

a An inability to obtain a clear view of the diverticulum (may not be realised until the endoscopy is performed, or may be predicted in patients with a short neck, severe kyphosis, decreased hyomental distance and/or a high body mass index)
b Small pouches (<2 cm) with a small cricopharyngeus muscle ridge or bar
c Anatomical factors that preclude adequate rigid endoscopy (e.g. upper teeth protrusion, inadequate jaw opening or insufficient neck mobility)

Transoral flexible endoscopic cricopharyngeal myotomy has been described avoiding a general anaesthetic. The cricopharyngeus is commonly divided using a needle knife (though other tools have been described). Some techniques have recommended the use of a soft diverticuloscope to stabilise the septum, improve visualisation and further guide the instrument of incision. This technique is suitable for patients with poor neck extension and/or limited jaw retraction, because the scopes used are more flexible and smaller in diameter, and does not require a general anaesthetic.

Open approach

The open (transcervical) approach to Zenker's diverticulum is a technically demanding procedure, but involves a full cricopharyngeal myotomy to be performed as well as sac inspection and excision or inversion to be performed depending on size. It is a definitive procedure with a minimal risk of recurrence and therefore arguably a better option for younger patients but often requires a longer hospital stay, nasogastric feeding and carries a higher risk of anastomotic leak.

Larger pouches and recurrent pouches have been reported to be associated with the rare occurrence of cancer [16].

The open approach is indicated:

a In small sized pouches and younger patients
b As a secondary therapy when an endoscopic approach has not relieved the patient's symptoms (up to 20%)

Inadequate cricopharyngeus myotomy is considered to be the major cause for recurrent and/or persistent symptoms. An open cricopharyngeal myotomy alone without excision of pouch has been reported with good results. The open surgical approach is considered a distinct advantage, and performing an extended myotomy better addresses the pathophysiological cause.

Outcomes and complications

A systematic review of endoscopic and open approaches as the treatment of pharyngeal pouch, found failure rates of open and endoscopic approaches were 4.2% and 18.4%, respectively, and corresponding complication rates were 11% and 7% [17]. Within endoscopic techniques, failure rates were 18.9% for stapler diverticulotomy and 21.7% for laser diverticulotomy. Corresponding complication rates were 4.3% and 7.9%. Interestingly flexible endoscopy techniques had a higher failure rate (14.3%). Most reported complications from transcervical techniques related to the recurrent nerve 3.4% and salivary fistula 3.7%, and for the endoscopic group emphysema 3.0% and mediastinitis 1.2%. Operation-related deaths occurred in both groups, but were more frequent with the open approach (0.9% vs 0.4%).

Postoperative ward rounds should specifically exclude hypopharyngeal perforation with the following:

- Any complaint of chest or inter-scapular pain
- Any resting persistent tachycardia or pyrexia
- The presence of surgical emphysema

Salivary fistulas are primarily managed conservatively with antibiotics and nasogastric feeding and may take several weeks to spontaneously resolve. A contrast swallows performed when the inflammation has settled (2 weeks) may give some guidance to reassure the patient.

The potential advantages of the transoral approach include low morbidity, short length of hospital stay, and similar medium-term outcome compared with the open diverticulectomy and cricopharyngeal myotomy. The higher long-term recurrence rate of symptoms is offset by the lower morbidity and the ease by which the procedure can be successfully repeated.

■ Hypopharyngeal neoplasms

Hypopharyngeal cancer represents 5%–10% of upper aerodigestive tract malignancies (~450 cases per year in UK). These tumours are strongly associated with tobacco and alcohol consumption. As with other head and neck cancer subsites, >90% of tumours are squamous cell carcinoma (SCC). Most patients present with advanced disease (>80% at stage III or IV). The hypopharynx has a rich lymphatic supply which predisposes that tumours have a tendency for extensive three dimensional submucosal spread and the high rates of metastatic lymphadenopathy at presentation. Synchronous secondary primary tumours (head and neck, lung, or oesophageal) are found in 5%–10% of patients.

History

These tumours tend to occur in the elderly patient (>65 years) and >75% are male. Presenting symptoms include:

- Sore throat (especially if lateralised)
- Ipsilateral otalgia (referred via the vagus nerve)
- Neck lump (>50% have metastatic lymphadenopathy at presentation)
- Hoarseness
- Progressive dysphagia
- Weight loss

Past medical history

Syndromes associated with this cancer include:

- Plummer–Vinson syndrome
- Fanconi's anaemia (a rare genetic disease causing bone marrow failure and predisposes to head and neck cancer)
- Previous neck irradiation

The patients co-morbidity status at the time of diagnosis has been shown to be a major determining factor in the selection of any likely treatment [18].

Examination

- Neck examination will reveal any cervical lymphadenopathy. Absence of laryngeal crepitus suggests invasion of the prevertebral fascia (Muir's crackle/Bocca's sign).

Table 10.9 UICC (8th edition 2017) T classification for hypopharyngeal carcinoma.

TX	Primary tumour cannot be assessed
T0	No evidence of primary tumour
Tis	Carcinoma in situ
T1	Tumour limited to one subsite of the hypopharynx and ≤2 cm in greatest dimension
T2	Tumour invades more than one subsite of the hypopharynx or an adjacent site or >2 cm but ≤4 cm in greatest dimension without fixation of hemilarynx
T3	Tumour >4 cm in greatest dimension or there is fixation of hemilarynx
T4a	Tumour invades thyroid/cricoid cartilage, hyoid bone, thyroid gland, oesophagus or central compartment soft tissue (including prelaryngeal strap muscles and subcutaneous fat)
T4b	Tumour invades prevertebral fascia, encases carotid artery or involves mediastinal structures

- Flexible nasendoscopy will identify the majority of tumours (phonation or Valsalva can open the piriform fossae for better visualisation). Vocal cord fixation is vital to staging the primary tumour (see **Table 10.9**).

Investigation

- Fine needle aspiration cytology should be undertaken. It has a sensitivity and specificity of at least 90% in diagnosing cervical metastases.
- Blood tests: Full blood count (FBC), urea and electrolytes (U&E), liver function test (LFT) (anaemia, malnutrition and deranged electrolytes are common).
- Rigid panendoscopy under general anaesthetic allows full assessment of the extent of the tumour. It may reveal tumours at the piriform apex not seen on FNE or in the post-cricoid. It is required to obtain a histological diagnosis and exclude a second primary tumour in the upper aerodigestive tract.
- Imaging: Ideally prior to biopsy, a CT and/or MRI neck (preference varies according to the local multidisciplinary team) is required to complete local and regional staging. A CT chest excludes distant metastases. The routine use of PET-CT should be considered for patients who are likely to be suitable for primary surgical treatment, or cases who have been treated non-surgically with curative intent and are being considered suitable for salvage surgical management.

- Staging combines radiological, endoscopic and clinical findings according to the Union for International Cancer Control (UICC) tumour, node, metastasis (TNM) classification (see **Table 10.10**). This is used most widely to stage primary tumour disease. An alternative staging system based on gross tumour volume and metabolic tumour volume is reported to be more predictive of patient clinical outcome, and may be better so for patients selected for non-surgical management [19,20].

Table 10.10 Stage groupings (UICC 8th edition 2017) combining the radiological, endoscopic and clinical findings after confirming the tumour to be a squamous cell carcinoma, early disease (stage I/II) and advanced disease (stage III/IV).

Stage	T	N	M
Stage 0	Tis	N0	M0
Stage I	T1	N0	M0
Stage II	T2	N0	M0
Stage III	T3 T1, T2, T3	N0 N1	M0
Stage IVA	T1, T2, T3 T4a	N2 N0, N1, N2	M0
Stage IVB	T4b Any T	Any N N3	M0
Stage IVC	Any T	Any N	M1

Management

- Treatment decisions are made with the patient after discussion at the multidisciplinary team meeting [21,22].
- The largest studies of outcomes of treatment of hypopharyngeal carcinoma show no survival advantage for primary radiotherapy or surgery with or without adjuvant radiotherapy, but these are by no means definitive. Only one randomised controlled trial comparing surgery vs. non-surgical management of hypopharyngeal cancer has been reported in the later 1990's but has attracted much criticism [23].

Early disease

Surgical options include endoscopic laser/ robotic excision or open partial laryngopharyngectomy with or without reconstruction with unilateral or bilateral selective neck dissection levels II–V.

Non-surgical treatments comprise radiotherapy (intensity-modulated radiotherapy where available). An example regime is 70-Gy in 35 daily fractions to the primary tumour and involved lymph nodes whilst 50-Gy in 25 daily fractions is delivered to at risk nodal sites.

Advanced disease

Transoral (laser or robotic) surgery have been reported.

Open surgery involves partial or total laryngopharyngectomy with flap reconstruction, bilateral neck dissection and adjuvant radiotherapy.

Recommended surgical margins are 1.5 cm superiorly, 3 cm inferiorly and 2 cm laterally [22]. Obtaining this is often challenging due to the rates of submucosal extension and anatomical limitations (e.g. adjacent common carotid artery).

Reconstruction in laryngopharyngectomy refers mainly to free tissue transfer [24]. Most popular options include:

Myocutaneous

a The radial forearm flap: Appropriate for partial laryngopharyngectomy.

b. The tubed anterolateral thigh flap: This is a perforator flap with low donor site morbidity and withstands postoperative radiotherapy.

Viscus

a The jejunal flap: More prone to radiotherapy-induced strictures and can produce problematic natural secretions. It also involves opening a second body cavity.

b The gastro-omental flap: Similar disadvantages but omentum does appear to possess anti-inflammatory and pro-healing properties useful in salvage surgery.

Non-surgical treatment comprises primary concomitant chemoradiotherapy. This usually takes the form of cisplatin (carboplatin in those with reduced creatinine clearance) given as 100 mg/m^2 every three weeks or weekly doses of 30–40 mg/m^2. This offers an absolute survival benefit of $\sim$6.5% over radiotherapy alone [25]. Patients with a performance status (or age >70 years) do not benefit from chemotherapy.

Radiotherapy is offered as mentioned earlier, though adjuvant radiotherapy is a total of 66 Gy.

Targeted therapies (e.g. cetuximab) are indicated for those in whom platinum-based treatments are contraindicated. Neoadjuvant chemotherapy currently remains unproven for routine patient treatment for hypopharyngeal cancer.

Much of the treatment, currently non-surgical, used to treat hypopharyngeal cancer was derived from experience with laryngeal cancer in the 1990s, using randomised controlled trials, which selected patients on strict criteria, in an optimum treatment environment not seen by most clinicians in daily practise. While many larynges have been preserved by the use of combination chemoradiotherapy regimens (CRT), increasing concerns arise about late toxicity and poor survival, which might be (partially) attributed to inappropriate patient section [25]. It has recently been admitted that extrapolation of data from CRT trials on larynx cancer may not be appropriate to hypopharyngeal cancer and that there is a paucity of data from adequately powered trials to inform management recommendations [26,27].

Outcomes and recurrence

Early disease – >60% 5-year survival

Advanced disease – <30% 5-year survival

Less than 15% present early. Up to 60% of patients develop loco-regional recurrence in the first year following treatment. Prognostic factors are listed in **Box 10.1**.

Persistence (diagnosed <3 months) or recurrent (diagnosed >3 months) cancer is a major problem in patients with hypopharyngeal cancer following treatment. Appropriate selection of suitable patients for treatment would seem the key to reducing such events. Recurrence in cases of incomplete excision or positive margins is most likely to occur even if treated by postoperative radiotherapy. In patients initially treated by CRT for 'cure' – currently there is only criteria for likely surgical treatment cure – so patients who recur following CRT should have been suitable for the liklehood of a surgical cure before embarking on salvage surgery.

Palliation

Palliative treatment can be offered to those unfit for curative treatment, or those with metastatic or recurrent disease [28]. Options include a tracheostomy or insertion of gastrostomy to relieve obstruction and aid nutrition. Palliative radiotherapy can be offered to relieve bleeding or pain, and in some suitable and selected patients targeted therapy such as cetuximab or immunotherapy can be offered.

Table 10.11 Complication of hypopharyngeal cancer surgery.

Laryngopharyngectomy	Neck dissection
Flap failure Pharyngeal fistula Wound infection Neopharyngeal stenosis	Bleeding CN XI, X, VII and XII injury Chyle leak

Note: If the patient has had previous radiotherapy, they are at a higher risk of all complications.

Complications of surgery

See **Table 10.11**.

Flap failure or salivary fistula formation can be initially managed conservatively with antibiotics and antimuscarinics to reduce salivary flow. Return to theatre may be required for washout, debridement and further flap reconstruction to reduce the risk of carotid blowout.

Follow-up

The role and frequency of follow-up of all patients treated for head and neck cancer, and more so patients with hypopharyngeal cancer, remains an area of controversy and variability. The most common time interval for the manifestation of loco-regional recurrence is within the first 2 years. Most cancer patients are followed up for at least 5 years, with the frequency of follow-up reducing as time goes on. The risk of a metachronus cancer in patients treated should also be

---

Box 10.1 Negative prognostic factors in hypopharyngeal carcinoma

Clinical	Histopathological
Increasing age Decreasing Karnofsky status Increased tumour or nodal stage Increased tumour or nodal mass on scan Multiple nodal metastases Low neck disease	Extracapsular nodal spread Poorly differentiated carcinoma Perineural/intravascular/lymphatic invasion

screened for possible lung and oesophageal cancer for the remainder of the patients life.

Key questions to ask regard:

- Swallowing
- Voice
- Weight loss

A change in these may indicate a stricture requiring endoscopic dilatation and exclusion of recurrent disease.

Neck pain/otalgia is highly suspicious for recurrent disease and MRI should be performed along with direct visualisation where possible. PET-CT should be considered in cases with persistent symptoms.

Chest symptoms or joint/back pain can indicate metastatic disease and should be investigated with cross-sectional imaging (CT) sooner rather than later.

Examination should include:

- Oral cavity – to exclude a local recurrence or second primary tumour
- FNE
- Neck
- Nutritional status

Top tip: most episodes of recurrence are highlighted to the clinician by the patient so make sure you listen!

TRAUMA

Isolated hypopharyngeal trauma is relatively uncommon and is most often part of neck/laryngeal trauma. Iatrogenic trauma during tracheal intubation (anaesthetic) or during examination of the pharynx or oesophagus (diagnostic or therapeutic) being the most common cause (**Figure 10.3**). Trauma can be described as follows: abrasion (mucosal and intermediate layer), haematoma (mucosal and intermediate layer), laceration (involving the mucosal and intermediate layer), and penetration (involving all 4 layers – associated with surgical emphysema).

Blunt trauma represents a risk to the airway due to subsequent oedema and/or haematoma. Symptoms include sore throat, odynophagia, dysphagia, haemoptysis, altered voice, noisy breathing and a globus sensation.

Penetrating trauma (including iatrogenic perforation) presents a risk of cervical sepsis and mediastinitis. Any history of chest or inter-scapular pain is a red flag symptom.

▌ History

Patients often present with trauma to the head and neck. If unconscious, a low index of suspicion is paramount.

▌ Examination

Stridor should alert you to impending airway disaster!

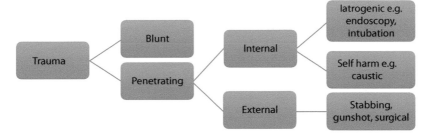

Figure 10.3 An algorithm illustrating a simple classification of laryngopharyngeal trauma.

Examine the patient being mindful of the high risk of associated cervical spine injury (i.e. after immobilisation if necessary).

Signs include laryngeal tenderness, ecchymosis and deviation of the larynx.

An otherwise unexplained pyrexia or resting tachycardia is concerning for a perforation and the presence of surgical emphysema in the neck should be considered pathognomonic.

FNE should be performed in a place of safety (i.e. in the case of a stridulous patient, in theatre with appropriate anaesthetic and surgical staff and support present).

▌ Investigation

A contrast swallow will confirm the presence of perforation.

Suspected spinal injuries need to be assessed with a CT of the neck. Penetrating neck injuries often require CT angiography as well to assess any vascular injury.

Endoscopy is advocated by some as having a higher sensitivity than contrast swallow for identifying hypopharyngeal perforation.

▌ Management

These patients often require a team approach including neurosurgeons, trauma surgeons, anaesthetists speech and language therapists and dieticians. Call for help early!

The airway must be secured and the cervical spine immobilised as a priority.

We will briefly discuss the management of these injuries in isolation.

Blunt trauma

When there is only minor laryngeal injury these can often be managed conservatively with:

- Steroids
- Humidification
- Anti-reflux treatment
- Voice rest

Formal swallowing assessment is required with nasogastric feeding if there is aspiration present. When airway compromise is more severe, the airway must be secured and nutrition established (via nasogastric tube if necessary). Tracheotomy is often required. Occasionally, massive haematomas may require surgical exploration and drainage.

Penetrating trauma

Where identified these need to be managed with a minimum of:

- Nasogastric feeding
- Anti-reflux treatment
- Antibiotics

Exploration and drainage of any collection is mandated in those failing to improve with primary repair being advocated by some. Often the haemodynamic stability, co-existing injuries and plan for their management influence treatment decisions accordingly.

Iatrogenic hypopharyngeal perforation

Iatrogenic hypopharyngeal perforations whilst rare are most frequently associated with a clinical manoeuvre – diagnostic or therapeutic (e.g. nasogastric tube placement, endotracheal intubation, or endoscopy [rigid or flexible]) [29].

Patients with neoplasms, diverticula or stenosis may be more difficult, and the use of dilatators/bougies is likely to increase the possibility of mucosal abrasions, tears and/or perforations. A perforation or tear must be suspected if the procedure which has been undertaken has resulted in bleeding in the hypopharynx.

History

Symptoms or signs may develop between 1.5 hours and 38 hours following procedure. Pain is the most common presenting complaint, and can occur anywhere in the neck, chest or epigastrium. Other symptoms include vomiting, haematemesis, dysphagia and breathlessness [29,30].

Examination

The most common signs are tachycardia, fever, subcutaneous emphysema and tachypnoea.

Investigation

Detection of a possible perforation should be made as early as possible, and once suspected a chest or neck radiograph may show surgical emphysema or free air in the mediastinum, the diagnosis will be confirmed by a contrast swallow study. High-risk patients are cases with a difficult or traumatic procedure, poor visibility, bleeding, mucosal tare, foreign body or food bolus.

Management

A conservative approach may be commenced with NPO (nil per oral intake) and intravenous antibiotics with close nursing monitoring of patients' vital signs. It has been suggested that patients who have eaten between time of perforation and diagnosis, have been 24 hours or more between injury or endsocopy and diagnosis or show signs of systemic toxicity are at higher risk of failing conservative management and a surgical consultation should be urgently sought to consider drainage.

REFERENCES

1 Frenz D, Smith RV. Surgical anatomy of the pharynx and esophagus. In: H. Vdwtras, ed. *Otolaryngology: Basic Science and Clinical Review*. Thieme Medical Publishers Inc; 2006.

2 Kendall KA, Leonard RJ, McKenzie SW. Sequence variability during hypopharyngeal bolus transit. *Dysphagia*. 2003;18(2):85–91.

3 Hendrix TR. Art and science of history taking in the patient with difficulty swallowing. *Dysphagia*. 1993;8(2):69–73.

4 Manabe N, Tsutsui H, Kusunoki H, Hata J, Haruma K. Pathophysiology and treatment of patients with globus sensation – From the viewpoint of esophageal motility dysfunction. *J Smooth Muscle Res*. 2014;50:66–77.

5 Bradley PJ, Narula A. Clinical aspects of pseudo-dysphagia. *J Laryngol Otol*. 1987;101(7):689–94.

6 Patel R. Assessment of swallowing disorders. In: G. Mankekar, ed. *Swallowing – Physiology, Disorders, Diagnosis and Therapy*. Springer; 2015.

7 Bastian RW. Videoendoscopic evaluation of patients with dysphagia: An adjunct to the modified barium swallow. *Otolaryngol Head Neck Surg*. 1991;104(3):339–50.

8 Abou-Nader L, Wilson JA, Paleri V. Transnasal oesophagoscopy: Diagnostic and management outcomes in a prospective cohort of 257 consecutive cases and practice implications. *Clin Otolaryngol*. 2014;39(2):108–13.

9 Goel A, Bakshi SS, Soni N, Chhavi N. Iron deficiency anemia and Plummer-Vinson syndrome: Current insights. *J Blood Med*. 2017;8:175–84.

10 Grant PD, Morgan DE, Scholz FJ, Canon CL. Pharyngeal dysphagia: What the radiologist needs to know. *Curr Probl Diagn Radiol*. 2009;38(1):17–32.

11 Lee BE, Kim GH. Globus pharyngeus: A review of its etiology, diagnosis and treatment. *World J Gastroenterol*. 2012;18(20):2462–71.

12 Karkos PD, Wilson JA. The diagnosis and management of globus pharyngeus: Our perspective from the United Kingdom. *Curr Opin Otolaryngol Head Neck Surg*. 2008;16(6):521–4.

13 Kocdor P, Siegel ER, Tulunay-Ugur OE. Cricopharyngeal dysfunction: A systematic review comparing outcomes of dilatation, botulinum toxin injection, and myotomy. *Laryngoscope*. 2016;126(1):135–41.

14 Little RE, Bock JM. Pharyngoesophageal diverticuli: Diagnosis, incidence and management. *Curr Opin Otolaryngol Head Neck Surg*. 2016;24(6):500–4.

15 Law R, Katzka DA, Baron TH. Zenker's diverticulum. *Clin Gastroenterol Hepatol*. 2014;12(11):1773–82; quiz e111–2.

16 Khan AS, Dwivedi RC, Sheikh Z et al. Systematic review of carcinoma arising in pharyngeal

diverticula: A 112-year analysis. *Head Neck.* 2014;36(9):1368–75.

17 Verdonck J, Morton RP. Systematic review on treatment of Zenker's diverticulum. *Eur Arch Otorhinolaryngol.* 2015;272(11):3095–3107.

18 Bradley PJ. Symptoms and signs, staging and co-morbidity of hypopharyngeal cancer. *Adv Otorhinolaryngol.* 2019;83:15–26.

19 Yang CJ, Kim DY, Lee JH et al. Prognostic value of total tumor volume in advanced-stage laryngeal and hypopharyngeal carcinoma. *J Surg Oncol.* 2013;108(8):509–15.

20 Roh JL, Kim JS, Kang BC et al. Clinical significance of pretreatment metabolic tumor volume and total lesion glycolysis in hypopharyngeal squamous cell carcinomas. *J Surg Oncol.* 2014;110(7):869–75.

21 Kwon DI, Miles BA, Education Committee of the American Head and Neck Society. Hypopharyngeal carcinoma: Do you know your guidelines? *Head Neck.* 2019;41(3):569–76.

22 Pracy P, Loughran S, Good J, Parmar S, Goranova R. Hypopharyngeal cancer: United Kingdom National Multidisciplinary Guidelines. *J Laryngol Otol.* 2016;130(S2):S104–10.

23 Lefebvre JL, Chevalier D, Luboinski B, Kirkpatrick A, Collette L, Sahmoud T. Larynx preservation in pyriform sinus cancer: Preliminary results of a European Organization for Research and Treatment of Cancer phase III trial. EORTC Head and Neck Cancer Cooperative Group. *J Natl Cancer Inst.* 1996;88(13):890–9.

24 Van der Putten L, Spasiano R, de Bree R, Bertino G, Leemans C Rene, Benazzo M. Flap reconstruction of the hypopharynx: A defect orientated approach. *Acta Otorhinolaryngologica Italica.* 2012;32:288–96.

25 de Bree R. The current indications for non-surgical treatment of hypopharyngeal cancer. *Adv Otorhinolaryngol.* 2019;83:76–89.

26 Siddiq S, Paleri V. Outcomes of tumour control from primary treatment of hypopharyngeal cancer. *Adv Otorhinolaryngol.* 2019;83:90–108.

27 Forastiere AA, Weber RS, Trotti A. Organ preservation for advanced larynx cancer: Issues and outcomes. *J Clin Oncol.* 2015;33(29):3262–8.

28 Bradley PJ, Fureder T, Eckel HE. Systematic therapy, palliation and supportive care of patients with hypopharyngeal cancer. *Adv Otorhinolaryngol.* 2019;83:148–58.

29 Zenga J, Kreisel D, Kushnir VM, Rich JT. Management of cervical esophageal and hypopharyngeal perforations. *Am J Otolaryngol.* 2015;36(5):678–85.

30 Daniel M, Kamani T, Nogueira C et al. Perforation after rigid pharyngo-oesophagoscopy: When do symptoms and signs develop? *J Laryngol Otol.* 2010;124(2):171–174.

11
LARYNX

James Moor and Amit Prasai

INTRODUCTION

The larynx sits at the junction of the upper and lower respiratory tracts. Its functions are:

- To protect the lower airway from penetration of ingested food and fluids
- To act as the organ of phonation

ANATOMY

The laryngeal skeleton is made up of paired and unpaired cartilages. The movements of the cartilage are hinged by intrinsic and extrinsic ligaments and muscles (see **Table 11.1**).

Special mention must be made of the posterior cricoarytenoid muscle which acts to abduct the vocal cords and is therefore essential in the maintenance of a patent airway.

The glottis, or rima glottidis, is the aperture or space bounded by the vocal cords and arytenoid cartilages, and is not an anatomical structure as such but provides a practical division of the larynx into supraglottic, glottic and subglottic areas. Clinically relevant spaces within the larynx include the paraglottic space, which is lateral to the vocal cords, and the pre-epiglottic space, which is anterior to the epiglottic cartilage. The laryngeal ventricle is a cavity bounded by the false cords superiorly and the true cords inferiorly (**Figure 11.1**) and extends superiorly a variable distance.

Histologically the vocal cords are covered with stratified squamous cell epithelium (mucosa), and submucosal glands are absent or rare. Deep to this layer lies the lamina propria with superficial, intermediate and deep layers; the superficial layer of lamina propria is referred to as Reinke's space and the intermediate and deep layers form the vocal ligament. Deep to the deep layer of lamina propria lies the vocalis muscle, which constitutes the main body of the vocal cord.

During phonation the mucosa and vocal ligament are under passive control, but the mechanical properties of the vocalis muscle are regulated both passively and actively. Elsewhere in the larynx the epiglottic mucosa is stratified squamous type similar to the oral cavity with modified salivary glands that secrete

Table 11.1 Anatomical features of the larynx.

			Function
Cartilages	Paired	Arytenoid Corniculate Cuneiform	Laryngeal skeleton
	Unpaired	Epiglottis Cricoid Thyroid	Vocal cord mobility and closure of laryngeal sphincter
Ligaments	Intrinsic	Quadrangular membrane, conus elasticus, cricothyroid membrane	Forms the vocal cord
	Extrinsic	Thyrohyoid membrane and cricothyroid ligament	
Muscles	Intrinsic		Mobility of vocal cord
	Extrinsic		Laryngeal elevation/depression

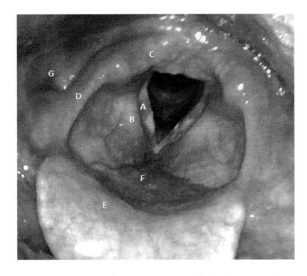

Figure 11.1 Endoscopic view of the larynx demonstrating leukoplakia affecting right vocal cord, biopsy confirmed moderate dysplasia. The discolouration affecting the left vocal cord is a contact lesion. A: vocal (true) cord; B: false cord; C: arytenoid cartilage; D: aryepiglottic fold; E: epiglottis; F: petiole of epiglottis; G: piriform fossa.

thick mucous. The rest of the supraglottic mucosa is ciliated columnar epithelium with modified salivary glands. In the subglottis the mucosa resembles that of the trachea and major bronchi.

▓ Innervation

Mucosal sensation and motor innervation of all muscles are from branches of the vagus nerve. Mucosal sensation above the level of the glottis is via the internal branch of the superior laryngeal nerve, and via the recurrent laryngeal nerve below the glottis. The cricothyroid muscle is supplied by the external branch of the superior laryngeal nerve and all other muscles by the recurrent laryngeal nerve.

▓ Vasculature

Arterial supply is from the superior and inferior laryngeal arteries, which are branches of the superior thyroid artery and thyrocervical trunk respectively. Venous drainage follows the course of these arteries and veins take the same names as their corresponding arteries.

▓ Lymphatic drainage

Lymphatic drainage from the level of the glottis is regarded as minimal, and consequently the risk of regional metastasis from small volume glottic carcinomas is small. Conversely, the supraglottic larynx has been shown to have a rich lymphatic drainage to ipsilateral and contralateral lymph nodes located in the superior deep cervical chain. Infraglottic lymphatics drain to paratracheal and inferior deep cervical chain nodes.

PHYSIOLOGY

At birth the larynx occupies an elevated position within the neck; there is direct communication from the nasopharynx to the laryngeal inlet which channels air inspired through the nose directly into the trachea and lower respiratory tract. This arrangement permits simultaneous breathing and feeding and is evident until 18–24 months of age. After that time the larynx descends and in adults sits low in the neck. This laryngeal descent causes potential compromise of the lower airway from ingested matter, from vomitus or refluxate since the laryngeal inlet (comprising epiglottis, aryepiglottic folds and arytenoid cartilages) can be regarded as a defect in the anterior pharyngeal wall.

The mechanisms in place to prevent aspiration include:

● Cessation of breathing during swallowing
● Temporary elevation of the larynx to approximate the epiglottis to the arytenoid, corniculate and cuneiform cartilages

● Opposition of the vocal cords to close off the laryngeal sphincter

Once a swallow has successfully been achieved, descent of the larynx to its resting position occurs along with lateralisation of the vocal cords and return to normal respiration.

Phonatory sounds are generated by passage of inhaled air across adducted vocal cords. Various physiological events at the level of the glottis cause the airflow to develop a wave form, the frequency of which varies among males (100–120 Hz), females (180–220 Hz) and children (250–300 Hz). The sound wave generated at the glottis is then modulated through the structures of the supraglottis, oropharynx and oral cavity, which results in resonate, articulated and amplified speech.

MALIGNANT PATHOLOGY

▉ Laryngeal squamous cell carcinoma

Aetiology

Squamous cell carcinoma (SCC) is the most common malignant tumour of the larynx; the standardised incidence in England is approximately 3.0/100,000 population with a male to female ratio of 6:1 [1]. The strongest aetiological factor is tobacco use [2]. In Asia and parts of Africa the chewing of betel nut is commonplace. It is highly carcinogenic, and head and neck cancer is far more common due to this habit. Alcohol is not definitively proven to be an individual risk factor for head and neck cancer but appears to act synergistically with smoking to raise relative risk [2, 3].

Recent years have seen a reduction in incidence followed by a plateau to current levels, which may be reflective in changes to smoking habits across the United Kingdom [4].

Laryngeal carcinoma is divided into three distinct subgroups based on the location at which the tumour arises: glottis, supraglottis or subglottis.

History

Glottic carcinoma

Glottic carcinoma (**Figure 11.2**) usually presents with hoarseness, which is constant in nature and tends to be progressive as the lesion enlarges.

Larger tumours can present with stridor, dysphagia, odynophagia and referred otalgia. This usually indicates the tumour spreading beyond the glottis well into the supraglottis and even beyond.

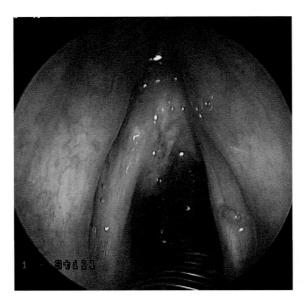

Figure 11.2 SCC affecting left anterior vocal cord crossing anterior commissure to affect anterior portion of right vocal cord. Intra-operatively the tumour was seen to have a significant sub-glottic component. Tumour stage was T1bN0M0.

Primary tumour behaviour is heterogeneous as some tumours can be seen to be relatively superficial and creep along the mucosal surfaces, invading into the laryngeal ventricle and onto the free edge of the false cord or inferiorly towards the subglottis. Others may tend to burrow deep into the submucosal structures and invade into the vocal ligament, vocalis muscle and paraglottic space.

Once the deep structures of the larynx become involved, progressive reduction in mobility and ultimately fixation of the vocal cord is seen and reflected in the T staging of the primary tumour.

Supraglottic carcinoma

Supraglottic carcinomas have less well-defined presenting symptoms.

Early tumours may be asymptomatic or present with mild dysphagia and throat discomfort.

Higher stage tumours may cause a more significant history of dysphagia and aspiration, odynophagia and pain both in the throat often unilateral, and referred otalgia.

Presentation with neck lumps due to cervical lymph node metastasis, or stridor and airway compromise are both not uncommon. Progression of disease that has arisen from either the glottis or supraglottis and then spread to other subsites can make categorisation of tumours difficult.

Subglottic carcinoma

Primary subglottic squamous cell carcinoma is very rare. The most frequent symptoms are stridor and dyspnoea due to mechanical obstruction [5].

Weight loss, change in diet to accommodate dysphagia or pain are all red flag symptoms for malignancy.

Examination

Clinical assessment begins as the patient is called into the consultation room when an overall view of their body habitus, mobility, appearance and general persona can be made. Tobacco staining may be evident on the skin of the distal phalanx of the hands or on the patients' hair, and clothing may emit aromas of tobacco smoke.

Examination of the neck is undertaken to assess for enlargement of cervical lymph nodes.

The larynx is palpated to assess for shape and form of the thyroid cartilage (large volume laryngeal tumours can splay the posterior edges of the thyroid cartilage laterally, as if a book being opened); for normal elevation of the larynx on swallowing and for normal laryngeal crepitus the larynx can be rolled side to side over the prevertebral fascia (loss of laryngeal crepitus can indicate invasion of tumour into the prevertebral space).

The oral cavity and oropharynx are inspected with good illumination and fibre-optic nasendoscopy is performed to view the larynx. Each of the subsites of the visable oropharynx (base of tongue, vallecula, lateral pharyngeal walls), supraglottis (supra- and infrahyoid epiglottis, aryepiglottic folds, arytenoid cartilages, false vocal cords) and glottis (vocal cords, anterior commissure, posterior commissure, entrance to laryngeal ventricle) and hypopharynx (piriform fossae, posterior pharyngeal walls) are systematically examined and the vocal cords are assessed for mobility. All findings are documented in the medical records, ideally with photo documentation.

Investigation

Radiological staging is required of the larynx, cervical lymph nodes, mediastinum, lungs and liver for all but T1a tumours that do not involve the anterior commissure, as these are rarely seen on cross-sectional imaging. Modern 64 slice multi-planar CT can acquire images of the larynx in under one second and so negates the influence of movement of the larynx and soft tissues of the neck from respiration, phonation and carotid pulsation when compared to the longer scan acquisition times required for MRI. Cartilage involvement is better assessed using MRI, but routine practice in the UK currently relies upon CT scanning for assessment of both the primary laryngeal tumour and the lung fields.

A panendoscopy and biopsy under general anaesthetic is mandated. This allows full examination of areas of the upper aerodigestive tract (UADT) that are unable to be assessed in the outpatient clinic (post-cricoid area, proximal oesophagus and trachea) to ensure there is no synchronous primary tumour. The risk of a second synchronous head and neck cancer is estimated to be 5%–10% [6,7]. Microlaryngoscopy is then performed with the laryngoscope in suspension and assessment of the distribution of the tumour made using 0°, 30° and 70° rigid endoscopes. An appropriate photographic record is made, and biopsies taken for histological diagnosis.

Clinical staging is performed prior to management (see **Table 11.2**).

Management

All relevant data is considered in discussion of the management of the patient at the multidisciplinary team (MDT) meeting or equivalent.

As with all diseases, when considering treatment options the following must be taken into account:

- Patient factors (e.g. patient choice, comorbidities, performance status)

- Tumour factors (e.g. stage, accessibility)
- Clinician/MDT factors (e.g. surgical/oncology expertise, equipment availability, local MDT protocols)

Always consider treatment of the primary tumour and potentially involved cervical lymph nodes.

T1–T2a glottic carcinoma (T1a/b/2a N0 M0)

Primary tumour

Primary tumours can be treated with either transoral laser microsurgery (TLM) or radiotherapy (RT) with either treatment option yielding similar rates of local control (T1a 90%–93%, T1b 85%–89%). T2a tumours also have similar response rates to both TLM and RT.

Some may argue that tumours involving the anterior commissure area should be recommended for RT, as resection of the anterior commissure may cause webbing (scarring) and significant dysphonia. However, TLM may appeal to some patients, as it can usually be offered as a day-case procedure and provides a quicker, simpler journey for the patient with a lower risk of aspiration and can even be repeated if a metachronous tumour appears in the future.

RT is given as an outpatient procedure and schedules vary from 50–52 grey (Gy) in 16 fractions to 53–55 Gy in 20 fractions over 3–4 weeks.

Neck

Due to the paucity of lymphatic tissue in the vocal cords it is rare to see lymph node metastasis in these tumours and elective treatment of the neck is not necessary by surgery or RT (therefore RT fields should be restricted to the larynx).

T2b–T3 carcinoma of the glottis (T2b/3 N0/+ M0)

Primary tumour

Tumours of this stage can be offered surgery (TLM or partial laryngeal surgery) or primary non-surgical treatment (RT with or without chemotherapy) [8,9]. The surgical options for this require technical

Table 11.2 TNM 8 staging for laryngeal carcinoma primary tumours.

Subsite	T stage	Definition
Supraglottis	1	Tumour limited to one subsite
	2	Tumour extends to greater than one adjacent subsite of supraglottis, or to the glottis, or to an adjacent site outside the supraglottis, without fixation of the vocal cord
	3	Tumour limited to the larynx with fixation of the vocal cord, and/or invades any of the following: post-cricoid, pre-epiglottic tissues, paraglottic space and/or with minor thyroid cartilage erosion (inner cortex)
	4a	Tumour invades through thyroid cartilage and/or invades soft tissues beyond the larynx (e.g. trachea, soft tissues of neck, deep muscles of tongue, strap muscles, thyroid, oesophagus)
	4b	Tumour invades prevertebral space, mediastinum or encases carotid artery
Glottis	1a	Tumour limited to one vocal cord, normal vocal cord mobility
	1b	Tumour involves both vocal cords, normal vocal cord mobility
	2a	Tumour invades into supraglottis and/or subglottis with normal vocal cord mobility
	2b	Tumour invades into supraglottis and/or subglottis with impaired vocal cord mobility
	3	Tumour limited to larynx with vocal cord fixation, and/or extension to paraglottic space, and/or with minor thyroid cartilage erosion
	4a	Tumour invades thyroid cartilage or invades tissues beyond the larynx (e.g. trachea, soft tissues of neck, strap muscles, thyroid, oesophagus)
	4b	Tumour invades prevertebral space, mediastinum or encases carotid artery
Subglottis	1	Tumour limited to the subglottis
	2	Tumour extends to the vocal cord(s) with normal or impaired vocal cord mobility
	3	Tumour limited to larynx with vocal cord fixation
	4a	Tumour invades through cricoid or thyroid cartilage and/or invades tissue beyond the larynx (e.g. trachea, soft tissues of neck, deep muscles of tongue, strap muscles, thyroid, oesophagus)
	4b	Tumour invades prevertebral space, mediastinum or encases carotid artery

expertise and experienced speech and swallowing therapy input.

Neck

In patients without evidence of lymph node metastasis, bilateral elective treatment of levels II, III and IV is recommended, be that with RT or surgery with postoperative RT. Where nodal involvement is evident at time of diagnosis, ipsilateral treatment of nodes in levels II–V is recommended [10].

T1–2 supraglottic carcinoma (T1–2 N0/N+ M0)

Primary tumour

RT, TLM or transoral robotic surgery (TORS) are all suitable treatment options for patients with these tumours.

Neck

The supraglottic larynx has much greater lymphatic supply than the glottis, and consequently elective treatment of the neck level II-IV bilaterally is recommended, either surgically or with RT. In the node-positive neck, ipsilateral II–V treatment is recommended.

T3 supraglottic carcinoma (T3 N0/+ M0)

Primary tumour

Most tumours will be suitable for non-surgical treatment offering an organ preservation strategy (RT with or without chemotherapy), but selected cases may be suitable for TLM, TORS or open partial laryngeal surgery where appropriate expertise exists.

Neck

Elective treatment of the neck to levels II, III and IV is recommended in patients staged N0, and ipsilateral treatment to levels II–V for patients with N+ disease.

T4 glottic and supraglottic carcinoma (T4a/b N0/+ M0)

Primary tumour

Laryngeal tumours with anything more than minor erosion of the thyroid cartilage (i.e. beyond the inner cortex of the cartilage) should be managed with total laryngectomy [8–10]. Total laryngectomy as a radical treatment (as compared to total laryngectomy in the context of palliation, a rare indication) should only be considered when the surgical team is confident that excision with clear surgical margins can be achieved.

Neck

In the N0 neck, elective treatment to levels II–IV is recommended, whilst in the node-positive neck, ipsilateral II–V.

Treatment decision making and organ preservation strategies

For each of the aforementioned tumour stages more than one treatment option may represent appropriate treatment; however, not all options are always suitable to be offered. Part of the process of managing and treating patients with laryngeal cancer is to be able to recognise which patients genuinely have a choice of treatments and which do not. This is not an easy or quick skill to learn, and a significant part of the process involves effective communication of the potentially life changing, and mutilating, treatments in the search of oncological cure. This should never be the remit of one individual; instead it is important that appropriate team members have the time and skill set to lead patients through the process.

Organ preservation refers to the retention of the larynx with an oncological cure in advanced laryngeal cancer, and was established by the Veterans Affairs (VA) study that demonstrated that induction chemotherapy and RT produced equivalent overall survival when compared to total laryngectomy and RT, but also demonstrated a laryngeal preservation rate of 64% at 2 years [8]. The Radiation Therapy Oncology Group (RTOG) 91-11 trial found concurrent chemoradiotherapy was superior to radiotherapy alone or induction chemotherapy [9].

It may be intuitive to assume that a patient with a cure from laryngeal cancer and who has retained their larynx in situ has a better quality of life compared to a patient who has a cure but gone through a laryngectomy to achieve that cure. However, laryngeal dysfunction following chemoradiotherapy is unpredictable at best, and up to 10% of patients following treatment require laryngectomy for intractable aspiration despite being disease-free [11,12]. An unknown number of further patients are unfit for surgery.

It is also important to remember that the aforementioned trials relied upon low volume disease with minimal cartilage invasion to make up their locally advanced tumours. This is a key reason why surgery is still the recommended treatment of choice for T4 tumours.

Partial laryngectomy procedures for advanced laryngeal cancer will also cause laryngeal dysfunction, and patients who require adjuvant post-op RT are likely to demonstrate worse functional outcomes than those where post-op RT is not required – case selection is paramount. It is worth bearing in mind that swallowing rehabilitation after partial laryngeal surgery may be prolonged, especially in the setting of salvage surgery following previous RT or chemo RT. Treatment decision-making in the context of advanced laryngeal carcinoma represents a significant challenge for patients and healthcare professionals alike.

Transoral laser microsurgery

The CO_2 laser has the necessary properties for undertaking resection of laryngeal tumours:

- Wavelength: 10,600 nm (easily absorbed by water in the tissues)
- Minimal surrounding tissue damage
- Narrow focus (precision cutting)
- Ability to be delivered down a narrow view (e.g. laryngoscope)

It is limited to use in patients without adequate access to their tumours; prominent upper incisors, retrognathia and a posteriorly placed larynx can all contribute to compromise the endoscopic view therefore making resections difficult or incomplete.

Steiner popularised the technique wherein typically the tumour is transected across its midpoint, relying on the surgeon's ability to observe the difference of the interaction of the laser with disorganised tumour tissue and organised non-tumour tissue [13]. Once the laser has transected through the tumour to reveal normal unaffected tissue at the deep margin, the surgeon completes the resection at that depth and the tumour is excised in anterior and posterior halves. The tumour is orientated and marked for the histopathologist before being formalin fixed. Tumours excised in this method will rarely have margins of normal tissue that approach adequacy, and therefore either intraoperative frozen section specimens or biopsy specimens from the residual larynx are used to confirm completeness of excision, but importantly this data is considered in the context of the operating surgeon's description of the case – neither should be considered independently.

Open partial laryngectomy

There are various procedures that fall under the broad heading of partial laryngectomy, and obviously the extent of the tumour determines which procedure is appropriate. The aim of any partial laryngectomy is oncological cure with preservation of respiration via the upper airway, maintenance of oral nutrition without long-term tube feeding and voice rehabilitation. Therefore it is essential to consider what structures are intended to be left behind that will facilitate these aims; at least one functional (i.e. innervated) crico-arytenoid unit must be preserved. Equally as important as surgical expertise is case selection, patients need to be highly motivated to rehabilitate from the surgery, which they will only be able to do with the input and close supervision of dedicated speech and language therapists with an interest in swallowing rehabilitation.

Follow-up

Patients require more frequent follow-up in the first 2 years, as this is the time where most recurrences occur. Traditionally they are reviewed for 5 years before being regarded as cured.

Complications of surgery

TLM has relatively low rates of complications. These include damage to the teeth or gums, dysphonia, a rare risk of airway fire (and subsequent tracheostomy) and the need for further surgery dependent on margins. Larger tumours, especially supraglottic tumours, may affect swallowing function.

Open surgery carries the general risk of infection, bleeding and those relating to anaesthetic. The main concern for these patients is pharyngocutaneous fistula (a salivary leak from the pharyngeal anastomosis). This is usually conservatively managed initially and if it does not resolve may require surgery with a pectoralis major flap (PMF) used to close the fistula. In salvage open laryngeal surgery, a PMF is often performed prophylactically due to the higher risk of pharyngocutaneous fistula in these patients [14].

Neck dissection carries additional specific risks to the internal jugular vein, accessory nerve, hypoglossal nerve, marginal mandibular nerve, vagus nerve and thoracic duct (leading to chyle leak).

PREMALIGNANT PATHOLOGY

■ Laryngeal dysplasia

Aetiology

Dysplasia is characterised by presence of architectural and cytological atypia within the surface epithelium above the level of the epithelial basement membrane. It is regarded as a premalignant condition. This means that the affected tissue has been subject to chronic local irritation (or may be a local manifestation of a systemic disease) and is at an increased risk of cancerous transformation [15,16].

The risk factors for developing this are not as clearly defined as in head and neck cancer, but are thought to include tobacco use, alcohol, vocal abuse and perhaps laryngopharyngeal reflux [15].

History

Dysphonia is the most common presenting symptom. Risk factors as described earlier need to be elucidated. Any history of immune-modulating medications may also be significant.

Examination

Fibre-optic nasendoscopy (FNE) is required to assess the larynx. This often reveals the presence of areas of leukoplakia (Figure 11.1) or erythroplakia (defined as white or red patches of mucosa that can not be removed by wiping) within the larynx. Biopsy for histological analysis for diagnostic purposes is always needed.

Investigation

Biopsy is needed to acquire histological diagnosis. This is generally required to be performed under general anaesthetic. Imaging is not required.

Management

There are different grading systems in use for categorisation, management and prognostication

Table 11.3 Classification systems used for staging or grading dysplasia.

Classification	Stages	Definition
Ljubljana	Simple hyper-plasia	Benign
	Abnormal hyperplasia	Benign
	Atypical hyper-plasia	Potentially malignant
	Carcinoma in situ	Malignant
WHO	Squamous cell hyperplasia	Benign
	Mild dysplasia	Benign
	Moderate dysplasia	Potentially malignant
	Severe dysplasia	Potentially malignant
	Carcinoma in situ	Malignant

Source: Hellquist H et al. *Histopathology*. 1999;34:226–33; Barnes L et al. *Pathology and Genetics: Head and Neck Tumors*. IARC Press; 2005, p. 177–80.

purposes, with the Ljubljana and World Health Organization (WHO) systems most commonly used in clinical practice (see **Table 11.3**).

Patients diagnosed with laryngeal dysplasia should be managed by clinicians routinely involved with managing patients with head and neck cancer or by designated laryngologists.

Progression of any dysplastic lesion to invasive carcinoma is estimated to occur in 8%–16% of patients [19,20]. This risk is higher in those with severe dysplasia (up to 30%) compared to mild dysplasia [4,21].

Lifestyle changes in terms of stopping smoking must be encouraged. The role of laryngopharyngeal reflux is unclear, but there is some limited evidence that the incidence of reflux is high in patients with premalignant disease [22].

Isolated lesions can be treated in an equivalent manner to T1a SCC, e.g. with transoral laser excision.

In patients where there is demonstrable evidence of widespread field change across the larynx amounting to severe dysplasia or carcinoma in situ, some centres may offer RT treatment in selected patients [23].

BENIGN PATHOLOGY

▐ Reinke's oedema

Aetiology

Accumulation of oedema within the superficial layer of lamina propria can cause florid vocal cord swelling. It is more commonly seen in women and smokers. Voice abuse and reflux have been implicated.

History

Hoarseness is typically constant and of particular distress to women, as it tends to result in a deeper voice.

Less commonly, stridor can present in severe oedema.

Examination

FNE generally reveals bilateral vocal cord swelling **(Figure 11.3)**, though unilateral swelling may be seen occasionally.

Investigation

No imaging is required. If there is any concern over dysplasia (this is uncommon in Reinke's oedema) or malignancy, a biopsy is essential.

Management

Conservative measures include smoking cessation, anti-reflux medication, and speech and language therapy.

Surgery is indicated in those refractory cases. Usually the redundant mucosa can be resected via an

Follow-up

These patients require long-term follow-up akin to patients who have been treated for laryngeal cancer to observe any potential transformation. Patients should be educated as to the symptoms of malignancy (see earlier) so as to encourage early presentation of any tumour.

endoscopic lateral cordotomy approach. Improvement of voice is unlikely without cessation of exposure to tobacco smoke, despite speech therapy input.

▐ Vocal cord polyps

Aetiology

The aetiology of polyps arising from the vocal cords is not well understood. They tend to occur at the free edge of the vocal cords. The incidence is low in the general population (<1.0/100000) and there are a variety of clinical factors that may be contributory such as voice abuse, reflux, smoking and alcohol

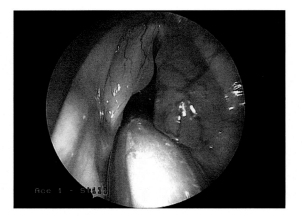

Figure 11.3 Intra-operative photo of the larynx showing typical appearance of Reinke's oedema of the vocal cords in a 54 year old female smoker. The changes are more marked on the left vocal cord, treatment comprised incision of the mucosa, aspiration of the oedematous fluid, redraping of the mucosa over the vocal cord and excision of excess 'redundant' mucosa.

exposure, but these are very variable. Mucous secreting glands are rarely seen at the glottis, and histological findings tend to show epithelial hyperplasia, oedema, vessel proliferation and hyperkeratosis.

History

The hoarseness is often preceded by an acute episode of vocal trauma (shouting, singing, etc.), though it can also occur as a result of chronic irritation.

Examination

Vocal fold polyps (**Figure 11.4**) can be either sessile or pedunculated, or unilateral or bilateral. Vocal quality often correlates with the size and location of the polyp(s) [24].

Investigation

No imaging is required.

Management

Surgery to excise the polyp, either with cold steel microdissection or transoral laser resection, is required to improve the dysphonia, alongside

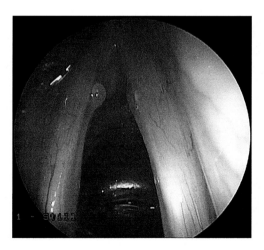

Figure 11.4 Intra-operative photo showing small sub-epithelial polyp affecting left vocal anterior vocal cord causing dysphonia in a male teacher. Note the contact lesion at the equivalent site on the right vocal cord.

attention to the aforementioned clinical factors that may be considered contributory. Voice therapy to prevent any triggers may be of use and can be commenced preoperatively and continued afterwards.

▇ Vocal cord nodules

Aetiology

Nodules of the vocal cords are benign mucosal lesions that typically occur bilaterally at the midpoint of the membranous vocal cord (the posterior third of the vocal cord is the vocal process of the arytenoid cartilage). This site represents the maximal amplitude of the mucosal wave and is therefore subject to maximal phono-traumatic force [25]. Disproportionately high mechanical shear on the free edge of the vocal cord damages the superficial layer of the lamina propria and results in micro-vascular changes and subsequent epithelial hyperplasia and hyalinisation. This results in the well-circumscribed nodules [26].

They occur in patients with a history of excessive voice use, be that as a child (screamer's nodules), a singer (singer's nodules), teacher, lawyer, broadcaster, call-centre worker or any other profession regarded as a 'high-end voice user'.

History

Hoarseness, which is worse after voice use, never remits completely. A social and occupational history is essential to elucidate the voice misuse factors. Patients may also complain of lack of projection and/or strength in voice.

Examination

FNE allows diagnosis of most cases, though stroboscopy provides a clearer view that can allow subtle lesions, and their impact on the mucosal wave of the vocal cord during phonation to be identified.

Investigation

No imaging is required.

Biopsy is not required as the diagnosis is clinical.

Management

Assessment and input from specialist speech and language therapists is required to address the patient's vocal habits, which are usually sufficient to initiate and sustain improvement in vocal performance with surgery to excise the nodules only rarely considered in refractory cases.

■ Laryngeal granulomas

Aetiology

Laryngeal granulomas are benign, chronic, inflammatory lesions arising in the posterior cartilaginous third of the vocal fold (the vocal process) [27]. These lesions are usually thought to arise as a result of trauma or irritation of the posterior glottis. This includes reflux of gastric contents into the laryngopharynx; trauma from endotracheal intubation is also considered an aetiological factor. Chronic coughing or throat clearing has also been implicated.

History

These can present with hoarseness, pain, cough or a globus-type sensation. Symptoms of reflux may be present, and a history of recent intubation is important to elicit.

Examination

FNE is essential. Laryngeal granulomas can vary in appearance, and so complete a UADT examination as well as a neck examination because the differential examination includes malignancy.

Laryngeal granulomas are unilateral, pale swelling often with overlying ulceration.

Investigation

A biopsy is often required due to the variable appearance to exclude cancer.

Management

Where the diagnosis is suspected but biopsy has been undertaken, intra-granuloma injection of steroid can be administered. Where the diagnosis is confidently made, a conservative approach can be taken using voice therapy, anti-reflux medication and possibly the use of inhaled steroids. Surgery is usually reserved for refractory cases or when debulking is required, either with cold steel or CO_2 laser [28].

■ Laryngeal papillomatosis

Aetiology

More common in the paediatric population than adults, laryngeal papillomatosis is frequently due to exposure to human papillomavirus (HPV) types 11 and 6. In paediatric patients, this exposure may occur during passage through the birth canal, as both HPV subtypes are known to be associated with genital warts.

It has a bimodal incidence with peaks in children (3–4 years) and a second peak in adults (3rd–4th decade). It affects approximately 2 per 100,000 [29].

History

Progressive dysphonia is typical. Left untreated, stridor can develop. Paediatric laryngeal papillomatosis can cause florid lesions to develop and can prove to be fatal due to airway obstruction if not managed expediently.

Examination

FNE should reveal the diagnosis as the macroscopic appearance is easy to recognise (**Figure 11.5**).

Investigation

Imaging is not routinely required. However, monitoring and recording of disease site and status is recommended using photography, especially to assess disease activity over time.

Management

Malignant transformation is rare and has been associated with HPV type 11. The mainstay of treatment is endoscopic excision. This can be performed with a microdebrider or CO_2 laser to maintain a patent airway and minimise dysphonia.

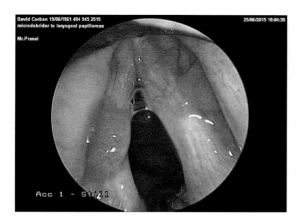

Figure 11.5 Macroscopic appearance of laryngeal papillomatosis by FNE.

Disease may be lifelong and recurrence is expected. Repeated surgical excision is required. Surgery tends to be conservative, in terms of always opting to preserve laryngeal structures and attempting to minimise scarring.

Disease activity tends to regress spontaneously over a number of years but is highly variable. The same disease in adults tends to be less florid and presents a much-reduced risk to airway patency.

Adjuvant therapies such as injection of intralesional cidofovir has also been reported and may have a role in difficult-to-manage cases, but the risk–benefit profile is unclear [30]. Bevacizumab (a monoclonal antibody) has been described in small case series as an effective treatment [31].

▉ Laryngopharyngeal reflux (LPR)

Aetiology

LPR is defined as retrograde flow of stomach contents to the laryngopharynx [32]. Estimates make this a highly prevalent condition and up to 50% of dysphonic patients have been purported to have evidence of LPR present. LPR has been implicated in many head and neck diseases including laryngitis, subglottic stenosis and even carcinoma with little definitive evidence of a causative role [33].

LPR is thought to be due to a failure of the protective barriers to stomach contents. These include the lower oesophageal sphincter, oesophageal peristalsis, saliva, gravity, and the upper oesophageal sphincter. Whilst acid reflux is a contributor to the effects of LPR, non-acid reflux with pepsin and/or bile salts are also damaging to laryngopharyngeal mucosa [33].

It can seem that all ear, nose and throat conditions are blamed on LPR. There is little definitive evidence for this approach!

History

The most common symptoms are:

- Hoarseness (variable, worse in the morning)
- Excessive throat clearing
- Coughing
- Globus pharyngeus

Belafsky et al. developed a nine-item questionnaire (Reflux Symptom Index) that is quick and simple (see **Table 11.4**) [34]. Scores >13 indicate LPR.

Examination

The findings on FNE of LPR are sometimes vague, subjective and non-specifi (**Figure 11.6**). Belafsky et al. also streamlined these findings into a specific list (Reflux Finding Score) where a score of 7 or more indicates reflux (see **Table 11.5**) [35]. However, there is not a strong correlation between clinical findings and response of symptoms to anti-reflux treatment.

Investigation

pH monitoring has not been found to provide definitive evidence of LPR that correlates to clinical findings and treatment response, though some units would advocate it [36].

Contrast swallows or cross-sectional imaging play no role in this diagnosis. Panendoscopy under general anaesthesia (GA) does not play a diagnostic role.

Table 11.4 Reflux symptom index.

How did the problems listed below affect you in the last month?	0 = no problem 5 = severe problem
1. Hoarseness 2. Throat clearing 3. Excess mucus/postnasal drip 4. Difficulty swallowing fluids, solids or tablets 5. Coughing after eating/lying down 6. Breathing difficulties or choking episodes 7. Cough 8. Sensation of lump in throat 9. Burning, heartburn, chest pain, indigestion or acid coming up (reflux)	
Total:	

Table 11.5 Reflux finding score.

Subglottic oedema	0 = absent 2 = present
Ventricular obliteration	0 = absent 2 = partial 4 = complete
Erythema	0 = absent 2 = arytenoid 4 = diffuse
Vocal fold oedema	0 = absent 1 = mild 2 = moderate 3 = severe 4 = polypoid
Laryngeal oedema	0 = absent 1 = mild 2 = moderate 3 = severe 4 = obstructive
Posterior commissure hypertrophy	0 = absent 1 = mild 2 = moderate 3 = severe 4 = obstructive
Granuloma	0 = absent 2 = present
Thick mucus	0 = absent 2 = present

Management

A clear explanation of the underlying cause is required. This can take some time.

Lifestyle changes include:

- Weight loss
- Smoking cessation
- Dietary changes (avoiding trigger foods or eating late at night)
- Alcohol avoidance

Medical management involves regular alginates with or without proton pump inhibitors. In those with strong clinical diagnosis of acid reflux, H2-receptor antagonist can be added. A trial of treatment is regarded by some as a diagnostic test [36]. Once malignancy has been excluded by FNE and treatment commenced, the patient can be discharged.

▌ Laryngeal leukoplakia

Aetiology

Leukoplakia is simply a clinical description. It literally refers to a 'white plaque'. It is generally regarded as a plaque present on a mucous membrane which cannot be rubbed/scraped off. The fact that it cannot

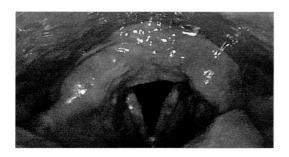

Figure 11.6 Endoscopic view of the posterior larynx demonstrating generally inflamed mucosa with oedema affecting the posterior commissure area and inter-arytenoid mucosa. The patient had a history consistent with LPR.

be easily removed implies it is a lesion arising from the underlying tissue rather than an overlying deposit such as those found in candidiasis.

It is not a diagnosis.

It is often used incorrectly to imply a diagnosis, such as dysplasia, but this can only be confirmed histologically. At the point of histological diagnosis, the term leukoplakia should no longer be used.

The underlying cause of the plaque can be varied. A meta-analysis by Isenberg et al. found the following in decreasing order of frequency [37]:

- No dysplasia (54%)
- Mild to moderate dysplasia (34%)
- Severe dysplasia to carcinoma in situ (15%)

Non-dysplastic lesions include hyperkeratosis and simple hyperplasia.

History

Voice change is the most common symptom. A history to stratify patient risk of malignancy should be taken (i.e. smoking, alcohol intake, previous radiotherapy, caustic injury, etc.).

Examination

FNE allows diagnosis of a white plaque. Complete UADT examination and neck examination should be performed.

Investigation

Examination under GA and biopsy are mandated to obtain histological diagnosis.

Management

Excision biopsy is usually performed, often with a CO_2 laser. Follow up is required on the basis of histological diagnosis. Interestingly Isenberg's meta-analysis suggested that even in the absence of dysplasia there is a 3.7% risk of developing invasive carcinoma. This is a relatively low risk, and the relationship of clinical risk factors to this risk is not clear. Where there is low clinical concern and no histological evidence of dysplasia, patients can likely be discharged with education on seeking re-referral in the advent of recurrent/deteriorating symptoms.

REFERENCES

1 Price G, Roche M, Crowther R, Wight R. *Profile of Head and Neck Cancers in England: Incidence, Mortality and Survival.* Oxford Cancer Intelligence Unit; 2010.

2 Menvielle G, Luce D, Goldberg P, Bugel I and Leclerc A. Smoking, alcohol drinking and cancer risk for various sites of the larynx and hypopharynx. A case-control study in France. *Eur J Cancer Prev.* 2004;13:165–72.

3 Brennan P, Boffetta P. Mechanistic considerations in the molecular epidemiology of head and neck cancer. *IARC Sci Publ.* 2004:393–414.

4 Spielmann PM, Palmer T, McClymont L. 15-Year review of laryngeal and oral dysplasias and progression to invasive carcinoma. *Eur Arch Otorhinolaryngol.* 2010;267:423–7.

5 Ferlito A, Rinaldo A. The pathology and management of subglottic cancer. *Eur Arch Otorhinolaryngol.* 2000;257:168–73.

6 Schwartz LH, Ozsahin M, Zhang GN et al. Synchronous and metachronous head and neck carcinomas. *Cancer.* 1994;74:1933–8.

7 Jain KS, Sikora AG, Baxi SS, Morris LG. Synchronous cancers in patients with head and neck cancer: Risks in the era of human papillomavirus-associated oropharyngeal cancer. *Cancer.* 2013;119:1832–7.

8 Department of Veterans Affairs Laryngeal Cancer Study Group, Wolf GT, Fisher SG et al. Induction chemotherapy plus radiation compared with surgery plus radiation in patients with advanced laryngeal cancer. *N Engl J Med.* 1991;324:1685–90.

9 Forastiere AA, Goepfert H, Maor M et al. Concurrent chemotherapy and radiotherapy for organ preservation in advanced laryngeal cancer. *N Engl J Med.* 2003;349:2091–8.

10 Jones TM, De M, Foran B, Harrington K, Mortimore S. Laryngeal cancer: United Kingdom National Multidisciplinary guidelines. *J Laryngol Otol.* 2016;130:S75–S82.

11 Theunissen EA, Timmermans AJ, Zuur CL et al. Total laryngectomy for a dysfunctional larynx after (chemo)radiotherapy. *Arch Otolaryngol Head Neck Surg.* 2012;138:548–55.

12 Hutcheson KA, Alvarez CP, Barringer DA, Kupferman ME, Lapine PR, Lewin JS. Outcomes of elective total laryngectomy for laryngopharyngeal dysfunction in disease-free head and neck cancer survivors. *Otolaryngol Head Neck Surg.* 2012;146:585–90.

13 Steiner W. Experience in endoscopic laser surgery of malignant tumours of the upper aero-digestive tract. *Adv Otorhinolaryngol.* 1988;39:135–44.

14 Sayles M, Grant DG. Preventing pharyngocutaneous fistula in total laryngectomy: A systematic review and meta-analysis. *Laryngoscope.* 2014;124:1150–63.

15 Blackwell KE, Calcaterra TC, Fu YS. Laryngeal dysplasia: Epidemiology and treatment outcome. *Ann Otol Rhinol Laryngol.* 1995;104:596–602.

16 Blackwell KE, Fu YS, Calcaterra TC. Laryngeal dysplasia. A clinicopathologic study. *Cancer.* 1995;75:457–63.

17 Hellquist H, Cardesa A, Gale N, Kambic V, Michaels L. Criteria for grading in the Ljubljana classification of epithelial hyperplastic laryngeal lesions. A study by members of the Working Group on Epithelial Hyperplastic Laryngeal Lesions of the European Society of Pathology. *Histopathology.* 1999;34:226–33.

18 Barnes L, Eveson J, Reichart P, Sidransky D. *Pathology and Genetics: Head and Neck Tumors.* IARC Press; 2005, p. 177–80.

19 Weller MD, Nankivell PC, McConkey C, Paleri V, Mehanna HM. The risk and interval to malignancy of patients with laryngeal dysplasia; a systematic review of case series and meta-analysis. *Clin Otolaryngol.* 2010;35:364–72.

20 Bouquot JE, Gnepp DR. Laryngeal precancer: A review of the literature, commentary, and comparison with oral leukoplakia. *Head Neck.* 1991;13:488–97.

21 Karatayli-Ozgursoy S, Pacheco-Lopez P, Hillel AT, Best SR, Bishop JA, Akst LM. Laryngeal dysplasia, demographics, and treatment: A single-institution, 20-year review. *JAMA Otolaryngol Head Neck Surg.* 2015;141:313–8.

22 Lewin JS, Gillenwater AM, Garrett JD et al. Characterization of laryngopharyngeal reflux in patients with premalignant or early carcinomas of the larynx. *Cancer.* 2003;97:1010–4.

23 Mehanna H, Paleri V, Robson A, Wight R, Helliwell T. Consensus statement by otorhinolaryngologists and pathologists on the diagnosis and management of laryngeal dysplasia. *Clin Otolaryngol.* 2010;35:170–6.

24 Martins RH, Defaveri J, Domingues MA, de Albuquerque e Silva R. Vocal polyps: Clinical, morphological, and immunohistochemical aspects. *J Voice.* 2011;25:98–106.

25 Won SJ, Kim RB, Kim JP, Park JJ, Kwon MS, Woo SH. The prevalence and factors associate with vocal nodules in general population: Cross-sectional epidemiological study. *Medicine (Baltimore).* 2016;95:e4971.

26 Martins RH, Defaveri J, Custodio Domingues MA, de Albuquerque ESR, Fabro A. Vocal fold nodules: Morphological and immunohistochemical investigations. *J Voice.* 2010;24:531–9.

27 Bohlender J. Diagnostic and therapeutic pitfalls in benign vocal fold diseases. *GMS Curr Top Otorhinolaryngol Head Neck Surg.* 2013;12:Doc01.

28 Karkos PD, George M, Van Der Veen J et al. Vocal process granulomas: A systematic

review of treatment. *Ann Otol Rhinol Laryngol.* 2014;123:314–20.

29 Derkay CS, Wiatrak B. Recurrent respiratory papillomatosis: A review. *Laryngoscope.* 2008;118:1236–47.

30 Derkay CS, Volsky PG, Rosen CA et al. Current use of intralesional cidofovir for recurrent respiratory papillomatosis. *Laryngoscope.* 2013;123:705–12.

31 Sidell DR, Nassar M, Cotton RT, Zeitels SM, de Alarcon A. High-dose sublesional bevacizumab (avastin) for pediatric recurrent respiratory papillomatosis. *Ann Otol Rhinol Laryngol.* 2014;123:214–21.

32 Ford CN. Evaluation and management of laryngopharyngeal reflux. *JAMA.* 2005; 294: 1534–40.

33 Campagnolo AM, Priston J, Thoen RH, Medeiros T, Assuncao AR. Laryngopharyngeal reflux: Diagnosis, treatment, and latest research. *Int Arch Otorhinolaryngol.* 2014;18:184–91.

34 Belafsky PC, Postma GN, Koufman JA. Validity and reliability of the reflux symptom index (RSI). *J Voice.* 2002;16:274–7.

35 Belafsky PC, Postma GN, Koufman JA. The validity and reliability of the reflux finding score (RFS). *Laryngoscope.* 2001;111:1313–7.

36 Joniau S, Bradshaw A, Esterman A, Carney AS. Reflux and laryngitis: A systematic review. *Otolaryngol Head Neck Surg.* 2007;136:686–92.

37 Isenberg JS, Crozier DL, Dailey SH. Institutional and comprehensive review of laryngeal leukoplakia. *Ann Otol Rhinol Laryngol.* 2008;117:74–9.

12 NASOPHARYNX

Jay Goswamy

INTRODUCTION

The functions of the nasopharynx are:

- A gateway for nasal airflow
- The portal to ventilation of the middle ear

ANATOMY

The nasopharynx is the superiormost of the three elements of the pharynx, acting as a posterior continuation of the nasal cavity and descending into the oropharynx. Whilst five of the six borders (see **Table 12.1**) of the area are fixed, the inferior aspect is in a continual state of motion, most noticeable during the acts of speech and swallowing.

During nasal inhalation, the nasopharynx (an open space) leads to the oropharynx. During speech, this is partially obscured by the soft palate, which then completely occludes the space during normal swallowing, due to the action of the muscles surrounding the torus, which then act to open the Eustachian tube for middle ear pressure equalisation. Hence, the logic behind swallowing repeatedly on the descent of a flight to raise the pressure in the middle ear to that of the surrounding environment.

▌ Lymphatic drainage

Lymph fluid drains in a medial and lateral direction from the nasopharynx. Drainage medially is to the central retropharyngeal lymph nodes (the echelon lymph node) and laterally to the lateral retropharyngeal, and through the superior constrictor to the deep cervical and the posterior triangle lymph nodes (see **Box 12.1**) [1].

▌ Innervation

The dorsum sellae of the sphenoid separates the nasopharynx from the sphenoid sinus, which in turn is medial to the cavernous sinuses, home to the internal carotid arteries and the ophthalmic and maxillary nerves, V1 and V2. The maxillary nerve,

Table 12.1 The anatomical relations of the nasopharynx.

Boundary	Anatomy
Anterior	Posterior choanae (divided by a strip of bone made up of the perpendicular plate of the ethmoid superiorly and the vomer inferiorly).
Superior	The basal aspect of the sphenoid, the dorsum sellae joins the clivus of the basal aspect of the occiput in a postero-inferior graduation.
Posterior	The atlas, the axis (C1 and C2).
Lateral	The torus tubarius (formed by the cartilaginous Eustachian tube), anterior to the torus opens the Eustachian tube. Posterior to the torus lies the fossa of Rosenmüller. Inferior to the torus, an anterior fold contains the salpingopalatine muscle and posteriorly a fold contains the salpingopharyngeus muscle.
Inferior	The soft palate.

Note: To orientate one's self within the nasopharynx visualise a Viking helmet.

Box 12.1 Useful knowledge in clinic

Most children at the start of nursery, subjected to the first major insult to their immune system, develop upper respiratory tract infections, usually centred on the nasopharynx, and as such have palpable lymph nodes in the posterior triangles of their necks, which can be alarming to those not anticipating such changes.

Remembering the lymphatic drainage of the nasopharynx explains these nodes.

in combination with the glossopharyngeal nerve (ninth cranial nerve, CN IX), supplies sensation to the nasopharynx. The glossopharyngeal nerve also serves a dual function, combining with the vagus (CN X) to form the pharyngeal plexus located on the surface of the middle constrictor, supplying all of the muscle fibres located in the nasopharynx apart from tensor veli palatini, which receives its supply from the third branch of the trigeminal, V3, the mandibular nerve.

NASOPHARYNGEAL CARCINOMA

▌ Aetiology

Whilst exceptionally rare in Europe, nasopharyngeal cancer (NPC) is common in South East Asia (Southern China, Singapore, Vietnam, Malaysia and the Philippines). Interestingly, people of Chinese descent who move to another geographic area reduce their risk of NPC, but they still remain at higher risk than non-Chinese people from Western areas. This is thought to be partly related to genetic factors and partly to the dietary predilection for salted fish [2,3].

Epstein–Barr virus (EBV) has been implicated in the aetiology of NPC, particularly the undifferentiated subtype, but is rarely found in normal nasopharyngeal epithelial tissues [4]. Whilst EBV does not directly cause NPC, infection in pre-malignant nasopharyngeal epithelial cells and expression of latent viral genes are crucial features in the development of NPC [5].

Smoking and alcohol may increase the risk of this cancer. It is also approximately twice as common in men compared to women.

▌ History

Early symptoms are often vague and non-specific. This is due to over 50% of tumours originating in the fossa of Rosenmüller. This is located in posterolateral pharyngeal recess posterosuperior to the torus tubarius. This allows space for a tumour to grow to considerable size before it is symptomatic. Due to this, often patients will present with a neck mass as their primary complaint.

Given the proximity to the skull base, sphenoid sinus and parapharynx, tumours are often locally advanced at presentation as well.

Red flags for NPC include:

- Ethnicity
- Unilateral otitis media with effusion (OME)
- Unilateral nasal obstruction
- Posterior epistaxis
- Headaches
- Trismus
- Cranial nerve palsies (e.g. facial numbness, diplopia)
- Neck lump

▌ Examination

Flexible nasoendoscopy is key to evaluating the nasopharynx. However, a tumour may be submucosal and therefore subtle in appearance.

Otoscopy may reveal an effusion, and neck examination is essential for assessment of potential nodal disease.

▌ Investigation

In patients presenting with unilateral otitis media with effusion, the traditional approach was to perform blind biopsy of the fossa of Rosenmüller and insert ventilation tube into the affected ear.

Now, MRI prior to biopsy can reliably identify any intra or extracranial lesions and combined with rigid endoscopic evaluation of the nasopharynx allowing for a precision biopsy, false negative rates are reduced [6]. Where the index of suspicion for NPC is high, ventilation tube insertion should be avoided,

as radiotherapy is a key part of treatment and can lead to a persistently discharging ear if the tympanic membrane is breached.

Cross-sectional imaging is essential in the work up of NPC. MRI offers better soft tissue definition of any spread into dura, orbit, parapharyngeal space, masticator space or infratemporal fossa. Computed tomography (CT) determines bony erosion of the paranasal sinuses, clivus or choanae. Both are required for accurate staging (see **Table 12.2**).

▌ Management

Given the technical difficulty of achieving sufficient surgical margins within the nasopharynx and the relative radio-sensitivity of NPC, the primary modality for NPC is radiotherapy. Surgery is hence reserved for recurrence or residual disease and is associated with significant postoperative morbidity.

Chemotherapy has been shown to have a small but significant benefit for overall and event-free survival in advanced stage (III and IV) disease when administered concomitantly with radiotherapy [8].

Radiotherapy fields will be modified dependent on the radiological staging but will include the nasopharynx and bilateral neck levels II to V given the propensity for bilateral lymphatic drainage. Intensity modulation has improved the morbidity associated with primary radiation therapy [9]. Radiation to the skull base in particular can result in hypopituitarism [10].

Numerous surgical approaches to the nasopharynx have been described (see **Table 12.3**). It is a challenging area to gain optimal access to and the approach will be dictated by tumour size and extension, patient fitness for surgery, and habitus as well as surgeon experience.

A variety of open approaches have been traditionally used. These include lateral rhinotomy, midfacial degloving, the Caldwell-Luc approach, transpalatal, Le Fort I and the infratemporal fossa approach. Those with intraorbital or intracranial extension

Table 12.2 TNM 8 staging system for nasopharyngeal carcinoma.

T Stage	Description	N Stage	Description	M stage	Description
Tx	Cannot be assessed	Nx	Cannot be assessed	M0	No distant metastasis
T0	No evidence	N0	No regional nodes		
Tis	Carcinoma in situ	N1	Unilateral metastasis in cervical node(s) and/or uni-/bilateral metastasis in retropharyngeal nodes, up to 6 cm, above caudal border of cricoid cartilage	M1	Distant metastasis
T1	Confined to nasopharynx/oropharynx/nasal cavity				
T2	Parapharyngeal extension	N2	Bilateral metastasis in node(s), up to 6 cm above the caudal border of cricoid cartilage		
T3	Involvement of skull base, cervical vertebra or paranasal sinuses	N3	Above 6 cm and/or extension below caudal border of cricoid cartilage		
T4	Intracranial extension, involvement of cranial nerve, hypopharynx, orbit, extensive soft tissue involvement (beyond the lateral surface of the lateral pterygoid muscle, parotid gland)				

Source: Pan JJ et al. *Cancer*, 2016;122:546–58.

may necessitate a combined open and endoscopic approach.

An open medial maxillectomy can be used for tumours not extending into the lateral infratemporal fossa and is approached by a midfacial degloving. A lateral rhinotomy is employed if the superior ethmoids are involved. The sequence of bony cuts is:

1 Osteotomy below inferior orbital rim
2 Osteotomy antrum to vestibule
3 Osteotomy across frontal process of maxilla
4 Osteotomy along floor of nose
5 Osteotomy through lacrimal bone
6 Osteotomy vertically through posterior end of medial antrum

A Le Fort I procedure is an alternative whereby the palate is downfractured following a horizontal osteotomy above the maxillary dental roots after pre-plating of the maxilla. This should be avoided in adolescents due to the impact on subsequent midfacial growth. Of note, this procedure will result in dental denervation.

Table 12.3 List of different surgical approaches to the nasopharynx.

Tumour size	Surgical approaches
Smaller	Endoscopic transnasal Transpalatal Transantral
Larger	Lateral rhinotomy Midfacial degloving Maxillary swing Le Fort I osteotomy Infratemporal fossa approach (Fisch type C) Transmaxillary, transpalatal Transmandibular, transpalatal Craniofacial approach

Note: No one approach is definitively better for all tumours and each tumour is assessed individually.

A transpalatal approach requires removal of the horizontal plate of the palatine bone after a soft tissue incision to separate the hard and soft palate.

A maxillary swing is accessed via a Weber Ferguson incision and is described in the NPC subsection of this chapter.

The infratemporal approach requires removal of the zygoma and reflection of the temporalis muscle. A hemicoronal incision is made from below the zygoma in the preauricular area and extends behind the hairline. Dissection proceeds in the lateral superficial to the temporals fascia. Anteriorly, a fat pad on the muscle protects the superior branch of the facial nerve. At this point, dissection proceeds deep to the fascia and fat pad. From the posterior margin of the muscle, incise the muscle 1 cm below the superior temporal line down to deep fascia in order to mobilise the muscle inferiorly. Incise the deep fascia along the superior surface of the zygoma. Remove the zygomatic arch after pre-plating in order to facilitate reconstruction on completion of tumour dissection. Inferior dissection is medial to the coronoid process of the mandible.

◼ Follow-up

Follow-up after completion of radiation therapy with or without concurrent chemotherapy should be with a rigid or flexible nasendoscope and should also include three-dimensional imaging at 3 months to assess response to treatment in the form of a CT, MRI or PET-CT [11]. Thereafter patients are reviewed at regular intervals (e.g. every 3 months) in clinic with direct visualisation of the upper aerodigestive tract (UADT) and neck examination for 5 years. Symptoms of recurrence can be vague – they may present with paraesthesia, pain or numbness due to neural or intracranial spread. A low threshold to assess locoregional status using cross-sectional imaging should be observed.

JUVENILE NASAL ANGIOFIBROMA (JNA)

Benign tumours of the nasopharynx are rare. Non-epithelial, vascular tumours (JNA) account for 50% of these tumours [12]. They are discussed in more detail in Chapter 11.

ADENOIDAL HYPERTROPHY

◼ Aetiology

Adenoidal lymphoid tissue is part of Waldeyer's ring of lymphoid tissue, the other contents of the ring include the lingual tonsil, covering the tongue base, which persists into adulthood, and the pharyngeal tonsils between the palatoglossal and palatopharyngeal arches. At birth, there is minimal lymphoid

Table 12.4 Causes of adenoidal hypertrophy.

Causes of adenoidal hypertrophy	Examples
Inflammation	Allergic rhinitis
Infection	Rhinosinusitis, recurrent tonsillitis, HIV, Epstein–Barr virus
Neoplastic	Lymphoma, vascular tumour, encephalocele

tissue in the nasopharynx but hypertrophy occurs rapidly over the first year of life and varies in maximal size but can completely occlude the posterior nasal cavity. At birth, neonates are obligate nasal breathers explaining the lack of lymphoid tissue in this area at this stage of development. The peak size of adenoidal lymphoid tissue is usually around the age of 5 years, followed by natural atrophy, which should be complete by 16 years (though nasal symptoms and rates of OME should improve by 7 years).

Adult adenoidal hypertrophy is less common [13]. The causes are listed in **Table 12.4**.

History

The main presenting symptom is nasal obstruction, usually bilateral. This may lead to snoring and even obstructive sleep apnoea. Due to obstruction of the Eustachian tube and subsequent otitis media with effusion, patients may complain of their ears feeling blocked, otalgia, hearing loss or disequilibrium.

General symptoms of weight loss, neck lumps, night sweats, fatigue and lethargy are all red flags for malignancy.

Examination

Using a cold metal spatula beneath the nares observe for misting, in unilateral obstruction only one side will mist, a false negative may be seen in the presence of a septal perforation. Anterior rhinoscopy

may reveal mucopus, oedematous nasal mucosa and engorged inferior turbinates.

Fibre-optic nasendoscopy is essential to assess the nasopharynx. Obstructive adenoids may preclude the passage of the endoscope beyond the posterior choanae. Given however that lymphoid tissue is pliable and soft, passage into the oropharynx should be attainable.

It is essential to examination the entire UADT as well as the neck to exclude any lymphadenopathy.

Investigation

Blood tests to exclude infections such as glandular fever and HIV should be performed.

MRI will assess the extent of disease and in rare instances of malignant causes will prevent artefacts caused by biopsy. It will also reveal any rare encephalocele or vascular lesions, preventing inappropriate biopsy.

Management

Following imaging, endoscopic biopsy provides histological diagnosis and allows debulking for symptomatic relief. This may also be performed as a per oral curettage adenoidectomy in patients with a low index of suspicion as long as the adenoids are still sent for histological examination.

Alternative tools for adenoidectomy such as monopolar suction diathermy or coblation may be used, but sufficient representative samples must be sent for histological diagnosis.

REFERENCES

1 Ho FC, Tham IW, Earnest A, Lee KM, Lu JJ. Patterns of regional lymph node metastasis of nasopharyngeal carcinoma: A meta-analysis of clinical evidence. *BMC Cancer.* 2012;12:98.
2 Yu MC. Nasopharyngeal carcinoma: Epidemiology and dietary factors. *IARC Sci Publ.* 1991;(105):39–47.

3 Jia WH, Luo XY, Feng BJ et al. Traditional Cantonese diet and nasopharyngeal carcinoma risk: A large-scale case-control study in Guangdong, China. *BMC Cancer.* 2010;10:446.

4 Tsang CM, Deng W, Yip YL, Zeng MS, Lo KW, Tsao SW. Epstein-Barr virus infection and persistence in nasopharyngeal epithelial cells. *Chin J Cancer.* 2014;33:549–55.

5 Tsang CM, Tsao SW. The role of Epstein-Barr virus infection in the pathogenesis of nasopharyngeal carcinoma. *Virol Sin.* 2015;30:107–21.

6 Leonetti JP. A study of persistent unilateral middle ear effusion caused by occult skull base lesions. *Ear Nose Throat J.* 2013;92:195–200.

7 Pan JJ, Ng WT, Zong JF et al. Proposal for the 8th edition of the AJCC/UICC staging system for nasopharyngeal cancer in the era of intensity-modulated radiotherapy. *Cancer.* 2016;122:546–58.

8 Baujat B, Audry H, Bourhis J et al. Chemotherapy as an adjunct to radiotherapy in locally advanced nasopharyngeal carcinoma. *Cochrane Database Syst Rev.* 2006;(4):CD004329.

9 Chen J, Liu P, Wang Q, Wu L, Zhang X. Influence of intensity-modulated radiation therapy on the life quality of patients with nasopharyngeal carcinoma. *Cell Biochem Biophys.* 2015;73:731–6.

10 Ratnasingam J, Karim N, Paramasivam SS et al. Hypothalamic pituitary dysfunction amongst nasopharyngeal cancer survivors. *Pituitary.* 2015;18:448–55.

11 Simo R, Robinson M, Lei M, Sibtain A, Hickey S. Nasopharyngeal carcinoma: United Kingdom National Multidisciplinary Guidelines. *J Laryngol Otol.* 2016;130:S97–103.

12 Fu YS, Perzin KH. Non-epithelial tumors of the nasal cavity, paranasal sinuses, and nasopharynx: A clinicopathologic study. I. General features and vascular tumors. *Cancer.* 1974;33:1275–88.

13 Rout MR, Mohanty D, Vijaylaxmi Y, Bobba K, Metta C. Adenoid hypertrophy in adults: A case series. *Indian J Otolaryngol Head Neck Surg.* 2013;65:269–74.

13

SINONASAL TUMOURS

Yujay Ramakrishnan and Shahzada Ahmed

INTRODUCTION

Sinonasal tumours represent an extremely varied group of rare tumours that can be difficult to manage. They account for between 3% and 5% of head and neck malignancies and typically present at an advanced stage due to non-specific early symptoms. Their close proximity with vital structures like the eye and brain can make management extremely challenging, potentially resulting in significant morbidity to patients.

Despite only occupying a relatively small area, the sinonasal tract is the epicentre of a variety of sinonasal tumours (>70) which are histologically diverse. According to the World Health Organization (WHO) classification, sinonasal neoplasms are classified into benign and malignant, and further subdivided based on their tissue origin, i.e. epithelial and mesenchymal

(see **Table 13.1**) [1]. Epithelial tumours are the most common and originate from the epithelial lining, accessory salivary glands, neuroendocrine tissue and olfactory epithelium, whilst mesenchymal tumours derive from the supporting tissue.

Currently, due to the low incidence and diverse histology, there is limited high-level evidence for management of sinonasal tumours. Based on the existing evidence base, national guidelines have been recently published on the work-up and management of sinonasal tumours [2]. The treatment plan of sinonasal malignancy should be discussed at a specialist skull based multidisciplinary team meeting [3]. The integration of multimodality treatment in high-grade and advanced tumours has been shown to improve survival rates.

EPIDEMIOLOGY

Sinonasal tumours commonly affect males and usually present in the fifth and sixth decades. Certain tumours like olfactory neuroblastoma have a bimodal distribution with a second, smaller peak

in the second decade. There is a wide geographical distribution. They are more common amongst males due to occupational risk exposure, which will be discussed later.

Table 13.1 Classification of sinonasal tumours.

Benign		Malignant	
Epithelial	Sinonasal papilloma ● Inverted ● Exophytic ● Oncocytic	Epithelial	Squamous cell carcinoma
	Salivary gland–type adenoma ● Pleomorphic adenoma ● Myoepithelioma ● Oncocytoma		Adenocarcinoma ● Intestinal type ● Non-intestinal type
			Salivary gland ● Adenoid-cystic carcinoma ● Acinic cell carcinoma ● Mucoepidermoid carcinoma
			Melanoma
			Olfactory neuroblastoma
			Sinonasal undifferentiated carcinoma
Mesenchymal	Bone and cartilage ● Osteoma ● Ossifying fibroma ● Fibrous dysplasia ● Chondroma	Mesenchymal	Bone and cartilage Osteosarcoma Chondrosarcoma
	Chordoma Juvenile angiofibroma Schwannoma Neurofibroma Myxoma Meningioma Haemangioma		Soft-tissue sarcoma ● Rhabdomyosarcoma ● Leiomyosarcoma ● Fibrosarcoma ● Liposarcoma ● Angiosarcoma ● Myxosarcoma ● Hemangiopericytoma
			Lymphoreticular ● Lymphoma ● Plasmacytoma ● Giant cell tumour
		Metastasis	Renal cell carcinoma Breast cancer Lung carcinoma

Source: Barnes L et al. *Pathology and Genetics: Head and Neck Tumors.* IARC Press; 2005.

Although tumours of the nasal cavities are equally divided between benign and malignant types, most tumours of the paranasal sinuses are malignant. Approximately 55% of sinonasal tumours originate from the maxillary sinuses, 35% from the nasal cavities, 9% from the ethmoid sinuses, and the remainder from the frontal and sphenoid sinuses [2]. Squamous cell carcinoma represents the most common malignancy (70%–80%), followed by adenocarcinoma and adenoid cystic carcinoma (10% each) [4]. In the paediatric setting, rhabdomyosarcoma is the most common tumour [5].

PATHOPHYSIOLOGY

Unlike other head and neck tumours, smoking is not thought to play a significant aetiological role. Occupational factors like wood dust, leather tanning and exposure to metals (nickel, chromium) play a key role in the pathogenesis of squamous cell carcinoma and adenocarcinoma. Hardwood such as oak and beech confer the highest risk of developing sinonasal adenocarcinomas, making this disease common amongst carpenters and furniture makers [6]. The molecular mechanism underlying wood dust leading to cancer is as yet unknown. As wood dust is not mutagenic, it is postulated that prolonged exposure and irritation by wood dust particles must result in chronic inflammation. Other suspected occupational carcinogens include formaldehyde, diisopropyl sulphate and dichloroethyl sulphide [1,7].

A number of studies have also explored the role of human papillomavirus (HPV) in sinonasal tumours with no definitive link being demonstrated [8].

HISTORY

The symptoms of sinonasal tumours are often non-specific and overlap with various benign conditions like rhinosinusitis. The signs and symptoms of sinonasal tumours can be understood by examining the close relationship of the sinuses with the surroundings structures. The symptoms can be divided as follows:

a *Nasal*: Obstruction, epistaxis
b *Eye*: Pain, unilateral epiphora, diplopia, proptosis, loss of vision
c *Oral cavity*: Palatal fullness, lump or ulceration, loose dentition, ill-fitting dentures, trismus (involvement of the pterygoid muscles or motor trigeminal nerve Vc)
d *Ear*: Hearing loss (Eustachian tube obstruction and secondary serous otitis media)
e *Facial*: Cheek fullness, pain and infraorbital nerve anaesthesia
f *Intracranial*: Headache, nausea and vomiting
g Neck lump

Tumours of the nasal cavity tend to be diagnosed earlier due to symptoms of nasal obstruction and/or epistaxis. In contrast, tumours arising in the sinuses present more insidiously and usually are at an advanced stage when diagnosed.

Red flag symptoms such as a unilateral nasal mass, facial swelling, diplopia or blurred vision, proptosis, and cranial neuropathy should raise a high index of suspicion and merit urgent assessment. Regional and distant metastasis are relatively rare, with the incidence of neck metastasis less than 10%. Distant metastasis is less frequent.

EXAMINATION

A thorough examination comprising the head, neck and cranial nerves, and nasal endoscopy should be performed. Physical examination of the nose should evaluate the extent of the mass (including spread to the opposite nasal cavity); eyes for diplopia, proptosis and visual loss; mouth for lumps/ulceration, loose dentition or ill-fitting dentures; neck lump; as well as altered sensation (numbness or hyperesthesia) of the cheek.

INVESTIGATIONS

Imaging should be performed pre-biopsy to prevent distortion of tumour margins.

Both computer tomography (CT) scanning and magnetic resonance imaging (MRI) have complementary roles.

CT allows detection of bony destruction and remodelling, while MRI is better at detecting mucosal, skin invasion, orbital or intracranial involvement. A contrast-enhanced CT will reveal tumour enhancement compared to the surrounding normal tissue, tumour vascularity and relationship to the carotid vessels. CT imaging can be performed quickly, but there is exposure to ionising radiation to patients.

MRI with contrast (gadolinium) provides superior soft tissue detail, differentiating tumour from secretions in an opacified sinus, and demonstrates orbital and intracranial spread as well as perineural spread (in adenoid cystic carcinoma). MRI has the advantage of not being affected by dental artefact and requires no exposure to ionising radiation, but does take longer to perform. Additionally, it may not be suitable for claustrophobic patients.

A staging CT scan of the head, neck and chest should be performed. The abdomen is also included in sinonasal adenocarcinoma.

Positron emission tomography–computed tomography (PET-CT) imaging is not routinely utilised in the staging of sinonasal tumours. However, they have been shown to be useful in staging aggressive sinonasal malignancies (sarcoma, malignant melanoma, sinonasal undifferentiated carcinoma, neuroendocrine carcinoma) where widespread metastasis is expected. PET-CT may also be useful in detecting the primary site of metastasis to the sinonasal tract (e.g. adenocarcinoma).

It is mandatory that a representative biopsy be taken. This can be performed in the outpatient setting under local anaesthetic. If profuse bleeding is anticipated, the biopsy should be performed in the controlled environment of the operating theatre. Where biopsies have been reported elsewhere, a second histopathologic opinion is vital for confirming the correct diagnosis. Up to 19% of sinonasal tumours have a change in the primary diagnosis following a second pathological opinion [9].

▍ Staging

The tremendous histological diversity amongst sinonasal tumours combined with its low incidence makes the development of a uniform staging system that is prognostically relevant difficult. Currently, the American Joint Committee on Cancer (AJCC) tumour, node, metastasis (TNM) staging system (based on anatomical involvement) is widely used for certain epithelial tumours of the nasal cavity and ethmoid sinus (see **Table 13.2**). A different staging system that incorporates histological grading is used for mesenchymal tumours like sarcoma, as this is the most significant prognostic factor. Sinonasal melanomas also have their own unique staging system (see **Table 13.3**).

TREATMENT

The optimal management is determined through a multidisciplinary approach.

One has to determine whether curative intent is achievable or palliation would be appropriate.

In general, surgery tends to be the mainstay of treatment (except lymphoma) and the role of radiation with or without chemotherapy is reserved for adjuvant treatment or palliation. Some studies have shown that induction chemotherapy can be used to treat advanced

Table 13.2 AJCC staging system for sinonasal tumour.

Nasal cavity and ethmoid sinus	
T1	Tumour restricted to one subsite, with or without bony invasion.
T2	Tumour invades two subsites in a single region or involves an adjacent region within the nasoethmoidal complex, with or without bony invasion.
T3	Tumour invades the medial wall or floor of the orbit, maxillary sinus, palate or cribriform plate.
T4a	Tumour involves any of the following: anterior orbital contents, skin of nose or cheek, minimal extension to anterior cranial fossa, pterygoid plates, sphenoid or frontal sinuses.
T4b	Tumour involves any of the following: orbital apex, dura, brain, middle cranial fossa, cranial nerves other than V2, nasopharynx or clivus.
Maxillary sinus	
T1	Tumour limited to the maxillary sinus mucosa without bony destruction.
T2	Tumour causing bone destruction including erosion into the hard palate and/or middle nasal meatus, except extension to posterior maxillary wall and pterygoid plates.
T3	Tumour invades any of the following: bone of the posterior wall of the maxillary sinus, subcutaneous tissues, floor or medial wall of the orbit, pterygoid fossa or ethmoid sinuses.
T4a	Tumour invades anterior orbital contents, skin of cheek, pterygoid plates, infratemporal fossa, cribriform plate, sphenoid or frontal sinuses.
T4b	Tumour invades any of the following: orbital apex, dura, brain, middle cranial fossa, cranial nerves other than V2, nasopharynx or clivus.

Table 13.3 Staging sinonasal melanoma.

Sinonasal melanoma	
Primary tumour (T)	
Tx	Primary tumour cannot be evaluated
T3	Confined to mucosa
T4a	Invades deep soft tissue, cartilage, bone or skin
T4b	Invades brain, dura, cranial nerves, carotid artery, prevertebral space or mediastinum
Regional lymph node (N)	
Nx	Regional lymph nodes cannot be evaluated
N0	No evidence of regional nodal metastases
N1	Regional lymph node metastases
Distant metastasis (M)	
M0	No distant metastases
M1	Distant metastases

tumours [10]. Heavy ion therapy like proton or carbon ion beams has also shown promise in the postoperative setting or stand-alone treatment [11].

▌ Surgery

Surgery is performed for curative and occasionally palliative intent to improve the nasal airway. It can be performed via an endoscopic or open approach.

Open approaches consist of different incisions to obtain access to the maxilla, ethmoid and frontal sinuses and even the nasopharynx if needed (see **Table 13.4**). Depending on the extent of the disease, different approaches can be taken and the method of resection individually tailored. Those involving the cribriform plate or anterior cranial fossa will require neurosurgical input and often a combined approach from the cranium and the face (craniofacial resection). See Chapter 12 for more information on open approaches to this region.

Endoscopic approaches have become more popular as technology and skills have progressed in the last two decades. In general, tumours involving the medial maxillary sinus wall, ethmoids, sphenoid and clivus can all be accessed endoscopically and removed piecemeal (see **Figure 13.1**). Endoscopic approaches can also be used in procedures involving neurosurgeons.

Clear margins are the aim of surgery and need to be obtained regardless of the approach.

One of the key advantages of the endoscopic endonasal approach (EEA) is the enhanced visualisation and superior illumination; compared to open approaches, the endoscope eliminates line of sight issues and therefore offers an improved panoramic view and magnification. The use of angled scopes and instruments also minimises removal of uninvolved structures, thereby reducing morbidity, ultimately leading to faster recovery. Compared to the traditional transcranial approaches, endoscopic also offers a more direct approach to the skull base thereby avoiding brain retraction.

However, endoscopic surgery may be unsuitable in certain cases. These include anatomical restrictions (dural involvement beyond medial aspect of the orbital roof, extensive brain infiltration and skin or soft tissue involvement), certain tumour histologies and the surgical team experience. In these cases, an open approach may be more suitable.

The biggest risks with EEA remain extraocular muscle damage, internal carotid artery injury, cerebrospinal fluid (CSF) leak and skull base reconstruction.

Expansion of the endoscopic endonasal approach leaves behind larger skull base defects. The use of pedicled local flaps to close skull base defects has reduced the rate of postoperative CSF leaks. These include the Hadad-Bassagaisteguy nasoseptal flap, the lateral nasal wall flap, middle turbinate flap, galeal-pericranial flap (inserted through a frontal slot sinosotomy or nasionectomy) and temporoparietal fascia flap. Interestingly, recent use of multilayered non-vascularised grafts (iliotibial tract and fascia lata) by Castelnuovo et al can achieve comparable CSF leak rates. This highlights the importance of meticulous closure of skull base defects, regardless

Table 13.4 Different incisions used to access sinonasal tumours in open surgery.

Incision	Access obtained
Lateral rhinotomy	Nasal cavity, ethmoid sinuses and medial maxilla
Weber-Ferguson With Diffenbach extension	Complete maxillectomy, ethmoidectomy and nasal cavity Improved access to lateral orbit and malar eminence
Midfacial degloving incision	Medial and inferior maxillectomy
Bi-coronal scalp flap	Allows access for intracranial extension of tumour in combined approach craniofacial resection

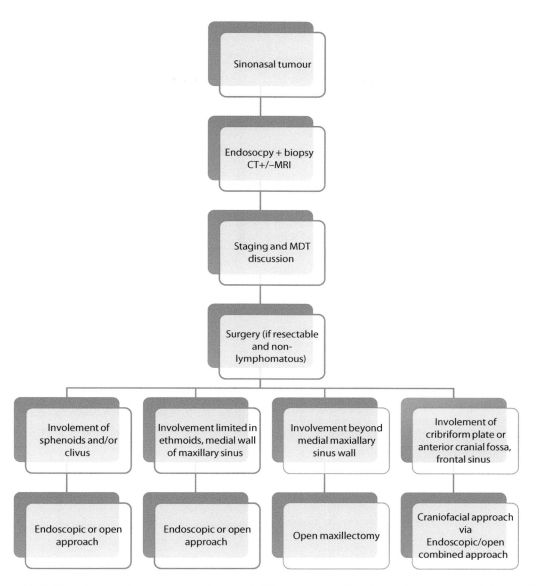

Figure 13.1 Flow chart to demonstrate work up and different approaches depending on extent of disease [12].

of whether a vascularized or non-vascularised flap is used [13–15].

▇ Management of the orbit

Orbital exenteration refers to complete removal of the contents of the orbit including the eyelids. Orbital clearance refers to removal of the globe, muscles and periorbita, whilst the eyelids and palpebral conjunctiva are preserved [16]. Orbital clearance is more commonly performed.

The degree of orbital invasion requiring orbital exenteration has been a controversial issue. A grading system for orbital invasion (see **Table 13.5**) has been developed. The authors opinion is that the orbit has to be sacrificed for invasion of the extraocular

Table 13.5 Grading system for degree of orbital invasion.

Grade	Degree of orbital invasion
I	Erosion of medial orbital wall
II	Extraconal invasion of orbital fat
III	Invasion of medial rectus, optic nerve, ocular bulb or skin of eyelid

Source: Iannetti G et al. *J Craniofac Surg.* 2005;16(6): 1085–91.

muscles, intraconal fat, globe or orbital apex [4]. If the periorbital is involved but can be resected with clear margins, orbital preservation can be achieved. Key aspects to consider during orbital preservation include oncological margins and the function of the preserved eye (see **Figure 13.2**).

Orbital clearance/exenteration also needs to be considered pre-emptively in cases where the orbit is going to receive radiotherapy (either directly or within the margins of the primary treatment area). Radiotherapy causes blindness through retinopathy/optic neuropathy, causes disabling and irreversible diplopia through fibrosis of the extraocular muscles, and can cause crippling pain. As a result, many patients may be better off having clearance/exenteration performed.

▌▌ Radiation

Radiation is used to treat lymphoreticular tumours (curative intent) in the adjuvant setting postoperatively (curative intent) or palliatively for unresectable cases or poor surgical candidates.

The major side effect in irradiating the paranasal sinuses is damage to the adjacent structures. These include ocular toxicity (blindness, retinopathy and optic neuropathy), brain necrosis and osteoradionecrosis.

Proton therapy

In recent years, proton beam therapy has risen in popularity and shown to be beneficial in select pathologies. This is a form of external beam radiotherapy that involves a beam of protons to target tumours. Proton

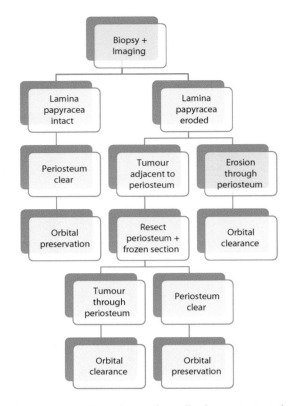

Figure 13.2 Flow chart to broadly demonstrate indications for orbital clearance/surgery [16].

beams have low scatter, meaning collateral damage is low, and the dose delivered is maximised only over a short specific distance reducing dose-related side effects and limiting damage to adjacent tissue. This is potentially very useful in sinonasal tumours due to the proximity of the brainstem, optic nerves and spine.

▌▌ Chemotherapy

The role of chemotherapy in paranasal cancer sinus tumours is considered within multimodality treatment with curative purposes (radiosensitiser) or in the palliative setting.

Chemotherapy may be delivered at different times:

- a As the primary treatment (usually concurrently with radiotherapy) for lymphoma and inoperable tumours.

b   Adjuvant chemotherapy – after surgery (usually concurrently with radiotherapy) to minimise recurrence in at-risk patients (e.g. positive margins after resection, perineural spread or extracapsular spread in regional metastases).

c   Neoadjuvant – or induction chemotherapy prior to definitive surgical or non-surgical treatment to shrink the tumour. Certain histological subtypes have been shown to respond to induction chemotherapy, e.g. neuroendocrine, sinonasal undifferentiated carcinoma, high-grade olfactory neuroblastoma and intestinal-type adenocarcinoma (with wild-type functional p53).

BENIGN TUMOURS

▮ Fibro-osseous lesions

Benign bony abnormalities are known collectively as fibro-osseous lesions. Osteoma, ossifying fibroma and fibrous dysplasia are three distinct entities that lie along a continuum from the most to least bony content.

Osteoma

Osteoma is the most common benign sinonasal tumour. It is a slow-growing bony tumour affecting mainly the frontal and ethmoid sinuses. The overall incidence of osteomas is 3% [17]. They typically present in patients in their 50s and 60s with a male-to-female ratio of 1.3:1 [17]. Most osteomas are isolated. Occasionally, they can be part of an autosomal dominant syndrome called Gardner syndrome. The triad of symptoms include osteomas (usually multiple), soft tissue tumours (such as epidermal inclusion cysts or subcutaneous fibrous tumours) and polyposis of the colon. Due to the high risk of malignant degeneration of these colonic polyps, a gastroenterology referral is advisable.

Clinical presentation

Patients are often asymptomatic and occasionally present with a bony lump or symptoms of a mucocele (lump, orbital proptosis and diplopia).

Investigations

A CT of the paranasal sinuses is usually adequate for diagnosis and evaluating the extent of disease.

Management

Asymptomatic tumours are treated conservatively, whilst if symptomatic or growing, the osteoma can be removed through an endoscopic or open approach.

Fibrous dysplasia

Fibrous dysplasia is commoner in females.

In fibrous dysplasia, the normal medullary bone is replaced by fibrous tissue. This usually presents in the first two decades of life.

There are two forms depending on the number of bones involved:

a   Monostotic (i.e. one bone) is more common (70%–85%).

b   Polyostotic (i.e. involving more than one bone).

McCune-Albright syndrome (the polyostotic form of fibrous dysplasia, precocious puberty, café-au-lait spots) is rare and preferentially affects young girls [18].

Clinical presentation

Patients can be asymptomatic and diagnosed incidentally. Some may present with bone pain, swelling and/or tenderness. A quarter of monostotic cases arise in the facial skeleton, particularly in the posterior maxilla and mandible. In polyostotic disease up to 75% of the body can be affected. Fibrous dysplasia leads to deformity (due to asymmetric/focal overgrowth) and fracture.

Investigations

CT identifies a typical ground glass appearance of the abnormal, fibrous bone.

Management

Treatment is based on symptoms and is usually reserved for visual loss or when there is significant cosmetic deformity. There are no medications capable of altering the disease course. Intravenous bisphosphonates may be helpful for treatment of bone pain. Malignant transformation is rare.

Ossifying fibroma

Ossifying fibroma is also a condition where normal bone is replaced by fibrous tissue. It is usually diagnosed in patients in their 30s and 40s. It preferentially affects the mandible (75%) or maxilla (10%–20%). The exact pathophysiology is not clearly understood [19].

Clinical presentation

It often presents as a rounded, painless swelling.

Investigations

On x-ray imaging, the lesions are initially radiolucent becoming more radiopaque as they mature.

Management

Like fibrous dysplasia, treatment is based on symptoms but the majority will have a surgical excision.

▌ Sinonasal inverted papilloma

A variety of sinonasal papillomas originate from the Schneiderian membrane. Based on microscopic appearances they are classified into inverted papilloma (endophytic growth), fungiform (exophytic) and oncocytic papilloma.

The most interesting of these is inverted papilloma due to its propensity for local tissue destruction, high recurrence and malignant transformation. It is the second most common benign nasal tumour (after osteoma) with an incidence of 0.5–1.6 cases/100,000 per year [20]. It commonly arises from the lateral nasal wall in the region of the middle meatus. This tumour is characterised by endophytic growth into the underlying stroma (intact basement membrane) with adjacent tissue destruction. Despite having the word 'papilloma' in its name, there is not definitive evidence this is caused by human papillomavirus.

Clinical presentation

The presenting symptoms are nasal obstruction, epistaxis, rhinorrhea and hyposmia.

Investigations

A CT reveals opacification and underlying bony erosion or hyperostosis. A characteristic feature of many inverted papillomas is focal hyperostosis at the origin of the tumour on CT.

MRI (on T2 and T1 contrast-enhanced sequences) often demonstrates characteristic mucosal infoldings, described as a convoluted cerebriform pattern, which distinguishes the tumour from the normal mucosal lining and mucus.

This tumour is staged by Krouse based on the extent of tumour involvement endoscopically and CT scan evaluation (see **Table 13.6**) [21].

Management

Surgery is the primary modality of choice. This is performed endoscopically in the vast majority of patients. Simple debridement of the lesion, as in benign polyp disease, leads to an unacceptable recurrence rate. The most important factors in preventing the recurrence of inverted papillomas are the determination of the location of the attachment and the completeness of resection during the primary surgery [22]. It is vital that complete resection of the affected and surrounding mucosa and mucoperiosteum with reduction of underlying bone be performed to minimise recurrence. The majority of inverted papillomas originate from the lateral nasal wall (see **Table 13.7**). This means a medial maxillectomy would be the minimum operation recommended for

Table 13.6 Krouse staging of sinonasal inverted papilloma.

Krouse stage	Disease extent
Stage I	Limited to the nasal cavity alone
Stage II	Limited to the ethmoid sinuses and medial and superior portions of the maxillary sinuses
Stage III	Involves the lateral or inferior aspects of the maxillary sinuses or extension into the frontal or sphenoid sinuses
Stage IV	Involves tumour spread outside the confines of the nose and sinuses, as well as any malignancy

Source: Krouse JH, *Laryngoscope.* 2000;110(6):965–8.

Table 13.7 Distribution of site of attachment of sinonasal inverted papilloma.

Site of attachment	Proportion of cases (%)
Maxillary sinus	42
Ethmoid sinus	18
Nasal cavity	15
Middle/superior turbinates	12
Frontal sinus	10
Sphenoid sinus	1.5
Cribriform plate	1.5

Source: Schneyer MS et al. *Int Forum Allergy Rhinol.* 2011;1(4):324–8.

these tumours, as these would obtain excision with mucosal and bony margins. The recurrence rate varies in the literature and can be anything up to 25% in definitive surgery and higher in cases where only a limited polypectomy has been performed [23].

Long-term follow-up is recommended to detect recurrence or transformation, as the disease can become quite extensive before it becomes symptomatic. In challenging inverted papilloma cases with multiple recurrences, 5-fluorouracil may have a place postoperatively [22]. The rates of synchronous and metachronous carcinomatous transformation of inverted papilloma are 7.1% and 3.6%, respectively. The mean time taken to develop a metachronous carcinoma in a systematic review was reported to be 52 months (range 6 to 180 months) [23].

Juvenile nasopharyngeal angiofibroma (JNA)

Juvenile nasopharyngeal angiofibroma (JNA) is an uncommon, benign, locally aggressive vascular lesion. In terms of pathogenesis, JNA is thought to be a vascular malformation rather than tumour. It arises from testosterone-sensitive cells in the vicinity of the pterygoid wedge, accounting for why JNA is only seen in males.

Clinical presentation

Found almost exclusively in young men, the early symptoms include nasal obstruction and epistaxis. As the tumour grows, facial swelling, visual or neurological deficits occur.

Investigations

The evaluation of patients with juvenile angiofibroma relies on diagnostic imaging. CT hallmarks include widening of the sphenopalatine foramen and pterygopalatine fossa, and anterior bowing of the posterior wall of maxilla. MRI typically reveals signal flow voids. The diagnosis is made radiologically; preoperative biopsy is not recommended due to the bleeding risk. Angiography providing information on the vascular supply of the tumour to assist surgical planning and providing a means by which to embolise the main feeding branches. The Pittsburgh staging system assesses two important tumour attributes: route of intracranial extension and extent of vascular supply from the internal carotid artery [25].

Management

The mainstay of treatment is complete resection, either endoscopically, open or combined approach. Preoperative embolisation reduces the vascularity of the tumour and is routinely performed in most units. When there is residual disease present, it is commonly in the basisphenoid due to invasion of the vidian canal, and this can lead to recurrence unless it is addressed intraoperatively. Postoperative contrast-enhanced CT or MR imaging is recommended to detect residual tumour. Radiotherapy and anti-androgenic therapies have significant side effects and are reserved for inoperable tumours.

▋ Neurogenic tumour

Both schwannoma (**Figure 13.3**) and neurofibroma fall into the neurogenic tumour group. Schwannomas arise from supporting cells around the nerve and rarely turn malignant. They occur along the branches of the trigeminal nerve and the autonomic nervous system. They arise from the ethmoid and maxillary sinuses, followed by the nasal cavity, sphenoid and frontal sinuses (see **Figure 13.4**).

Patients present with a mass lesion, obstruction, pain and, uncommonly, epistaxis [26].

Neurofibromas arise from within nerve fibres and usually occur as part of Von Recklinghausen's disease. They can undergo malignant change. These

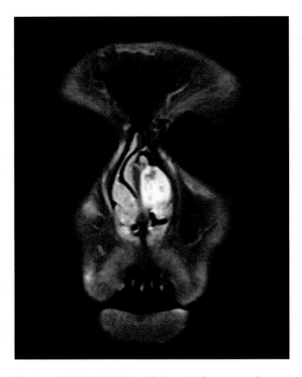

Figure 13.3 MRI (T1 gadolinium) showing enhancement of the schwannoma within the left anterior nasal cavity.

tumours should be completely excised unless vital surrounding structures are involved in which case subtotal resection is acceptable.

MALIGNANT TUMOURS

Primary epithelial tumours are more common than non-epithelial malignant tumours. Squamous cell carcinoma is the most common epithelial tumour, whilst lymphoma is the most common non-epithelial tumour.

▋ Squamous cell carcinoma (SCC)

Squamous cell carcinoma is the most common sino-nasal malignant tumour (>70%). The maxillary sinus is predominantly affected (70%), followed by the nasal cavity (20%) then ethmoid sinus [27].

It primarily affects males in their 60s. There are recognised occupational exposure risk factors for this disease. These include wood dust workers, leather dust workers, formaldehyde, farming and construction [7].

This tumour usually presents at an advanced stage with local invasion and occasionally metastasis (see **Figures 13.5** and **13.6**). The first echelon of nodal drainage is into the retropharyngeal nodes and then into the subdigastric nodes.

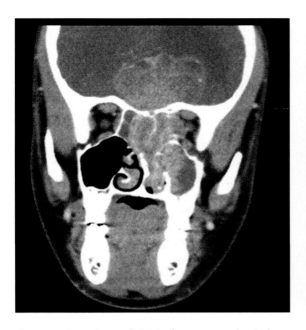

Figure 13.4 Coronal CT (soft tissue window) showing olfactory neuroblastoma extending intracranially, filling the nasal cavity, and eroding the lamina papyracea.

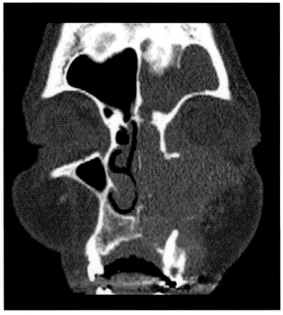

Figure 13.5 Coronal CT of squamous cell carcinoma eroding the various walls of maxillary sinus and extending into nasal cavity.

▌ Adenocarcinoma

Adenocarcinoma is the second most common malignant sinonasal tumour (5%–20%). These tend to be more superiorly located within the ethmoid sinuses. They are related to occupational wood dust exposure, with a much greater increased risk of developing this cancer compared to SCC, particularly of hardwood dusts. They have also been associated with leather dust, formaldehyde and the textile industry [7].

Histologically, they can be divided into salivary type (5%–10%), and non-salivary type. The non-salivary type can be further divided into intestinal type (ITAC) and non-intestinal type.

Of the two types of adenocarcinomas – intestinal and non-intestinal – only the former is associated with wood dust exposure. The tumour tends to be multifocal within the nasal cavity (particularly ITAC) due to bilateral exposure to carcinogens, so bilateral ethmoid resections are usually performed.

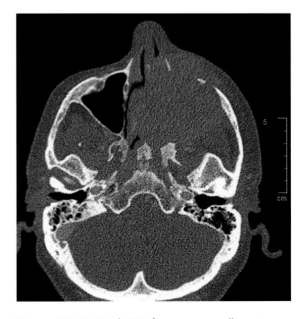

Figure 13.6 Axial CT of squamous cell carcinoma eroding the various walls of maxillary sinus and extending into nasal cavity, cheek and infratemporal fossa.

Adenoid cystic carcinoma

Adenoid cystic carcinoma arises within the minor salivary glands of the paranasal sinus. In general it tends to grow at an intermediate rate and has a low risk of lymphatic spread [28]. Perineural spread is common therefore accounting for delayed local recurrence and metastasis, despite aggressive surgery and radiotherapy. Distant metastases most commonly are found in the lungs. Though adjuvant radiotherapy is usually given, there is no definitive evidence it improves survival [28].

Melanoma

Sinonasal melanoma represents the most common mucosal site of melanoma in the head and neck (66%) [29]. They arise from melanocytes located in the respiratory epithelium. Mucosal melanomas represent approximately 1% of all melanomas. Their aetiology is poorly understood, due to their rareness. These tumours have a variable amount of pigmentation. Up to 30% of mucosal melanomas can be amelanotic leading to diagnostic challenges and incomplete clearance.

Like most sinonasal tumours, the presentation is non-specific. On CT, a polyp lesion may be visible with bony remodelling or erosion. On MRI, a high T1 signal may sometimes be seen due to paramagnetic melanin within the tumour. Biopsy and immunohistochemistry often reveal positivity for vimentin, S100 and melan-A. Mucosal melanomas are now recognised to have distinct molecular alterations compared to cutaneous or uveal melanomas; BRAF V600E mutations are rare (<6%) in mucosally derived melanomas compared to cutaneous melanomas (50%) [39].

A variant of the TNM system (see **Table 13.3**) is used to stage sinonasal mucosal melanoma, which reflects its universally poor prognosis. T1 and T2 disease do not exist for sinonasal melanoma. Treatment is primarily surgery with or without postoperative radiation therapy. This tumour type is not infrequently seen in older patients who are poor candidates for radical, curative treatment. They can be managed with debulking and palliative procedures to improve airway and epistaxis.

Olfactory neuroblastoma

Olfactory neuroblastoma (ONB) is a rare tumour originating from olfactory epithelium. ONB represents approximately 5% of all malignant sinonasal tumours. There is a wide age range (3–90 years); some authors report a bimodal peak in the second and sixth decades [30].

The hallmark of diagnosis is rosettes of the neuroblastoma cells, but due to the wide variation in histology, it is sometimes mistaken as undifferentiated carcinoma. Hyams grading and Kadish staging (see **Table 13.8**) are used to prognosticate and guide treatment decisions. There is significantly better survival for Hyams low-grade (I and II) disease than high-grade (III and IV) tumours (56% vs 25% respectively). Staging is performed using a system proposed by Kadish et al. (**Figure 13.4**) [31].

The primary treatment modality is surgery (open or EEA) followed by postoperative radiotherapy. Advanced lesions with extensive intracranial involvement (stage C) may require adjuvant chemotherapy.

Neuroendocrine carcinoma (NEC): Small cell (SmCC) and large cell types

These rare tumours are highly aggressive, presenting with systemic metastasis in a short space of

Table 13.8 Kadish staging for ONB.

Stage	Tumour extent
A	Limited to nasal cavity
B	Limited to paranasal sinuses and nasal cavity
C	Extends beyond the nasal cavity and paranasal sinuses

Source: Kadish S et al. *Cancer.* 1976;37(3):1571–6.

time. Recent data reported that neoadjuvant chemotherapy followed by surgical resection and adjuvant intensity-modulated radiotherapy (IMRT) can improve survival outcomes [32,33].

Sinonasal undifferentiated carcinoma (SNUC)

Sinonasal undifferentiated carcinoma (SNUC) is a rare aggressive tumour with an overall low incidence of 0.02 per 100,000 person. SNUC demonstrates a predilection for males: 3:1 male-to-female ratio. It tends to present in the 50s but has a broad age range [34]. It is rapidly progressive and typically presents late with local invasion and cervical neck nodes.

If the diagnosis is advanced stage, there is difficulty in achieving negative margins surgically, and a high rate of recurrence makes treatment very challenging. Despite multimodality treatment (surgery, radiotherapy $\pm$ chemotherapy), the prognosis is poor, with a median survival of less than 18 months and 5-year survival of less than 20%. In a recent study, no statistically significant differences in disease-free and overall survival were identified between patients treated with chemoradiation or surgery followed by adjuvant therapy [34].

Chondrosarcoma

Chondrosarcomas are malignant mesenchymal tumours with a cartilaginous origin. They can occur at any age. They commonly arise from the nasal septum or clivus. Patient typically present with nasal obstruction (septal involvement), or headaches, dizziness and diplopia (clival involvement). CT demonstrates a multilobulated, heterogeneous lesion consisting of a chondroid matrix with peripheral and scattered central calcifications. On MR imaging,

the high water content of the chondroid matrix presents with high signal on T2. However, calcifications of the chondroid matrix can result in signal voids. Management is by surgical resection with some evidence for adjuvant radiotherapy [35].

Lymphoma

Lymphomas are the second most common malignant tumours occurring in the sinonasal tract following carcinomas. They are divided into Hodgkin lymphoma (HL) and non-Hodgkin lymphoma (NHL). The term NHL has been replaced by the dominating cell type into B-, T- and natural killer (NK) cell lymphomas [36].

Sinonasal lymphoma is more common in Asia compared to the West. B-cell lymphoma is most common in the maxillary sinus and has a better prognosis compared to the T-cell lymphoma arising from the nasal septum. Though diagnosed by biopsy, they are not managed surgically [36].

Rhabdomyosarcoma

Although rhabdomyosarcoma is relatively rare, it is the most common soft tissue sarcoma in the paediatric population. It is a malignancy of the skeletal muscle. The embryonal subtype predominates in children, while the alveolar subtype predominates in adults [37].

These sinonasal tumours often spread to adjacent sites like the skull base and orbit. About 40% metastasise to lymph nodes, bones and lungs. The tumours are staged according to the Intergroup Rhabdomyosarcoma Study. The first treatment strategy is chemotherapy, with or without radiotherapy. Surgery is reserved for non-responders or recurrent disease [38].

CONCLUSION

The clinical management of sinonasal tumours has dramatically improved through advances in endoscopic techniques, irradiation modalities and induction chemotherapy. Despite this, outcomes are far

from optimal. The key factor in unlocking the appropriate treatment strategy is a more refined approach to tumour classification based on tumour genomics and molecular profiling, rather than the classic anatomical and histological grouping. This would open the possibility of new drug targets and personalized treatment.

Identifying the tumour at an early stage is vital. There should be greater awareness amongst patient and healthcare professionals of the non-specific nature of symptoms. For optimal treatment, patients should be treated by a multidisciplinary team within centres specialised in skull based pathologies.

REFERENCES

1 Barnes L, Eveson J, Reichart P, Sidransky D. *Pathology and Genetics: Head and Neck Tumors.* IARC Press; 2005.

2 Lund VJ, Clarke PM, Swift AC, McGarry GW, Kerawala C, Carnell D. Nose and paranasal sinus tumours: United Kingdom National Multidisciplinary Guidelines. *J Laryngol Otol.* 2016;130(S2):S111–S8.

3 Castelnuovo P, Lepera D, Turri-Zanoni M, Battaglia P, Bolzoni Villaret A, Bignami M et al. Quality of life following endoscopic endonasal resection of anterior skull base cancers. *J Neurosurg.* 2013;119(6):1401–9.

4 Iannetti G, Valentini V, Rinna C, Ventucci E, Marianetti TM. Ethmoido-orbital tumors: Our experience. *J Craniofac Surg.* 2005;16(6):1085–91.

5 Gerth DJ, Tashiro J, Thaller SR. Pediatric sinonasal tumors in the United States: Incidence and outcomes. *J Surg Res.* 2014;190(1):214–20.

6 Wolf J, Schmezer P, Fengel D, Schroeder HG, Scheithauer H, Woeste P. The role of combination effects on the etiology of malignant nasal tumours in the wood-working industry. *Acta Otolaryngol Suppl.* 1998;535:1–6.

7 Binazzi A, Ferrante P, Marinaccio A. Occupational exposure and sinonasal cancer: A systematic review and meta-analysis. *BMC Cancer.* 2015;15:49.

8 Syrjanen KJ. HPV infections in benign and malignant sinonasal lesions. *J Clin Pathol.* 2003;56(3):174–81.

9 Mehrad M, Chernock RD, El-Mofty SK, Lewis JS, Jr. Diagnostic discrepancies in mandatory slide review of extradepartmental head and neck cases: Experience at a large academic center. *Arch Pathol Lab Med.* 2015;139(12):1539–45.

10 Hanna EY, Cardenas AD, DeMonte F, Roberts D, Kupferman M, Weber R et al. Induction chemotherapy for advanced squamous cell carcinoma of the paranasal sinuses. *Arch Otolaryngol Head Neck Surg.* 2011;137(1):78–81.

11 Hadad G, Bassagasteguy L, Carrau RL et al. A novel reconstructive technique after endoscopic expanded endonasal approaches: Vascular pedicle nasoseptal flap. *Laryngoscope.* 2006;116(10):1882–6.

12 Lopez F, Grau JJ, Medina JA, Alobid I. Spanish consensus for the management of sinonasal tumors. *Acta Otorrinolaringol Esp.* 2017;68(4):226–34.

13 Majer J, Herman P, Verillaud B. 'Mailbox Slot' pericranial flap for endoscopic skull base reconstruction. *Laryngoscope.* 2016;126(8):1736–8.

14 Zanation AM, Snyderman CH, Carrau RL, Kassam AB, Gardner PA, Prevedello DM. Minimally invasive endoscopic pericranial flap: A new method for endonasal skull base reconstruction. *Laryngoscope.* 2009;119(1):13–8.

15 Mattavelli D, Schreiber A, Ferrari M et al. Three-Layer Reconstruction with Iliotibial Tract After Endoscopic Resection of Sinonasal Tumors. *World Neurosurg.* 2017;101:486–92.

16 Suarez C, Ferlito A, Lund VJ et al. Management of the orbit in malignant sinonasal tumors. *Head Neck.* 2008;30(2):242–50.

17 Earwaker J. Paranasal sinus osteomas: A review of 46 cases. *Skeletal Radiol.* 1993;22(6):417–23.

18 MacDonald-Jankowski D. Fibrous dysplasia: A systematic review. *Dentomaxillofac Radiol.* 2009;38(4):196–215.

19 MacDonald-Jankowski DS. Ossifying fibroma: A systematic review. *Dentomaxillofac Radiol.* 2009;38(8):495–513.

20 Lund VJ, Stammberger H, Nicolai P et al. European position paper on endoscopic management of tumours of the nose, paranasal sinuses and skull base. *Rhinol Suppl.* 2010;22:1–143.

21 Krouse JH. Development of a staging system for inverted papilloma. *Laryngoscope.* 2000;110(6):965–8.

22 Adriaensen GF, Lim KH, Georgalas C, Reinartz SM, Fokkens WJ. Challenges in the management of inverted papilloma: A review of 72 revision cases. *Laryngoscope.* 2016;126(2):322–8.

23 Mirza S, Bradley PJ, Acharya A, Stacey M, Jones NS. Sinonasal inverted papillomas: Recurrence, and synchronous and metachronous malignancy. *J Laryngol Otol.* 2007;121(9):857–64.

24 Schneyer MS, Milam BM, Payne SC. Sites of attachment of Schneiderian papilloma: A retrospective analysis. *Int Forum Allergy Rhinol.* 2011;1(4):324–8.

25 Snyderman CH, Pant H, Carrau RL, Gardner P. A new endoscopic staging system for angiofibromas. *Arch Otolaryngol Head Neck Surg.* 2010;136(6):588–94.

26 Azani AB, Bishop JA, Thompson LD. Sinonasal tract neurofibroma: A clinicopathologic series of 12 cases with a review of the literature. *Head Neck Pathol.* 2015;9(3):323–33.

27 Lund VJ, Wei WI. Endoscopic surgery for malignant sinonasal tumours: An eighteen year experience. *Rhinology.* 2015;53(3):204–11.

28 Amit M, Binenbaum Y, Sharma K et al. Adenoid cystic carcinoma of the nasal cavity and paranasal sinuses: A meta-analysis. *J Neurol Surg B Skull Base.* 2013;74(3):118–25.

29 Williams MD. Update from the 4th edition of the World Health Organization Classification of Head and Neck Tumours: Mucosal Melanomas. *Head Neck Pathol.* 2017;11(1):110–7.

30 Faragalla H, Weinreb I. Olfactory neuroblastoma: A review and update. *Adv Anat Pathol.* 2009;16(5):322–31.

31 Kadish S, Goodman M, Wang CC. Olfactory neuroblastoma. A clinical analysis of 17 cases. *Cancer.* 1976;37(3):1571–6.

32 Bell D, Hanna EY, Weber RS et al. Neuroendocrine neoplasms of the sinonasal region. *Head Neck.* 2016;38(Suppl 1):E2259–66.

33 Mitchell EH, Diaz A, Yilmaz T et al. Multimodality treatment for sinonasal neuroendocrine carcinoma. *Head Neck.* 2012;34(10):1372–6.

34 Xu CC, Dziegielewski PT, McGaw WT, Seikaly H. Sinonasal undifferentiated carcinoma (SNUC): The Alberta experience and literature review. *J Otolaryngol Head Neck Surg.* 2013;42:2.

35 Khan MN, Husain Q, Kanumuri VV et al. Management of sinonasal chondrosarcoma: A systematic review of 161 patients. *Int Forum Allergy Rhinol.* 2013;3(8):670–7.

36 Steele TO, Buniel MC, Mace JC, El Rassi E, Smith TL. Lymphoma of the nasal cavity and paranasal sinuses: A case series. *Am J Rhinol Allergy.* 2016;30(5):335–9.

37 Malempati S, Hawkins DS. Rhabdomyosarcoma: Review of the Children's Oncology Group (COG) Soft-Tissue Sarcoma Committee experience and rationale for current COG studies. *Pediatr Blood Cancer.* 2012;59(1):5–10.

38 Szablewski V, Neuville A, Terrier P et al. Adult sinonasal soft tissue sarcoma: Analysis of 48 cases from the French Sarcoma Group database. *Laryngoscope.* 2015;125(3):615–23.

39 Ozturk Sari S, Yilmaz I, Taskin OC, Narli G, Sen F, Comoglu S et al. BRAF, NRAS, KIT, TERT, GNAQ/GNA11 mutation profile analysis of head and neck mucosal melanomas: A study of 42 cases. *Pathology.* 2017;49(1):55–61.

14
THE SALIVARY GLANDS

Giri Krishnan and Neeraj Sethi

ANATOMY

There are three main pairs of salivary glands – the parotid, the submandibular and sublingual. There are numerous other minor salivary glands scattered throughout the mucosa of the upper aerodigestive tract.

■ Parotid gland

The parotid gland is the largest of the main salivary glands. It is positioned anterior and inferior to the ear, seated superficially on the ramus of the mandible, wrapping posteriorly and deeply to it. It extends from the lower border of the mandible and up to the zygomatic arch. It is enclosed within the split investing layer of deep cervical fascia.

The parotid duct (Stensen's duct) leaves the anterior edge of the gland, roughly midway between the zygomatic arch and the corner of the mouth. It crosses the medial border of the master muscle, then turns deeply piercing the buccinator muscle entering the mouth near the second upper molar tooth. It is roughly 5 cm long.

The facial nerve has an important relationship to the gland. It exits the skull through the stylomastoid foramen, passing into the parotid gland, where it divides into upper and lower trunks. These travel through the substance of the gland, creating the arbitrary surgical division between the deep and superficial lobes, before splitting into its five main terminal branches – the temporal, zygomatic, buccal, marginal mandibular and cervical branches.

Blood supply

The posterior auricular, maxillary and superficial temporal branches from the external carotid artery (ECA) supply the gland as they pass through the gland. It drains to the retromandibular vein, which is formed in the substance of the parotid gland by the superficial temporal and maxillary veins.

Lymphatic drainage

Lymph drains to the preauricular (parotid) nodes (of which there can be over 20) and then to the nodes of the upper group of deep cervical nodes [1].

Innervation

The auriculotemporal nerve (a branch of V3) provides sensory innervation to the parotid gland. This division of the trigeminal nerve exits the skull through the foramen ovale. The auriculotemporal nerve also carries parasympathetic secretomotor fibres to the parotid. They originate in the otic ganglion in the infratemporal fossa. The preganglionic parasympathetic fibres to the otic ganglion come from the glossopharyngeal nerve (CN IX) [2].

Submandibular gland

The submandibular gland is surgically divided into superficial and deep lobes relative to the mylohyoid muscle, the posterior, free edge of which it wraps around. The superficial part has a lateral surface that is grooved posteriorly by the facial artery, which hooks under the mandible to reach the face at the front of the masseter muscle. The superficial surface of the gland is covered by skin, platysma and the investing fascia. It is crossed by the facial vein, the cervical and marginal mandibular branches of the facial nerve. Caution needs to be taken during incision when resecting this gland to avoid diving these nerves.

There are submandibular lymph nodes in contact with the surface of the gland, but also within its substance, and therefore the lymph nodes as well as the gland are removed during neck dissections. The deep lobe of the gland is cushioned between the mylohyoid and hyoglossus, and has the lingual nerve running above it and the hypoglossal nerve running below it.

The submandibular duct (Wharton's duct) runs with the deep lobe of the gland between the mylohyoid and the hyoglossus, and opens in the floor of the mouth on the sublingual papilla adjacent to the frenulum of the tongue [2].

Blood supply

Blood supply is from the facial artery. Venous drainage is via the facial vein.

Lymphatic drainage

Lymphatic drainage is to the submandibular lymph nodes.

Innervation

Autonomic preganglionic fibres pass from cell bodies in the superior salivary nucleus in the pons via the nervus intermedius, facial nerve, chorda tympani and the lingual nerve. Postganglionic fibres pass to the submandibular gland and also to the lingual nerve for transmission to the sublingual gland. Sympathetic (vasoconstrictor) fibres come from the plexus around the facial artery [1].

Sublingual gland

The sublingual gland is the smallest of the major salivary glands. It sits in the sublingual fossa in the sublingual fascial space at the floor of the mouth, superficial to the mylohyoid muscle. It has as many as 20 short ducts (of Rivinus), which can occasionally combine to form a sublingual (or Bartholin) duct. This opens through the same opening as the submandibular duct into the oral cavity.

Blood supply

The sublingual and submental arteries supply the sublingual gland. These are branches of the lingual and facial arteries, respectively.

Lymphatic drainage

Lymph drains into the submandibular lymph nodes.

Innervation

The sublingual gland is innervated by the efferent (parasympathetic) fibres of the chorda tympani nerve and the submandibular ganglion of the facial nerve [2].

Minor salivary glands

There are up to 1000 minor salivary glands scattered throughout the oral cavity, sinonasal cavity, pharynx, larynx, trachea, lungs and middle ear. In the oral cavity, they are distributed in the submucosa of the buccal, labial, lingual mucosa, the soft palate, lateral parts of the hard palate and the floor of the

Table 14.1 Parasympathetic innervation of the salivary glands.

Preganglionic	Ganglion	Postganglionic	Glands
CN VII (greater petrosal nerve, nerve of pterygoid canal)	Pterygopalatine	CN V2	Minor salivary glands of oral cavity
CN VII (chorda tympani, lingual nerve)	Submandibular	CN V3	Submandibular gland Sublingual gland Minor salivary glands
CN IX (tympanic nerve, lesser petrosal nerve)	Otic	CN V3	Parotid gland

mouth. These glands have unnamed tiny ducts and blood supply dependent on location, as is their lymphatic drainage.

Innervation

In the oral cavity, minor salivary glands are innervated by the facial nerve (see **Table 14.1**) [2].

PHYSIOLOGY

The salivary glands are exocrine glands that produce and excrete saliva. The maximal rate of saliva production in humans is about 1 mL/min/g of glandular tissue. Saliva is formed via active transport processes that occur in the secretory unit, which are under the control of neuronal and hormonal signals.

Salivary gland structure

The basic unit of a salivary gland consists of an acinus, a secretory duct and a collecting duct.

- The *acinus* has a central lumen surrounded by pyramidal-shaped cells and myoepithelial cells. It produces the primary secretion. Acini are classified as serous (numerous cytoplasmic granules), mucous (clear cytoplasm) or mixed.
- The *secretory ducts* are composed of intercalated and striated ducts, which are intralobular. They make saliva hypotonic by taking in Na^+, releasing K^+ and excreting HCO_3^-.
- The *collecting ducts* are composed of two cell layers – the inner flat cells and the outer

columnar cells. When the myoepithelial cells contract, preformed secretions are expelled through the duct [3].

Saliva

Though saliva is 98% water, there are a plethora of other components in it. These are listed in **Table 14.2** [3].

The functions of saliva are:

- Lubrication (essential for speech, mastication and swallowing)
- Buffering and clearance of acids (due to slightly alkaline pH)
- Maintenance of tooth integrity (by influencing mineralisation, demineralisation and remineralisation)
- Antibacterial activity
- Taste
- Digestion (salivary amylase initiates digestion of carbohydrates) [4]

Table 14.2 Constituents of saliva.

Cells and particles	Epithelial cells, neutrophils, microorganisms (bacteria, viruses, candida and protozoa), microparticles, exosomes
Proteins and peptides	Mucin glycoproteins, statherin, proline-rich proteins, carbonic anhydrase 6, histatins, secretory component, secretory IgA, IgG, albumin, lysozyme, lactoferrin, matrix metalloproteinase-8, interleukin 8, nerve growth factor, leptin, LL37, alpha-defensin
Nucleic acid-containing molecules	DNA, mRNA, noncoding RNA, microRNA
Steroid hormones	Oestrogen, testosterone and cortisol
Lipids	Triglycerides, cholesterol
Small signalling molecules	Adenosine diphosphate
Electrolytes/ions	Na^+, Cl^-, Ca^{2+}

PATHOLOGY

▌ Sialosis

Sialosis refers to the bilateral, diffuse, symmetric, painless enlargement of the salivary glands, most commonly the parotids. It is associated with diabetes, alcohol, obesity, liver disease, malnutrition (and eating disorders) and medications such as ramipril [5].

History

Sialosis can present as a unilateral or bilateral swelling noticed by the patient. Past medical history should reveal any of the aforementioned conditions or medications.

Examination

An examination should reveal bilateral symmetric, non-tender parotid glands. The patient may only have noticed one side, but objective examination should reveal bilaterally, enlarged parotids.

Investigation

Blood tests will reveal no liver abnormality. Ultrasound (US) will confirm no detectable pathology is present.

Management

No specific treatment is needed for sialosis, but screening and lifestyle advice on the aforementioned risk factors is appropriate.

▌ Acute salivary gland infections

Acute infection of the salivary glands (acute sialadenitis) can be caused by a variety of viruses and bacteria. It most commonly affects the parotid gland, though it can affect any salivary gland [6].

Acute bacterial suppurative parotitis is caused most commonly by *Staphylococcus aureus* and mixed oral aerobes and/or anaerobes (see **Table 14.3**). It often occurs in the setting of debilitation, dehydration and poor oral hygiene. Paramyxovirus (mumps) is the most common viral cause of acute parotitis. It can be associated with other serious complications such as sensorineural hearing loss, aseptic meningitis, orchitis and pancreatitis.

History

History should include onset and duration of symptoms.

Table 14.3 Pathogens involved in acute parotitis.

Viral	Bacterial
Paramyxovirus, parainfluenza, Coxsackie, influenza A, cytomegalovirus, Epstein–Barr, human immuno-deficiency virus	*Streptococcus pyogenes, Streptococcus viridans, Streptococcus pneumoniae, Haemophilus influenzae, Peptostreptococcus, Bacteroides, Fusobacterium*

Mumps has an incubation period of 2–3 weeks followed by symptoms of low-grade fever, malaise and anorexia prior to signs of gland infection. In considering viral causes, a drug and immunisation history should also be taken.

Recurrent infection may raise suspicion of sialolithiasis with obstruction of the duct leading to secondary infection of the gland. Also ask about a recent operative history or recent dental work.

Acute suppurative sialadenitis is commonly seen in the hospital in patients who are unable to maintain oral hydration and hygiene independently.

Past medical history is important, as it is more common in patients with diabetes and renal failure.

Examination

Acute suppurative sialadenitis is characterised by the sudden onset of a firm, erythematous swelling of the affected gland with exquisite local pain and tenderness. A purulent discharge may be seen intraorally at the duct orifice. If the parotid gland is involved there may be trismus and dysphagia.

Facial weakness is an uncommon finding.

Fluctuance in the parotid may not be clinically evident until the abscess is quite advanced because of the overlying tense parotid fascia. Submandibular gland infections tend to show fluctuance earlier.

Systemic features such as fevers, chills and marked toxicity are generally present.

Investigation

Imaging studies can be used to differentiate between acute suppurative infection and frank abscess collection, and are useful to assess for inflammation or duct obstruction by a stone. Note that x-ray sialography, which requires the injection of contrast into the salivary duct, cannot be used during acute infection.

Ultrasound

Ultrasound (US) is a good initial imaging modality. It can detect stones in the duct or parenchyma, thereby differentiating between obstructive and non-obstructive sialadenitis. An abscess collection may be seen as a hypoechogenic area surrounded by an irregular echogenic rim within the gland parenchyma. It is, however, highly operator dependent and may be poorly tolerated during acute infection, which can be exquisitely tender.

Computed tomography (CT)

CT is a sensitive tool for differentiating cellulitis from frank abscess with rim enhancement and is a good supplement when US findings are not definitive. It allows for exclusion of spread of infection to the deep neck spaces. It can also identify calcifications, intraglandular masses and adjacent inflammatory stranding [7].

Microbiology

When purulent discharge is present, it should be collected for gram stain and culture. This must be interpreted with caution due to likely contamination with oral flora. The duct openings of each gland must be inspected whilst manually massaging the gland to see if pus can be expressed.

Management

Treatment of suppurative parotitis includes hydration and intravenous antibiotics. Antibiotic regimens for adults include flucloxacillin 2 g IV 6-hourly de-escalated, in an oral step-down regime if clinical improvement is made to oral dicloxacillin 500 mg 6-hourly. Oral clindamycin or IV lincomycin can also be used. Duration of therapy depends on the host immune status, severity and extent of infection and response to therapy.

Since suppurative parotitis may potentially spread to deep fascial spaces of the head and neck and is potentially life-threatening, outpatient management with oral antibiotics is not advised.

Surgical incision and drainage should be implemented if there is no clinical response after 48 hours of treatment with empiric intravenous antibiotics.

Prognosis/follow-up/complications

Progression of the infection may lead to massive swelling of the neck, respiratory obstruction, septicemia and osteomyelitis of the adjacent facial bone. Since the parotid space abuts the parapharyngeal space, suppurative parotitis is an important source of parapharyngeal space infection with potential for septic jugular thrombophlebitis (Lemierre's syndrome).

Other rare potential complications included facial nerve palsy or a fistula. CT sialography and fistulography can be performed to evaluate the extent of the fistula and to exclude the possibility of an underlying malignancy.

In rare instances, recurrent infection of the parotid gland may occur, particularly in patients with co-morbid conditions, such as diabetes mellitus. In such patients, a parotidectomy may be considered as a last resort.

▉ Obstructive salivary gland disease and sialolithiasis

Obstructive salivary gland disease is the most common non-neoplastic salivary gland disorder and may be caused by calculi, ductal stenosis, fibromucinous plugs, foreign bodies or anatomical variants of the ductal system.

Sialolithiasis is the main cause of obstructive sialadenitis. The submandibular gland is involved in 80%–90% of cases, followed by the parotid gland (95%–10%) and sublingual glands (<1%). Calculi vary in size and can be single or multiple. The formation of stones is associated with chronic sialadenitis [8].

History

Patients generally present with a history of recurrent pain and swelling of the affected salivary gland, typically post-prandial. The course of the disease is typically relapsing and remitting.

Examination

The gland should be palpated bimanually for the presence of calculi. Examine the ductal opening for purulence. Intraoral palpation should extend to the floor of the mouth and soft tissue of the tongue and cheek. All of the major salivary glands should be examined for masses, symmetry and the presence of discharge, and the neck should be palpated for lymphadenopathy. A quick cranial nerve examination should be conducted paying particular attention to CN VII and XII.

Investigation

Radiography

Conventional radiography is simple and cheap. Anteroposterior, lateral and oblique intraoral occlusal views are used and calculi are radiopaque in 70% of cases [8]. A disadvantage of this scan is that no anatomical information about the ductal system or soft tissues is available.

Sialography

Sialography can be used to evaluate sialoliths as well as other obstructive entities and inflammatory and neoplastic disease. Filling defects from calculi, retained secretions in chronic sialadenitis, strictures in inflammatory processes, irregular contoured borders in neoplasms and extravasation seen in Sjögren's disease are noted. This investigation is contraindicated in patients with an iodine allergy or in acute sialadenitis [8].

Ultrasonography

US can detect stones with a diameter of 2 or 3 mm, and can be used during acute attacks of sialadenitis [8].

CT scanning

CT can detect any size sialolith, but comes at the expense of higher radiation exposure to the patient. Location of the stone can be elucidated, which can help with surgical planning.

Management

The primary objective of salivary gland sialolithiasis treatment should be preservation of gland function, and minimisation of complication and discomfort for the patient.

Conservative treatment

Non-invasive conservative management with gentle gland massage, use of warm compresses, sialagogues and irrigation is the first-line approach. This has a high success rate when the stones are small and located in the duct. When infection is suspected, antibiotics should be commenced [9].

When conservative management is unsuccessful, invasive management is considered. This includes removal via sialendoscopy, extracorporeal shock-wave lithotripsy or open surgical removal.

Sialendoscopy

Stones up to 4 mm can be drawn out with sialendoscopy and basket retrieval if in a suitable position distal to the gland. This procedure can be carried out under general or local anaesthesia. The duct orifice is first dilated and then the endoscope introduced. A basket is passed behind the stone and activated to collect and retrieve the stone out of the duct [10].

Stones larger than 8 mm in the descending portion of the duct or locked behind strictures have been managed using what is described as 'sialendoscopy assisted surgery'. Briefly, this approach involves using sialendoscopy to locate the stone and then guide an open dissection onto the stone to enable its removal without requiring excision of the gland [11].

Lithotripsy

Moderately sized stones 5–8 mm in diameter can potentially be targeted with lithotripsy. Previously only extracorporeal shock-wave lithotripsy (ECSWL) was available but recently new intracorporeal devices have become available [12].

Stone excision

Stones that are visible or easily palpable superficially in the oral cavity may be excised transorally and the duct marsupialised.

Gland excision

For recalcitrant disease not amenable to or having failed all available alternative means described previously can be managed definitively with gland excision.

Follow-up

Following minimally invasive intervention or conservative management, patients should be encouraged to carry out gland massage several times a day combined with a sour diet and sialagogues to stimulate salivary flow.

Recurrence of sialoliths is uncommon and is estimated to occur in 1%–10% of patients [9].

▮ Benign salivary gland neoplasms

Salivary gland neoplasms are uncommon and are generally benign. It is useful to consider the 'rule of 70s' when approaching salivary gland tumours – approximately 70% of all tumours occur in the parotid, 70% of parotid tumours are benign and 70% of benign parotid neoplasms are pleomorphic adenoma. The proportion of tumours that are malignant rises progressively in submandibular glands, sublingual glands and minor salivary glands [13].

Pathology

Pleomorphic adenoma

Pleomorphic adenomas, also known as benign mixed tumours, are the most common salivary gland tumour. The tumours have epithelioid and connective tissue components. In the parotid gland,

90% occur in the superficial lobe, with some of these forming 'dumbbell tumours' that originate in the superficial lobe and stretch through the stylomandibular 'tunnel' to form a narrow isthmus connecting with more tumours in the deep lobe. Ten per cent originate completely within the deep lobe. Pleomorphic adenomas can also originate in minor salivary glands, most commonly in the palate and then the upper lip. Multiple pleomorphic adenomas are rare [14].

These tumours are unique among the subset of benign salivary tumours because their capsule has varying thickness or completeness with satellite nodules or pseudopodia being well described in the literature [15]. This is why when performing surgery to excise these tumours a surrounding cuff of tissue is mandated by some as essential to reduce the risk of recurrence.

Malignant transformation of pleomorphic adenoma occurs in long-standing tumours. The risk of transformation is 1.5% within the first 5 years and 10% if observed for >15 years [16,17].

Pleomorphic adenoma can uncommonly recur and typically does so at the periphery of the lesion. Multiple foci of recurrence continue to manifest over several years. Surgical excision remains the mainstay of management for recurrent disease and has an increased risk of facial nerve damage and risk of recurrence. Consider radiotherapy for elderly patients after first attempt at revision surgery, but for younger patients repeated surgical procedures can be considered.

Warthin's tumour (papillary cystadenoma lymphomatosum)

Warthin's tumour is the second most common benign salivary gland tumour. This tumour is almost exclusively found in the parotid. Histologically, it demonstrates papillae of eosinophilic epithelia projecting into cystic spaces with a lymphoid matrix [18].

In 10% of cases this tumour is bilateral. It tends to predominate in males and is associated with smoking [18].

Basal cell adenoma

Basal cell adenoma is characteristically encapsulated. It has an intact basement membrane, which differentiates it from pleomorphic adenoma. It can be difficult to distinguish from solid adenoid cystic carcinoma on biopsy [19].

Oncocytoma

Oncocytomas make up less than 1% of benign salivary gland tumours. They usually arise in the parotid but may arise in any other salivary glands.

Others

Other rare benign salivary gland neoplasms include canalicular adenoma and myoepithelioma.

History

Benign tumours of the salivary glands usually present as a slow-growing, painless lump. Patients are generally otherwise asymptomatic.

Warthin's tumour is usually a slow-growing mass, but unlike other benign salivary pathologies, it can present with pain, swelling and other inflammatory changes likely related to an immunologic response of the lymphoid element [18].

Examination

Benign tumours are usually well defined, non-tender and freely mobile. They are commonly found in the tail of the parotid gland, which can be confused as being a level II lymph node. Deep lobe parotid tumours may extend into the parapharyngeal space and may result in a medialised tonsil on inspection of the oropharynx. Benign tumours of the submandibular, sublingual and minor salivary glands are much rarer and therefore, lumps in these areas must be assessed for features that are suggestive of malignancy:

- Facial nerve palsy or paresis (for parotid tumours)
- Weakness or numbness of the ipsilateral tongue (indicating perineural extension in submandibular malignancies)

- Fixation of the mass to overlying skin or underlying structures
- Cervical adenopathy
- Pain (bearing mind that Warthin's tumours may be painful and that swelling due to sialadenitis and sialolithiasis is painful though it follows a different clinical course)

Investigation

Fine-needle aspiration cytology

Fine-needle aspiration cytology (FNAC) is an established first-line technique for diagnosis of salivary neoplasms. It has a greater than 85% specificity for differentiating benign and malignant disease [20]. It must be borne in mind the risk of a false negative result and therefore not regarded as a definitive diagnosis alone. The most common diagnostic error is inadequate sample, so ultrasound guidance is often recommended to improve diagnostic yield.

Imaging

Imaging does not necessarily change the decision for surgery, as parotidectomy is still regarded by many as 'the grand biopsy', but it can help stratify urgency, guide approach and highlight potentially challenging cases such as deep lobe tumours. In submandibular and minor salivary gland disease, imaging is essential.

Advantages of imaging:

- Accurate delineation of location/extent
- Relation to neurovascular structures
- Perineural spread
- Skull base invasion
- Intracranial extension
    - Ultrasound is inexpensive, non-invasive and free of complications. It differentiates solid and cystic tumours and, as already mentioned, enhances accuracy of FNA. The expertise of the operator immensely influences the outcome.
    - CT and MRI (magnetic resonance imaging) provide superior information to other imaging techniques or physical examination. The choice of which imaging modality tends to be influenced by institutional factors such as availability and cost. MRI provides better soft tissue tumour delineation without a dose of radiation, but CT is more widely available and cheaper.

Surgical management

The surgical principles of management of benign salivary gland tumours have remained constant for many years.

The key features for parotidectomy are:

- Complete excision with an adequate margin to avoid local recurrence.
- Type of resection (i.e. partial, superficial, total) depends on tumour size.
- Typically a modified Blair or rhytidectomy incision is used for lower or mid-gland regions of the parotid. The rhytidectomy incision can be extended in the hairline for further exposure.

Tips for identifying facial nerve branches distally during parotidectomy:

- *Marginal mandibular*: Below the lower border of the mandible as it crosses superficial to facial vessels
- *Buccal*: Underneath the parotid-masseteric fascia, coursing parallel to the parotid duct
- *Zygomatic*: Half-way between lateral canthus and tragus

Complications following parotidectomy

Facial nerve palsy

Facial nerve palsy following parotid surgery for benign disease is common. Fortunately, the vast majority are temporary. Temporary weakness occurs in up to half of patients, whilst permanent weakness is much lower and reported to be approximately <3% [21]. Permanent weakness is more likely in revision cases or where total parotidectomy is performed, and often can be predicted and the patient counselled appropriately with facial reanimation planned appropriately.

In the instance of facial nerve palsy, diligent eye care to avoid exposure keratitis is necessary. Artificial tears, lubricating ointment and protective dressings should be used.

Sensory deficits

Greater auricular nerve injury is common during this operation and in many instances it is not possible to save the posterior branch to the ear lobe. Patients may notice a loss in sensation or numbness in this nerve's sensory distribution, but for most it will not cause a significant decrease in quality of life.

Frey's syndrome (auriculotemporal syndrome)

Frey's syndrome presents with flushing or sweating of the ipsilateral face skin during mastication, also known as 'gustatory sweating'. Its true incidence is unknown but estimated to be up to 60% [22,23]. It is caused by aberrant cross-reinnervation between the postganglionic secretomotor parasympathetic fibres to the parotid and the postganglionic sympathetic fibres supplying the sweat glands of the skin. It can be tested with Minor's starch–iodine test, where the ipsilateral face is painted with iodine solution followed by covering the painted area with dust starch powder. When the patient chews a sialogogue there is an appearance of dark blue spots along the face confirming gustatory sweating.

Management options for Frey's syndrome include:

- Prevention – use a thick skin flap during partial superficial parotidectomy
- Watchful waiting (often it is a transient problem that resolves spontaneously)
- Antiperspirant over the skin
- Glycopyrrolate (1%)
- Injection of Botox A
- Tympanic neurectomy

Salivary fistulas/sialoceles

Salivary fistula can occur in up to 14% of patients [24]. It manifests with clear fluid discharge from the wound or as a fluid collection under the skin flaps. The vast majority are self-limiting, but for those that don't resolve, management includes repeated aspiration, pressure dressings, good wound care and patience. Oral anticholinergics such as glycopyrrolate may be helpful for temporarily reducing salivary flow.

▨ Malignant salivary gland neoplasms

Salivary gland malignancies make up only 3% of head and neck malignancies. They are diverse and heterogeneous in their histological appearance and behaviour. The most common primary salivary gland neoplasm is mucoepidermoid carcinoma, followed by adenoid cystic carcinoma. In Australia, the most common malignant parotid lesion is metastatic squamous cell carcinoma. Almost all benign salivary gland neoplasms have a malignant counterpart. Management is dependent on histological type and grade, and where lesions are resectable, surgery tends to be the mainstay, with or without adjuvant postoperative radiotherapy.

Pathology

Mucoepidermoid carcinoma

Mucoepidermoid carcinoma is the most common salivary gland cancer, with the majority arising in major salivary glands. It is more common in women.

Grading is important and correlates strongly with clinical behaviour:

- Low-grade predominantly cystic with abundant well-differentiated mucous cells, less aggressive with lower risk of cervical metastasis and recurrence
- High-grade more solid with squamoid and intermediate cells predominating [25]

Adenoid cystic carcinoma

Adenoid cystic carcinoma is notorious for its infiltrative growth and slowly progressive behaviour with a high rate of late recurrences and distant metastases, related to perineural invasion, and spread over a protracted course of many years. Patients with these malignancies therefore require follow-up for at least 20 years [26].

Histologically there are three growth patterns:

- *Tubular*: Small tubules, sitting in a pink, hyalinised, hypocellular stroma
- *Solid*: Rounded lobules of tumour cells with almost no gland-like structures (defined as >30% solid within a cribriform background)
- *Cribriform*: The classic 'Swiss cheese' variant; nests of cells arranged around gland-like spaces
  - Cells are markedly basaloid with little cytoplasm and round-to-oval nuclei
  - Uniform cell size with little mitotic activity (except solid type)

FNA demonstrates tumour cells with scant cytoplasm and round, regular nuclei in sheets and clusters. Clinical staging is more important than histologic grading [26]. These tumours can be extensive and extend into tissue that appears macroscopically normal at the time of surgery. Local control despite positive margins is usually achieved, but the risk of late metastasis remains.

Acinic cell carcinoma

Acinic cell carcinomas are tumours with cells showing differentiation toward cells of the normal salivary gland acini. They are uncommon, and more than 90% occur in parotid. They affect a wide age range of patients from children to the elderly [27].

Histology [27]:

- Highly variable
- Four patterns – solid/lobular, microcystic, papillary-cystic, follicular
- Two classical features
  - Acinic cell – blue cytoplasm with abundant serous-type granules and a small, round, eccentrically placed nucleus
  - Dense lymphoid infiltrate with germinal centres
- Periphery often not infiltrative but pushing
- No benign equivalent for this lesion

Recurrence occurs in one-third of patients and 10% metastasise locally or distantly. Survival is 90% at 5 years and 70% at 10 years. Dedifferentiation is associated with poor outcome [28].

Polymorphous low-grade adenocarcinoma

Polymorphous low-grade adenocarcinoma arises almost exclusively from minor salivary glands. It is the second most common minor salivary gland carcinoma and occurs most commonly on the palate [29].

Histology:

- Quite variable
- Well-circumscribed but unencapsulated with peripheral infiltration
- PNI is common

It is a low-grade malignancy and conservative resection is the treatment of choice. Local recurrence occurs in 10%–15%, and regional lymph node metastases are distinctly uncommon [29].

Malignant mixed tumour

The term 'malignant mixed tumour' encompasses three tumour types [30]:

- True malignant mixed tumour (carcinosarcoma)
  - Distinct carcinomatous and sarcomatous (chondro- or osteo-) components
- Carcinoma ex pleomorphic adenoma (the most common)
  - A pleomorphic adenoma in which a carcinoma is present
  - Extent of invasion is critical for prognostication
    - Non-invasive
    - Minimally invasive (<1.5 mm beyond capsule)
    - Invasive (>1.5 mm)
- Metastasising pleomorphic adenoma
  - Least common
  - Metastasise to local lymph nodes (30%) or distant sites such as bone (50%) and lung (30%)
  - Typically poor prognosis

Treatment involves wide local excision and postoperative radiotherapy.

History

Pain is more common in malignant cases than benign disease but is only present in 10% of cases. Episodic pain and swelling is more likely to indicate salivary gland obstruction and inflammation. Constant pain is more worrisome. It is important to ask for a history of previous skin cancer.

Examination

Parotid gland assessment

- Palpation of gland for tenderness or fixation to underlying structures
- Palpation of the neck for cervical adenopathy
- Assessment of overlying skin for involvement or fixation
- Bimanual palpation of buccal space including Stensen's duct
- Examination of the oropharynx for deep lobe involvement and medialised tonsil
- Facial nerve assessment – 10% present with VII palsy (a poor prognostic indicator); where present with a parotid mass it should be considered malignant until proven otherwise
- Complete cranial nerve exam for cranial nerve neuropathies secondary to a tumour extending to the post-styloid compartment
- Otoscopy to assess for an anterior bulge of the external auditory canal
- Skin inspection to identify concerning lesions or scars from previous excision

Submandibular/sublingual gland assessment

- Bimanual palpation of the gland to assess extent of tumour and fixation to skin or mandible
- Assess for signs of tumour involvement in closely related nerves:
  - Lingual nerve: Numbness of tongue
  - Hypoglossal nerve: Weakness of tongue
  - Facial nerve: Weakness of the lower lip

Cervical lymph node examination

Up to 20% of malignant salivary gland tumours and 16% of minor salivary gland cancers will present with clinically apparent nodal metastases [31,32].

Investigation

Fine-needle aspiration

See earlier discussion.

Core biopsy

Core biopsy can increase sensitivity and specificity, especially for lymphoma and inflammatory conditions. Accurate diagnosis enables avoidance of unnecessary surgery. However, the risk of seeding must be borne in mind (which remains important for benign tumours as well).

Frozen section

Frozen section is used less often as a first-line diagnostic option since the widespread adoption of FNA. It still plays a role in assessing extent of tumour spread to local or regional tissues, assessment of surgical margins, or confirmation or establishment of the diagnosis in cases where preoperative FNA was not diagnostic or was equivocal. On its own it is insufficient to make radical management decisions. It has no significant risk of tumour seeding, but widely overlapping histology usually necessitates biopsy or resection tissue for definitive diagnosis, especially for low-grade tumours.

Imaging

Ultrasound

Ultrasound is cheap, can depict the location of superficial tumours reliably and guide the needle for aspiration/biopsy. It has limited view of the deep parotid extension and is limited at distinguishing between benign and malignant tumours [33].

CT

CT is particularly useful for assessing cortical bone erosion from adjacent tumours, assessing intra-mass calcifications, and can identify the superficial and deep lobe tumour. It cannot distinguish definitively between benign and malignant tumours.

MRI

Benign and malignant lesions are well visualised on MRI with better soft tissue delineation. They typically have a low-intermediate T1 signal. T2 signal may be used to distinguish benign from malignant salivary gland neoplasms, with benign lesions demonstrating a high signal and malignant lesions demonstrating a low signal with poorly defined margins. MRI can also provide information on extent of tumour spread (i.e. deep vs superficial) and nodal disease [33].

PET

Positron emission tomography (PET) is not often used for the evaluation of salivary gland tumours and cannot reliably distinguish between benign and malignant disease, as Warthin's tumours are fluoro-deoxyglucose (FDG) avid.

Staging

Clinical staging is used for prognosis and treatment decisions.

Major salivary glands staging according to the eighth edition of the American Joint Committee on Cancer (AJCC) staging manual [30]:

- Tis: Tumour confined to the cells lining the salivary duct
- T1: <2 cm no extraparenchymal spread
- T2: 2–4 cm no extraparenchymal spread
- T3: >4 cm or extraparenchymal spread
- T4a: Invades skin, mandible, external auditory canal (EAC), VII
- T4b: Invades skull base, pterygoid plates, encases carotid artery

Minor salivary glands are staged as per their anatomic site of origin (e.g. oral cavity, sinus, larynx).

Management

Primary tumour resection

Resectable salivary gland malignancies are treated surgically with either parotidectomy, or submandibular or sublingual gland excision depending on which salivary gland is involved. The resection of minor salivary gland malignancies is dictated by the site of the tumour. As the palate is the most frequent location, transoral and transfacial approaches are most commonly used.

Resection of the facial nerve during parotidectomy depends on whether it is involved with the tumour. If it is frankly involved and preoperatively paralytic, then it must be sacrificed to negative margins. Otherwise the nerve is preserved wherever possible if fully functional beforehand. Routine resection of the facial nerve insignificantly affects locoregional control/distant metastasis.

Management of the deep lobe is another important consideration when planning parotidectomy. It does not need to be resected routinely and should be palpated at time of surgery to guide this decision.

Success in parotid surgery is generally assessed by:

- Adequacy of resection
- Facial nerve function
- Contour deformity
- Incisions

Management of the neck

The decision to treat a clinically node-negative neck is controversial. Most advocate that the neck should be treated only in patients with tumours that have poor prognostic features for metastasis, such as:

- High T stage
- High-grade tumour (i.e. high-grade mucoepidermoid carcinoma, salivary ductal carcinoma, carcinoma ex pleomorphic)
- Parotid tumour is actually a nodal metastasis (i.e. SCC)

Adjuvant therapy

Radiotherapy is good for clearing microscopic disease postoperatively and appears to improve locoregional control. Chemotherapy generally plays no role for curative treatment and is reserved for palliative management of locally advanced, unresectable, recurrent or metastatic disease.

Follow-up

Patients with malignant salivary gland disease required long term follow-up. Though clinical assessment is a vital part of this interval cross-sectional imaging (e.g. MRI) is commonly used to exclude any recurrence deep in the neck. This is particularly useful in patients with a history of malignant parotid disease and extensive surgical resection which may include overlying free flaps making assessment of the resection bed clinically very difficult. It is the author's practice to employ MRI imaging in these cases, initially at 6 months post-treatment and then 6 monthly for the first two years, and annually thereafter.

REFERENCES

1 McKean ME, Lee K, McGregor IA. The distribution of lymph nodes in and around the parotid gland: An anatomical study. *Br J Plast Surg.* 1985;38(1):1–5.

2 Standring S, editor. *Gray's Anatomy: The Anatomical Basis of Clinical Practice.* 41st ed. Elsevier; 2015.

3 Proctor GB. The physiology of salivary secretion. *Periodontol 2000.* 2016;70(1):11–25.

4 Mandel ID. The functions of saliva. *J Dent Res.* 1987;66 Spec No:623–7.

5 Scully C, Bagan JV, Eveson JW, Barnard N, Turner FM. Sialosis: 35 cases of persistent parotid swelling from two countries. *Br J Oral Maxillofac Surg.* 2008;46(6):468–72.

6 McQuone SJ. Acute viral and bacterial infections of the salivary glands. *Otolaryngol Clin North Am.* 1999;32(5):793–811.

7 Kessler AT, Bhatt AA. Review of the major and minor salivary glands, Part 1: Anatomy, infectious, and inflammatory processes. *J Clin Imaging Sci.* 2018;8:47.

8 Bodner L. Salivary gland calculi: Diagnostic imaging and surgical management. *Compendium.* 1993;14(5):572, 574–6, 578 passim; quiz 586.

9 Bull PD. Salivary gland stones: Diagnosis and treatment. *Hosp Med.* 2001;62(7):396–9.

10 Strychowsky JE, Sommer DD, Gupta MK, Cohen N, Nahlieli O. Sialendoscopy for the management of obstructive salivary gland disease: A systematic review and meta-analysis. *Arch Otolaryngol Head Neck Surg.* 2012;138(6):541–7.

11 Hills AJ, Holden AM, McGurk M. Sialendoscopy-assisted transfacial removal of parotid calculi. *Acta Otorhinolaryngol Ital.* 2017;37(2):128–31.

12 Capaccio P, Torretta S, Pignataro L, Koch M. Salivary lithotripsy in the era of sialendoscopy. *Acta Otorhinolaryngol Ital.* 2017;37(2):113–21.

13 Tian Z, Li L, Wang L, Hu Y, Li J. Salivary gland neoplasms in oral and maxillofacial regions: A 23-year retrospective study of 6982 cases in an eastern Chinese population. *Int J Oral Maxillofac Surg.* 2010;39(3):235–42.

14 Eveson JW, Cawson RA. Salivary gland tumours. A review of 2410 cases with particular reference to histological types, site, age and sex distribution. *J Pathol.* 1985;146(1):51–8.

15 Zbaren P, Stauffer E. Pleomorphic adenoma of the parotid gland: Histopathologic analysis of the capsular characteristics of 218 tumors. *Head Neck.* 2007;29(8):751–7.

16 Beahrs OH, Woolner LB, Kirklin JW, Devine KD. Carcinomatous transformation of mixed tumors of the parotid gland. *AMA Arch Surg.* 1957;75(4):605–13; discussion 613–4.

17 Spiro RH, Huvos AG, Strong EW. Malignant mixed tumor of salivary origin: A clinicopathologic study of 146 cases. *Cancer.* 1977;39(2):388–96.

18 Eveson JW, Cawson RA. Warthin's tumor (cystadenolymphoma) of salivary glands. A clinicopathologic investigation of 278 cases. *Oral Surg Oral Med Oral Pathol.* 1986;61(3):256–62.

19 Sowa P, Goroszkiewicz K, Szydelko J et al. A review of selected factors of salivary gland tumour formation and malignant transformation. *Biomed Res Int.* 2018;2018:2897827.

20 Jeong WJ, Park SJ, Cha W, Sung MW, Kim KH, Ahn SH. Fine needle aspiration of parotid tumors: Diagnostic utility from a clinical perspective. *J Oral Maxillofac Surg.* 2013;71(7):1278–82.

21 Sethi N, Tay PH, Scally A, Sood S. Stratifying the risk of facial nerve palsy after benign parotid surgery. *J Laryngol Otol.* 2014;128(2):159–62.

22 Rustemeyer J, Eufinger H, Bremerich A. The incidence of Frey's syndrome. *J Craniomaxillofac Surg.* 2008;36(1):34–7.

23 Motz KM, Kim YJ. Auriculotemporal syndrome (Frey syndrome). *Otolaryngol Clin North Am.* 2016;49(2):501–9.

24 Wax M, Tarshis L. Post-parotidectomy fistula. *J Otolaryngol.* 1991;20(1):10–13.

25 Ghosh-Laskar S, Murthy V, Wadasadawala T et al. Mucoepidermoid carcinoma of the parotid gland: Factors affecting outcome. *Head Neck.* 2011;33(4):497–503.

26 Garden AS, Weber RS, Morrison WH, Ang KK, Peters LJ. The influence of positive margins and nerve invasion in adenoid cystic carcinoma of the head and neck treated with surgery and radiation. *Int J Radiat Oncol Biol Phys.* 1995;32(3):619–26.

27 Al-Zaher N, Obeid A, Al-Salam S, Al-Kayyali BS. Acinic cell carcinoma of the salivary glands: A literature review. *Hematol Oncol Stem Cell Ther.* 2009;2(1):259–64.

28 Wahlberg P, Anderson H, Biorklund A, Moller T, Perfekt R. Carcinoma of the parotid and submandibular glands – A study of survival in 2465 patients. *Oral Oncol.* 2002;38(7):706–13.

29 Chatura KR. Polymorphous low grade adenocarcinoma. *J Oral Maxillofac Pathol.* 2015;19(1):77–82.

30 Amin MB, Greene FL, Edge SB et al. The Eighth Edition AJCC Cancer Staging Manual: Continuing to build a bridge from a population-based to a more 'personalized' approach to cancer staging. *CA Cancer J Clin.* 2017;67(2):93–9.

31 Armstrong JG, Harrison LB, Thaler HT et al. The indications for elective treatment of the neck in cancer of the major salivary glands. *Cancer.* 1992;69(3):615–9.

32 Lloyd S, Yu JB, Ross DA, Wilson LD, Decker RH. A prognostic index for predicting lymph node metastasis in minor salivary gland cancer. *Int J Radiat Oncol Biol Phys.* 2010;76(1):169–75.

33 Kessler AT, Bhatt AA. Review of the major and minor salivary glands, Part 2: Neoplasms and tumor-like lesions. *J Clin Imaging Sci.* 2018;8:48.

15

PAEDIATRIC NECK LUMPS

Mat Daniel

INTRODUCTION

Children's neck lumps are common. They can be divided into those that are congenital and those that are acquired. Although congenital ones are present from birth, they may not become clinically apparent until a later age, for example due to a sudden increase in size precipitated by infection. Congenital neck masses are the subject of a separate chapter.

The commonest acquired lump will be due to reactive lymphadenopathy. Malignancy in children is rare, but proportionally forms a higher number of certain neck lumps in children compared to the proportion in adults (e.g. the majority of clinicians need to keep that possibility in mind and tailor their investigations and management accordingly). Indeed, 12% of all malignant masses in children are detected in the head and neck [1].

ANATOMY

The anatomy of the neck is discussed in previous chapters.

AETIOLOGY

The broad categories for acquired paediatric neck lumps fall into inflammatory/infective and neoplastic. The location of the lump also helps guide working out the aetiology of it as shown in

Table 15.1. There are of course others including traumatic, but these tend to cause less difficulty as a diagnostic conundrum.

Table 15.1 Aetiology of common acquired paediatric neck lumps according to location.

Location	Aetiology	
	Inflammatory/infective	**Neoplastic**
Submental	Lymphadenitis Reactive lymphadenopathy Sialadenitis	Benign connective tissue tumour Malignant lymphadenopathy
Submandibular	Lymphadenitis Reactive lymphadenopathy Sialadenitis	Malignant lymphadenopathy Salivary gland tumour Benign connective tissue tumour
Level II–III	Lymphadenitis Reactive lymphadenopathy Fibromatosis colli	Benign connective tissue tumour Malignant lymphadenopathy
Level IV	Thyroid	Benign connective tissue tumour Malignant lymphadenopathy
Level V	Lymphadenitis Reactive lymphadenopathy	Benign connective tissue tumour Malignant lymphadenopathy

HISTORY

The patient's history, as always, will dictate and focus your examination, investigation, differential diagnosis and management. Key areas to be covered are discussed in the following sections.

▉ Age

Cervical masses in the neonatal period and early infancy are usually congenital (though these can present at a later age) [2]. Reactive lymphadenopathy usually occurs in children over 6 months of age. The age of the child may also provide information about a possible infectious source, for example acute otitis media in children under the age of 2 years. Reactive lymphadenopathy is common with 40%–55% of young children found to have palpable lymph nodes [2].

▉ Duration

Lumps that appear suddenly and last a few days would suggest infectious aetiology. Chronic lymphadenopathy with a lymph node present for longer than 3 or 4 weeks requires a different approach than the acute swelling.

▉ Progression

A lump that is progressively increasing in size would suggest a neoplasm. A lump that fluctuates or is reducing in size would be more typical of infection. Infantile haemangioma has a specific pattern of rapid growth, then involution phase, and finally involuted phase.

▉ Size

Lymph nodes smaller than 1 cm would be unlikely to be malignant [3]. However, neck lumps other than lymph nodes may require investigation even if smaller than 1 cm.

▉ Precipitating factors

Acute upper respiratory or ear infections would be a common precipitant of acute lymphadenopathy, often with associated fever, rhinorrhoea and sore throat. Skin conditions such as eczema would be a common cause of chronic lymphadenopathy. Trauma or local infections can also precipitate the appearance of a neck lump.

Associated symptoms

Acute upper respiratory infections may be associated with an increase in the size of a lump, or the new appearance of a lump. The lump may discharge, suggesting infection, or be painful. The presence of pit would suggest a congenital sinus. In the case of chronic lymphadenopathy, it is important to enquire about weight loss, night sweats, fevers, fatigue, or pain in chest/abdomen, as these may be the symptoms of lymphoma. Other swellings elsewhere in the body may also point to a neoplastic cause. Red flag features of presentation are listed in **Table 15.2**.

Contacts/travel/family history

These could give a clue as to a possible infectious agent such as tuberculosis or cat scratch disease.

Table 15.2 Concerning red flag clinical features of the paediatric neck lump.

Red flags
Weight loss
Night sweats
Widespread lymphadenopathy
Lymph node >3 cm
Location (thyroid, supraclavicular)
Persisting >4 weeks

Past medical history

Past infections may point to an infectious aetiology of a neck lump. Known history of malignancy should prompt formal exclusion of malignancy in the new lump.

EXAMINATION

Location

The anatomical position of the lump should be determined, as that gives clues to the likely aetiology. Midline lumps would commonly be thyroglossal cysts, dermoids or a lymph node. Lumps in the anterior triangle levels II, III, and IV would commonly be reactive lymph nodes, with other causes including congenital branchial cysts, neoplasia, or congenital vascular lesions. In the posterior triangle, lymphadenopathy may occur in the accessory chain (see **Table 15.1**). Supraclavicular lumps would be suspicious of malignancy. Thyroid masses need to be investigated due to the risk of malignancy.

Features

Distinguish lumps that are hard and matted and fixed from ones that are mobile and not attached.

Thyroid lumps move on swallowing. Thyroglossal cysts typically move on tongue protrusion. Non-tuberculous mycobacterial lymphadenopathy would be characterised by violaceous skin discolouration. Red discolouration and tenderness would suggest an acute infective process.

Ear, nose and throat examination

Look for other lumps and a possible source of infection.

General

Look for other lymphadenopathy, hepatosplenomegaly or other systemic abnormality.

INVESTIGATION

In many children, a diagnosis can be made on clinical grounds alone, and no investigations are required.

▮ Blood tests

When investigating neck lymphadenopathy, the following blood tests can help guide further management: full blood count, serology for toxoplasma, cytomegalovirus, and Epstein–Barr virus. *Bartonella henselae* serology (cat scratch disease) is no longer available in the UK, although it is possible to test any excised tissue.

▮ Imaging

Ultrasound

An ultrasound scan can help describe the nature and location of the lump, and is particularly useful in the case of a suspected abscess. Ultrasound alone is not able to diagnose lymphoma, but can accurately measure the size of a lymph node and identify features that would distinguish a benign from a malignant node.

On ultrasound, normal or reactive lymph nodes are well defined and reniform in shape, with fatty echogenic hila and a hypoechoic cortex relative to muscle [4]. Sonographic features of malignant lymphadenopathy include size >1 cm, rounded shape, absence of echogenic hilum, hypoechoic parenchyma and aggregation of lymph nodes [5].

Additionally, colour Doppler can be used to highlight malignant features such as subcapsular vessels, displacement of hilar vasculature and absence of nodal vessels [6].

Ultrasound scan is, however, highly operator-dependent.

Radiography

A chest radiograph can be useful when investigating neck lymphadenopathy, as a means of establishing the presence of mediastinal lymphadenopathy, especially if a general anaesthetic is planned.

Cross-sectional imaging

Cross-sectional imaging is able to describe anatomical relations, and can be useful when planning surgery or identifying deep neck space infection or venous thrombosis. Magnetic resonance imaging (MRI) tends to be better than computerized tomography (CT) for defining soft tissue lesions and it avoids the need for radiation. However, it requires that a child lie still in a claustrophobic environment for 20–30 minutes, so a general anaesthetic may often be required. On the other hand, CT is quick and a general anaesthetic can thus be avoided.

PATHOLOGY

▮ Chronic cervical lymphadenopathy

Chronic neck lymphadenopathy, with nodes persisting more than 3 to 4 weeks or so, is common in otherwise well children. The majority are due to reactive lymphadenopathy, but it is important to exclude an underlying neoplastic cause (principally lymphoma). It may be difficult to reassure patients and differentiate between benign and malignant lymphadenopathy (see **Table 15.3**).

History

Important aspects to cover are:

● History of recent upper respiratory infection, as a trigger for the lymphadenopathy
● Skin conditions, especially affecting the scalp
● Progression and fluctuation, with progressive size increase indicating neoplasm and fluctuation typical of reactive nodes

Table 15.3 Clinical features that help distinguish benign/reactive nodes from ones that are more likely to be malignant.

Probable reactive node	Malignancy should be excluded
Size ≤1 cm	Size >2 or 3 cm
Size fluctuates	Supraclavicular location
Mobile	History of malignancy
Appears with upper respiratory tract infection	Progressive increase in size
Tender	Fixed
No systemic symptoms	Matted
	Systemic symptoms

- Weight loss, drenching night sweats, fevers, rash, itching, and abdominal and chest pain may indicate lymphoma
- Past medical history of neoplasm or conditions that may predispose to malignancy

Examination

- Accurate documentation of the size and distribution of enlarged nodes is important for follow-up and as a criterion for excision biopsy.
- Look for a possible source of infection including ears/nose/throat/scalp/dentition.
- Examination of the axillae and groins for lymph nodes, and of the abdomen for liver and spleen may also lead to findings that suggest serious pathology. Request the help of a paediatrician if you do not feel comfortable to do this yourself and the suspicion of pathology is high.
- Skin discolouration and cold abscess formation in a systemically well child suggests non-tuberculous mycobacterial infection.

Investigation

See earlier.

Management

Clearly benign nodes

Some lymph nodes are clearly reactive/benign requiring no further investigation. Clinicians should be able to reassure parents and discharge them with instructions to return if the nodes get progressively larger (rather than fluctuating in size).

Likely malignant nodes

Lymph nodes clearly suspicious of malignancy will require an urgent biopsy.

Indeterminate nodes

In a large number of children the diagnosis may not be clear, and this is the most difficult group to manage. These patients should have a chest x-ray and blood taken for a full blood count and serology for toxoplasma, cytomegalovirus and Epstein–Barr virus. The child should be reviewed in a fortnight with the test results. Consideration should be given to a trial of antibiotics during this time.

If the full blood count or chest x-ray report is abnormal, the nodes should be excised urgently for histology. If the serology is positive, the diagnosis is made and excision biopsy for histology is not required.

Most children will have negative serology, normal chest x-ray and normal full blood count. Unless the nodes are regressing in size, the only course of action that will lead to a definitive diagnosis at this point is excision biopsy.

It is often worth involving a paediatrician when investigating a child with lymphadenopathy, as they will have a different skill set than the ear, nose and throat surgeon and may be able to help guide management.

▌ Non-tuberculous lymphadenitis

Non-tuberculous mycobacterial (NTM) lymphadenitis was first recognised in the 1950s and is a common cause of unilateral persistent cervicofacial lymphadenitis in young children in industrialised countries. Atypical, or non-tuberculous, mycobacteria are a miscellaneous collection of acid fast, Gram-positive aerobes that are ubiquitous in the environment, existing in soil and water, and as pharyngeal flora in clinically well humans. Examples include *Mycobacterium avium intracellulare* complex, *M. chelonae* or *M. fortuitum.*

History

Infection occurs predominantly in children between the ages of 2 and 5, and is rare after the age of 12. Most children present with a subacute history (2–6 weeks) of firm, painless, discrete mass (usually submandibular or parotid area) that fails to respond to conventional antibiotics. There is no systemic upset or fever.

A common presentation is with a neck lump of a few weeks with violet skin discolouration in a well child. Oral antibiotics are given but fail to help, leading to an emergency admission with suspected abscess. The judicious clinician recognises the possibility of NTM and guides management accordingly, but the unwary proceeds to incision and drainage, and creates a chronically discharging fistula.

Examination

As the disease progresses, the mass enlarges and becomes fluctuant. The overlying skin develops violet discolouration and eventually breaks down, leading to chronic discharge and unsightly scarring. Without treatment, the infection tends to resolve naturally over a period of months to years.

Investigation

NTM lymphadenitis is usually diagnosed clinically; if the diagnosis is unclear, then the investigation pathway outlined in the section on chronic lymphadenitis should be followed.

Skin tests containing purified protein derivative can also be used, with specificity of around 94%, although lower sensitivity.

Imaging can distinguish a solid mass from a fluid collection but cannot diagnose NTM. It is more useful for any surgical planning than for diagnosis.

Needle aspiration can lead to skin breakdown, and culture is only positive in fewer than half of cases; in children, it should be avoided.

Management

Simple incision and drainage must be avoided as healing is protracted and scarring is unsightly.

The ideal scenario is to diagnose NTM early and perform full surgical excision before any skin involvement occurs. In reality, in the UK healthcare setting, diagnosis is usually only made once skin involvement is present, and suppuration or discharge occurs. Full surgical excision is then difficult or impossible due to high risk of damage to surrounding structures and poor skin quality.

The options for NTM with skin involvement/discharge are:

- Do nothing. Discharge is likely to stop spontaneously but may take months [7]. Resulting scarring is likely to be poor, but elective scar revision surgery is possible in the future.
- Curettage of abscess cavity. If skin has broken down and abscess is discharging, evidence suggests that formal curettage speeds up recovery.
- Prolonged oral antibiotics. Choice needs to be guided by microbiology advice. It is a significant undertaking, requiring long treatment duration, potential side effects, as well as concerns about side effects and emergence of resistance [7].
- Surgical excision. Again this is a significant undertaking, requiring a neck-dissection approach in many children. Unless identified early, NTM involvement of tissue and skin is extensive, making surgery challenging. However, when undertaken in appropriate patients speed of resolution of symptoms and cosmetic result may be improved, but plans need to be tailored to the individual patient [8,9].

It is worth noting here that there is only limited high-quality evidence guiding treatment. The literature trends towards surgical excision, but this is by no means definitive. Readers should be cautious when interpreting such publications. In the case of a self-resolving condition, the clinician needs to be sure that what is offered to patients is better than doing nothing. Conservative management should be an option, albeit with associated downsides too.

The best way of managing cervical NTM lymphadenitis is at present not known. Clinicians need to be wary of operating on the basis of parental pressure, case series or so that 'something is being done' for a condition that without treatment may resolve anyway. The risks and benefits of surgery should be discussed with parents and individual decisions made, taking into account stage of disease, research evidence and parental preference.

▌ Thyroid masses in children

Thyroid nodules in children are uncommon. They occur in up to 2% of children [10]. Up to 50% of thyroid nodules in children have been reported to be malignant [11]. Thyroid cancer is the most common endocrine malignancy in children [12]. The distribution of thyroid cancer in children is similar to that of adults with papillary thyroid carcinoma being the most common.

History

The majority present with an isolated non-compressive neck mass and are euthyroid [13]. Questions should be asked of the symptoms of hyper- or hypothyroidism. These masses tend to be slow growing. Compressive symptoms should be interrogated for dysphagia, hoarseness, and shortness of breath.

Risk factors for thyroid malignancy include:

- Prior history of thyroid disease (e.g. Hashimoto's disease)
- Exposure to radiation
- Genetic disease (e.g. multiple endocrine neoplasia type II)

Medullary thyroid carcinoma (MTC) forms 5% of paediatric thyroid malignancies. Approximately 20% of patients with MTC have familial cancer associated with a germline RET mutation [10]. Familial MTC may occur in isolation or as part of multiple endocrine neoplasia type IIa and type IIb (MEN II and MEN III in the new classification) [10]. Associations within these syndromes are shown in **Table 15.4**.

Non-medullary paediatric thyroid carcinomas can occur in conditions such as Carney's complex (multiple neoplasia and lentiginosis syndrome) or Cowden's syndrome (multiple hamartoma syndrome) [10].

Examination

Neck examination should include the thyroid and cervical lymph nodes, as metastatic lymphadenopathy in paediatric thyroid cancer is common. The size, consistency, tenderness and fixity of the thyroid should be assessed.

Investigation

Blood tests

Thyroid function tests should be performed. Anti-thyroid peroxidase antibodies can confirm thyroiditis.

Ultrasound

Ultrasound is the primary imaging modality for thyroid and essential in all patients. Ultrasound scan features associated with malignancy include:

- Solid nodules (rather than cystic)
- Multifocal lesions within an otherwise clinically solitary nodule

Table 15.4 Conditions associated with MTC within MEN.

Syndrome	Associated conditions with MTC	Proportion
MEN IIa (aka MEN II)	Bilateral phaeochromocytoma Parathyroid hyperplasia or adenoma	50% 35%
MEN IIb (aka MEN III)	Phaeochromocytoma Marfanoid habitus Mucosal neurofibromas	50%

- Nodule with hypoechogenic echostructure
- Subcapsular localisation
- Increased intranodular vascularity
- Irregular infiltrative margins
- Microcalcification
- Suspicious regional lymph nodes accompanying nodule [10,14]

Adult criteria are used to classify and describe paediatric thyroid nodules.

Fine-needle aspiration cytology (FNAC)

FNAC is very valuable in guiding decision making for surgery. It can only be used in appropriate patients who are mature enough to tolerate this procedure under local anaesthetic. The classification system for this is the same as in adults (see Chapter 6).

Molecular studies of FNAC, analysing the presence of a genetic mutation for RAS, BRAF, RET/PTC or PAX8/PPR on indeterminate cytology, has been demonstrated to increase the positive predictive value of FNAC to almost 100% [15].

Management

Surgery

Surgery remains the mainstay of management as well as providing tissue for definitive diagnosis. This should take the form of either lobectomy or total thyroidectomy. Where investigations are suspicious, the goal of surgery is to provide definitive diagnosis with a lobectomy. If there are bilateral nodules or confirmed malignancy on cytology, total thyroidectomy should be offered.

Table 15.5 Aetiology of paediatric salivary gland swellings.

	Congenital	Acquired
Benign	Juvenile recurrent parotitis Polycystic parotid Ranula Haemangioma	Viral sialadenitis Bacterial sialadenitis Obstructive sialadenitis Pleomorphic adenoma Warthin's tumours
Malignant	Sialoblastoma	Mucoepidermoid carcinoma Acinic cell carcinoma Adenoid cystic carcinoma

Total thyroidectomy also allows improved efficacy of radioiodine scanning and thyroglobulin monitoring as well as radioiodine ablation by minimising any thyroid tissue.

In differentiated thyroid carcinoma (DTC), neck dissection should only be performed where there is clinical or radiologic evidence of metastasis.

In MTC, children should have a total thyroidectomy and central neck dissection as the minimum operation. Lateral neck dissection must be performed in those with any evidence of lateral nodal metastases.

Radioactive iodine ablation

Radioactive iodine ablation is usually offered to all paediatric patients with DTC following surgery to ablate any residual thyroid tissue [16].

SALIVARY GLAND SWELLINGS

Salivary gland swellings are uncommon in children (excluding infective conditions such as mumps). These can be congenital or acquired, with the main aetiologies being infective/inflammatory and neoplastic (see **Table 15.5**).

As can be seen, the aetiology for salivary gland swellings is similar to those in adults. It is suggested that there is a higher proportion of malignant tumours that present in children with persistent salivary gland swellings compared to adults [17]. There is a similar distribution for the types of malignant tumours as found in adults with mucoepidermoid carcinoma being the most common. These should be investigated as for any paediatric neck lump and managed with primary surgery to obtain definitive diagnosis and to provide therapeutic clearance. Adjuvant therapies are used judiciously with children according to histopathological findings with regard to tumour subtype, margins and the presence of histologic aggressive features.

REFERENCES

1 Albright JT, Topham AK, Reilly JS. Pediatric head and neck malignancies: US incidence and trends over 2 decades. *Arch Otolaryngol Head Neck Surg*. 2002;128:655–9.

2 Smith A and Cronin M. Paediatric neck lumps: An approach for the primary physician. *Aust J Gen Pract*. 2019;48:289–93.

3 Soldes OS, Younger JG, Hirschl RB. Predictors of malignancy in childhood peripheral lymphadenopathy. *J Pediatr Surg*. 1999;34:1447–52.

4 Ludwig BJ, Wang J, Nadgir RN, Saito N, Castro-Aragon I, Sakai O. Imaging of cervical lymphadenopathy in children and young adults. *AJR Am J Roentgenol*. 2012;199:1105–13.

5 Toma P, Granata C, Rossi A, Garaventa A. Multimodality imaging of Hodgkin disease and non-Hodgkin lymphomas in children. *Radiographics*. 2007;27:1335–54.

6 Tschammler A, Ott G, Schang T, Seelbach-Goebel B, Schwager K, Hahn D. Lymphadenopathy: Differentiation of benign from malignant disease – Color Doppler US assessment of intranodal angioarchitecture. *Radiology*. 1998; 208: 117–23.

7 Lindeboom JA. Conservative wait-and-see therapy versus antibiotic treatment for nontuberculous mycobacterial cervicofacial lymphadenitis in children. *Clin Infect Dis*. 2011; 52: 180–4.

8 Timmerman MK, Morley AD, Buwalda J. Treatment of non-tuberculous mycobacterial cervicofacial lymphadenitis in children: Critical appraisal of the literature. *Clin Otolaryngol*. 2008;33:546–52.

9 Gonzalez CD, Petersen MG, Miller M, Park AH, Wilson KF. Complex nontuberculous mycobacterial cervicofacial lymphadenitis: What is the optimal approach? *Laryngoscope*. 2016;126:1677–80.

10 Guille JT, Opoku-Boateng A, Thibeault SL, Chen H. Evaluation and management of the pediatric thyroid nodule. *Oncologist*. 2015;20:19–27.

11 Hayles AB, Kennedy RL, Beahrs OH, Woolner LB. Management of the child with thyroidal carcinoma. *J Am Med Assoc*. 1960;173:21–8.

12 Fowler CL, Pokorny WJ, Harberg FJ. Thyroid nodules in children: Current profile of a changing disease. *South Med J*. 1989;82:1472–8.

13 Canadian Pediatric Thyroid Nodule Study Group. The Canadian Pediatric Thyroid Nodule Study: An evaluation of current management practices. *J Pediatr Surg*. 2008;43:826–30.

14 Saavedra J, Deladoey J, Saint-Vil D et al. Is ultrasonography useful in predicting thyroid cancer in children with thyroid nodules and apparently benign cytopathologic features? *Horm Res Paediatr*. 2011; 75: 269–75.

15 Buryk MA, Monaco SE, Witchel SF et al. Preoperative cytology with molecular analysis to help guide surgery for pediatric thyroid nodules. *Int J Pediatr Otorhinolaryngol*. 2013;77:1697–700.

16 Rivkees SA, Mazzaferri EL, Verburg FA et al. The treatment of differentiated thyroid cancer in children: Emphasis on surgical approach and radioactive iodine therapy. *Endocr Rev*. 2011;32:798–826.

17 Iro H, Zenk J. Salivary gland diseases in children. *GMS Curr Top Otorhinolaryngol Head Neck Surg*. 2014; 13: Doc06.

16

RECONSTRUCTION IN HEAD AND NECK SURGICAL ONCOLOGY

Kishan Ubayasiri and Andrew Foreman

BACKGROUND

Head and neck tumours often require ablative surgery that is mutilating and functionally debilitating. Not infrequently non-surgical treatments result in complications such as osteoradionecrosis or fistula formation that also require reconstructive surgery. Post-ablative defects require careful reconstructive consideration in order to provide the best cosmetic and functional results for patients, thereby maximising their quality of life. This chapter aims to give an insight into the principles, options, work-up and care involved in patients undergoing complex reconstruction in head and neck surgical oncology.

RECONSTRUCTIVE FRAMEWORKS: THE RECONSTRUCTIVE LADDER

The choice of reconstructive options depends on:

- Patient factors (e.g. co-morbidities, previous surgery or radiotherapy, social history, body habitus)
- Surgical factors (e.g. what types of tissue have been lost, vascularity, prior or planned irradiation, and donor site morbidity)

Despite more recent increasingly complex reconstructive frameworks, such as the 'reconstruction supermarket', where reconstructive surgeons shop for options on behalf of patients who ultimately foot the bill, the reconstructive ladder remains an age-old, tried, tested and easy-to-understand model (see **Table 16.1**) [1]. The reconstructive surgeon may need to employ multiple rungs on the ladder for any given single reconstruction and bypass lower rungs when appropriate. In the age of microvascular reconstruction, the 'ladder' concept, where the most simple available option is employed, has been

Table 16.1 The reconstructive ladder with its increasingly complex rungs, from bottom to top, along with potential complications that may afflict any reconstruction.

Rungs of the ladder	Potential pitfalls of all rungs
Prosthetics	Haematoma
Pre-fabrication	
Free flaps	Infection
Regional flaps	
Local flaps	Necrosis
Grafts	
Primary closure	Failure
Healing by secondary intention	

Table 16.2 Advantages and disadvantages of pedicled flaps in the head and neck.

Advantages	Disadvantages
Do not require two teams working	Constrained by rotational arc and length of flap pedicle
Are quicker, mainly because they involve no microvascular anastomosis, so are particularly useful for co-morbid patients at higher anaesthetic risk where shorter operative times are preferable	No satisfactory pedicled regional option for osseous reconstruction
Far less onerous postoperative care	Some regional flaps in the head and neck may still partially be in a previously operated or irradiated field
Provide a cost saving over free flap reconstruction	May not provide as functional or aesthetic a result as a free flap

overtaken by a focus on optimising outcomes with free tissue transfer when appropriate. Nevertheless, the reconstructive ladder remains an excellent aide-memoire for options available in reconstructing these defects.

▌ Pedicled flaps

A brief word on pedicled flaps: consigned by some to the past, they remain a stalwart of the armamentarium of the head and neck surgeon. **Table 16.2** lists some of the advantages and disadvantages of these flaps.

HEAD AND NECK SUBSITES

▌ Oral cavity (soft tissue)

Indications for oral cavity reconstruction include the need to seal the oral cavity from the neck; cover exposed areas of bone; and to maintain mobility of the oral tongue, floor of mouth and buccal mucosa. A limited number of defects can be closed primarily or allowed to heal by secondary intention (e.g. lateral tongue defects consisting of less than one-third of the tongue). Tumours crossing a combination of oral cavity subsites almost always require reconstruction. Reconstructive access is usually the same as that used for the resection (e.g. transoral, mandibulotomy or a lingual release).

Whilst reconstructive microsurgery is used for the majority of oral cavity soft tissue defects, other pedicled options exist, such as the buccinator myomucosal flap, naso and submental island flap or even melolabial flaps. These can be limited by length of pedicle, previous radiotherapy fields and size of tissue available. All of these can be overcome by the use of free flaps. The most commonly used free flaps for oral cavity soft tissue reconstruction are the radial forearm free flap (RFFF) and the antero-lateral thigh (ALT) flap. Less commonly used is the medial sural artery perforator (MSAP) flap (see **Table 16.3**).

Table 16.3 Comparison of advantages and disadvantages of common free flaps.

Free flap	Common subsite use	Advantages	Disadvantages
Radial forearm flap	Oral cavity soft tissue	Thin, pliable tissue Reliable Quick to harvest Long pedicle length (up to 15 cm) Multiple paddle variations (cutaneous, fasciocutaneous, fascial, adipofascial, osseo-fascial or osseo-cutaneous)	Cosmetically poor donor site Less tissue volume available
Anterolateral thigh flap	Hypopharynx Maxilla Oral cavity soft tissue	Large tissue volumes available Multiple paddle variations (fasciocutaneous, fasciomyocuta-neous or fascial flap) Good pedicle length (up to 7 cm) Donor site can usually be closed primarily Donor site morbidity is limited to a linear scar	Variable pedicle anatomy (can be more challenging to raise) Thick flap can be difficult to thin without damaging perforators
Fibular flap	Mandible Maxilla	Long length of bone Suitable for osteotomy and shaping Can be raised with skin or muscle for oral cavity lining and bulk	May lack adequate height Fixed bone length harvested Minimum bone segment length is 2 cm as dependent on periosteal blood supply Pedicle length can vary according to length of bone required Peroneal artery may be affected by artherosclerosis affecting suitability
Scapular flap	Mandible Maxilla	Arterial pedicle relatively unaf-fected by artherosclerosis Large or small bone segments can be harvested Large volume of skin and muscle can be harvested if required	Two-team working not possible Requires turning of the patient twice, prolonging theatre time

The RFFF is based on the radial artery and its two accompanying venae comitantes. Additionally, the cephalic vein is also frequently included in the flap where possible, giving a second venous drainage option reducing congestion and the risk of flap failure. Most RFFFs include skin and the donor site frequently requires skin grafting to close. This can be either a split skin graft usually taken from the thigh, or a full-thickness skin graft from the abdomen or more proximally from the forearm. V–Y closures have also been described to close small donor sites avoiding grafting altogether in some cases.

The ALT is a versatile flap based on the descending branch of the lateral circumflex femoral artery and its accompanying two venae comitantes.

Although free flap reconstruction is generally the primary reconstructive option for most defects of the head and neck, a free flap might not always be appropriate, for instance, due to patient co-morbidity and a consequent need for a shorter general anaesthetic. In these cases, alternative pedicled reconstructive options must be considered. The submental flap is based on the submental artery, a branch of the facial artery. It is best used in women, as in men a significant quantity of hair-bearing skin is transferred into the oral cavity. Other disadvantages include the proximity of the flap to the site of primary malignancy and its nodal drainage basin. Extreme care must be taken when selecting patients, as positive level Ib neck nodes can compromise the oncologic safety of this flap [2].

The buccinator myomucosal flap is based on buccal or facial artery and provides excellent match, bulk and coverage for the lateral tongue, floor of mouth and soft palate. Limitations include the frequent need for division of the pedicle approximately 6 weeks later and the limited size of defect that can be covered, although this can be increased by using bilateral flaps in appropriate patients [3].

▊ Mandible

Reconstruction of the mandible must address the site and size of the bony defect, associated soft tissue loss and potential dental rehabilitation. Free tissue transfer of bony flaps is the mainstay of mandibular reconstruction. This allows for the transfer of bone which can be fashioned to fit the desired shape, is well vascularised and is amenable to the future insertion of osseointegrated implants. The most commonly used flap by far is the fibular free flap (FFF). If the fibula cannot be used a scapular flap, iliac crest/deep circumflex iliac artery (DCIA) or osteocutaneous RFFF, can be considered.

The FFF allows for harvest of a long length of bone with which can be osteotomised as required to provide a bespoke contoured mandibular reconstruction, which is of adequate height for future osseointegration. Preoperative 3D modelling and planning significantly reduces operative time. In these cases, reconstruction plates can be either pre-bent on a 3D model or custom made. Custom saw guides can be manufactured so that all osteotomies are precisely tailored to the reconstruction plate.

An alternative to the FFF for mandibular reconstruction is the scapular flap, which provides good bone height. Two variations exist: the lateral scapular flap and the scapula tip flap. These bony segments have different blood supplies: the circumflex scapular artery via periosteal perforators and the angular artery off the thoracodorsal artery. Traditionally, the main disadvantage of this flap has been the inability for concurrent flap harvest. The tumour needs to be resected with the patient supine and the patient then needs to be turned into the lateral position to access the patient's back. After flap harvest and donor site closure, the patient needs to be turned supine once again for flap inset. This adds approximately 2–3 hours compared to a standard two-team free flap procedure. Recent adaptations in positioning enable the scapular tip variation, in particular, to be harvested simultaneously as the tumour ablation.

Dental rehabilitation is an increasingly important consideration in mandibular reconstruction. Preoperative assessment for postoperative dental rehabilitation should always occur, with osseointegrated dental implants being gold standard where appropriate.

In patients unsuitable for osseous free flap reconstruction, a plate bridging the gap, which is then covered with free or pedicled soft tissue, such as a pectoralis major flap, can be used as an alternative. The risk of plate extrusion with this approach has been reported to be as high as 30%, relegating it to an option only appropriate for the medically unfit patient. In certain cases, although not ideal, the mandible can be allowed to 'swing', meaning the mandibular defect is left totally unreconstructed but is covered by a soft tissue flap. This is most useful for lateral mandibular defects where the cosmetically important anterior mandibular arch is not violated. In addition it has a secondary benefit in reducing trismus if the pterygoid muscles have been involved in the tumour and require resecting. However, it has the disadvantages of taking dentulous patients out of occlusion over time and placing extra strain on the temporomandibular joint (TMJ) on the side of the intact mandible, which normally manifests as pain.

▊ Maxilla and midface

The two main options for addressing the maxillectomy defect are an obturator or free flap

Table 16.4 Summary of Brown's classification of maxillary and midface defects.

Class of defect	Definition	Reconstructive option
I	Purely maxillary with no oroantral fistula	Secondary intention Obturation Pedicled local flap (e.g. buccinator, temporalis)
II	Hemimaxillectomy not involving orbital floor or periorbita	Obturation Osseous free flaps to aid osseointegrated implantation option
III	Loss of orbital floor along with maxilla	Plates covered with vascularised tissue associated with a free flap (osseous or otherwise)
IV	Maxillectomies which include orbital floor resection and orbital exenteration	Plates covered with vascularised tissue associated with a free flap (osseous or otherwise)
V	Orbitomaxillary defect	Where orbital exenteration is required, free flap reconstruction is required
VI	Nasomaxillary defect including loss of facial skin	Free flap reconstruction

reconstruction. The correct option is best assessed by contemplating the class of the defect present shown in **Table 16.4** [4].

In class I (purely maxillary with no oroantral fistula) and class II (maxillary, extending into the nasal cavity) defects, obturation is a reasonable option. Obturation becomes a progressively less favourable option with orbital adnexal involvement (class III), orbital exenteration (class IV), orbitomaxillary (class V) or nasomaxillary (class VI) defects. In class V and VI defects, the palate and dental alveolus are often intact. Classes I–VI mainly describe the vertical component of the maxillectomy defect, while classes a–d describe the dental/alveolar and palatal components, which also represent increasing difficulty of defect obturation.

The nose

Great care has to be taken to reconstruct all three layers of the nose:

- The facial skin
- Structural support
- Internal nasal lining

The facial skin can be constructed with a combination of local flaps (e.g. cheek advancement flap, paramedian or glabella flaps) or a free flap (e.g. RFFF).

The structural layer of the nose, which is either cartilage or bone, can be reconstructed with any number of a combination of septal or auricular cartilage, costochondral cartilage (rib graft), split calvarial bone (especially when using a paramedian forehead flap) or septal hinge flap.

The internal nasal lining is often the hardest layer to reconstruct. The use of a local septal flap or a flap of facial alar skin can be used if appropriate. Where a paramedian forehead flap has been raised an underlying pericranial flap can also be raised for reconstructing nasal lining. However, it is prone to desiccation and consequent partial necrosis and should only be used when there is no other option.

Total rhinectomy can be rehabilitated with a prosthesis, allowing for negative margin confirmation and further additional resection, if required, prior to any tissue reconstruction. A prosthesis may be the best long-term solution for many patients. However, if a patient wants total nasal reconstruction, the deleterious effects of any postoperative radiotherapy on the reconstruction must be considered and whether delayed secondary reconstruction would be best. Complications due to postoperative radiotherapy on primary nasal reconstructions most commonly occur to the structural components reconstructing the nasal bones and overlying skin, as well as alar retraction and general thinning of the soft tissue envelope [5].

▌ Temporal bone

The aims of reconstruction should address the following issues:

- Protection for the brain where the dura has been breached
- The skin defect
- The auricular defect
- The tissue volume deficit
- Any mandibular defect
- Facial nerve dysfunction

Cerebral protection is of paramount importance and dural defects can be repaired with non-vascularised tissue, such as autologous fascia lata grafts, xenografts or synthetic materials [6].

Smaller skin defects with smaller volume loss can be reconstructed with local pedicled flaps (e.g. cervicofacial rotation, temporalis, supraclavicular or submental island flaps) or free flaps (e.g. radial forearm free flap). Many defects are larger and the anterolateral thigh (ALT) free flap is, thus, the workhorse for lateral skull base defect reconstruction. It provides a large quantity of skin, has minimal donor site morbidity, can be harvested with a vascularised nerve graft, and allows for harvest of fascia lata or the lateral cutaneous nerve of the thigh. ALTs also allow for two teams to work simultaneously.

Where mandibular reconstruction is also required, a chimeric flap, such as a scapular osteomyocutaneous flap, can be employed instead.

The ear canal is not reconstructed after lateral temporal bone resection. Instead, the soft tissue reconstruction is laid directly onto the head of the stapes forming a type III tympanoplasty.

Primary or secondary implant insertion should also be considered for ear prosthesis. Magnets or a bar can be secured onto the implants so that a prosthetic ear may be attached.

▌ Oropharynx

The use of transoral techniques for oropharyngeal resections, the defects from which are generally not reconstructed, result in better functional outcomes than when the oropharynx is reconstructed with a denervated non-sensate soft tissue flap. In most circumstances where the oropharynx needs reconstruction a mandibulotomy is required.

Tongue base reconstruction

Function of the tongue base can generally only be preserved if less that half the tongue base has been resected. When reconstruction is required, pedicled regional options include the pectoralis major, buccinator, submental island and supraclavicular flaps. Free flap options include the ALT or RFFF, either folded over or with the beaver tail modification.

Lateral pharyngeal wall reconstruction

Transoral resection without reconstruction might not always be appropriate for tumours of the lateral pharyngeal wall. This can occur when tumours are too large for transoral surgery, involve (or expose the mandible and during salvage surgery. Pedicled flaps such as the pectoralis major and submental island flaps are good locoregional reconstructive options. The RFFF is a good free flap choice for this area; ALTs are generally too bulky unless the mandible is also resected, in which case they provide excellent tissue replacement to maintain facial contour.

Soft palate reconstruction

Local flaps for a soft palate defect include the posteriorly based buccinator myomucosal flap, superior constrictor advancement rotation flap (SCARF) and superiorly based pharyngeal flap. Free flap options include the RFFF and MSAP. The functional implications of total soft palate resection are significant and the patient should be counselled about the accompanying dysphagia and velopharyngeal incompetence.

Hypopharynx

Reconstruction of partial and circumferential hypopharyngeal defects present major challenges. Modern chemoradiotherapy protocols, medical co-morbidity and poor nutritional status increase surgical morbidity. The aims of hypopharyngeal reconstruction are to:

- Restore swallowing
- Allow speech rehabilitation
- Limit morbidity and mortality

Partial hypopharyngeal defects with more than 3.5 cm width of unstretched remaining pharyngeal mucosa can be closed primarily. Where less than 3.5 cm width of remnant mucosa exists, a pharyngeal patch is generally required [7]. This can be a pedicled flap or a free flap. The most widely used pedicled options are the pectoralis major and supraclavicular flaps. The RFFF is the most widely used free flap for a pharyngeal patch. Any longitudinal strip of native pharyngeal mucosa that can be preserved is extremely useful, as it tends to reduce the stricture rate and improves functional outcomes of the neopharynx. Debate exists when less than 1 cm width of native pharyngeal mucosa remains, with some believing it better to excise this, thereby creating a circumferential defect allowing for easier flap inset. There are concerns about the viability of narrow strips of mucosa, particularly in the irradiated patient. Others believe that preserving even this small amount of mucosa may reduce stricture rates. Limited case series suggest speech and swallow outcomes may be improved with free compared to pedicled flaps but these are highly flawed and far from definitive.

Total circumferential hypopharyngeal defects superior to the clavicles

Total circumferential pharyngolaryngectomy defects can be reconstructed with any of the following free flaps:

- Tubed ALT
- Tubed RFFF

- Jejunal free flap
- Gastro-omental free flap

Low-level evidence suggests a salivary bypass tube may reduce fistula rates [8]. A size 12 or 14 salivary bypass tube is best. In a proportion of patients with significantly large and fat thighs, the ALT may not be a good choice to address the circumferential hypopharyngeal defect, as too much tissue may be introduced into the neck preventing primary closure of the neck incision. Thinning of the ALT flap puts perforators at risk. In these patients a tubed RFFF may be a more appropriate choice, although the size of the donor site defect will be unsightly, requiring a large skin graft in a readily visible area. If primary neck closure cannot be achieved, especially in the setting of prior radiotherapy, and an ALT flap is used, a separate skin paddle can be designed to close the external skin defect, otherwise a pectoralis major pedicled flap can be used. The pectoralis major can be harvested as a myocutaneous flap for this purpose or a muscle-only flap can be covered by a split-thickness skin graft. Jejunal free flaps are an alternative to fasciocutaneous flaps. However, there is concern over donor site morbidity and uncoordinated peristalsis leading to poorer swallowing and 'wet' sounding speech [9]. The jejunal and gastro-omental free flaps do have the advantage of containing omentum, which can be used to provide vascularised tissue coverage over the anastomosis in much the same way a pectoralis major pedicled flap would.

An alternative to a tubed flap reconstruction is a U-shaped one, with the ends sutured directly onto the prevertebral fascia. The advantage of this is that pedicled flaps can be used, generally a pectoralis major, which then do not require the extreme width necessary for tubing. Of course this can only be an option so long as the prevertebral fascia has not been resected as a margin.

All reconstructive options carry with them the risk of anastomotic leak, flap failure and donor site morbidity. Anastomotic stricture is a potential complication resulting in dysphagia and, with the tubed flaps, this generally occurs at the inferior anastomosis, whilst the superior anastomosis is more prone to leak.

Total circumferential hypopharyngeal/ oesophageal defects inferior to the clavicles

After circumferential resection of the distal hypopharynx/proximal oesophagus, including a 3 cm margin, the lower anastomosis for any tubed flap would be inferior to the clavicles. For this reason, a gastric pull up is the reconstruction of choice. This procedure carries significant morbidity due to the need to enter three visceral cavities (neck, thorax and abdomen). Gastric pull up carries a mortality rate of 5%–15%, morbidity of 30%–55% and reported fistula rates of 3%–23% [10,11]. Intraoperatively, the patient also experiences cardiac arrhythmia as the surgeon manually frees the oesophagus from the posterior surface of the heart.

Colonic transposition is a far less widely used alternative, which carries all the same complications as gastric pull up, but has a greater proximal reach, being able to reconstruct pharyngeal defects which extend as far as the oropharynx.

▋ Salvage surgery

Surgery in general and especially reconstructive surgery in the post-(chemo)radiotherapy era carries a higher complication rate due to scarred fibrotic tissue, reduced tissue vascularity and poor wound healing in the irradiated field [12]. Should it not be possible to close the neck incision because of poor quality or contracted skin, a myocutaneous pectoralis major, skin grafted muscle only pectoralis major or chimeric ALT may be used to resurface the neck, thereby providing additional skin.

Up to 50% of patients undergoing salvage total laryngectomy after chemoradiation will suffer from postoperative pharyngocutaneous fistulae. Introducing vascularised tissue from outside the radiation field as overlay to any pharyngeal repair or reconstruction can significantly reduce fistula rates [13]. The gold standard for this is a pectoralis major pedicled flap overlaid on the pharyngeal repair in these previously irradiated cases. Free flaps (e.g. temporoparietal free flap, RFFF or ALT) have also been reported as an alternative to the pectoralis major.

GENERAL CONSIDERATIONS

▋ Preoperative imaging

Fibula free flaps should have preoperative computed tomography angiograms (CTAs) of the lower limbs to confirm normal three-vessel run-off for the proposed leg. In some more advanced software, a magnetic resonance angiogram (MRA) may be indicated to model skin perforators to plan bony cuts.

▋ Intraoperative considerations

Tourniquet use

When using a tourniquet during free flap elevation, tourniquet pressure should be set to 100 mm Hg and 200 mm Hg above the patient's systolic blood pressure for the upper limb and lower limb, respectively. This is generally 250 mm Hg for the upper limb and 350 mm Hg for the lower limb.

Pedicle ligation

When ligating the vascular pedicle of a free flap immediately to transfer, Ligaclips should not be applied to the flap side. The flap can then be allowed to drain of blood prior to being moved to the site of the defect.

Osseous flap plating

Thought must be given as to what plating system to use. Multiple miniplates can be used instead of a larger reconstruction plate. This removes the need to adapt a reconstruction plate intraoperatively when no pre-bent plate is available, but probably reduces the overall stability of the initial reconstruction.

Microvascular anastamosis

Microvascular anastomoses can be undertaken either using at least 4.5 × magnification loupes or an operative microscope. The microscope provides superior magnification and illumination, and affords both the surgeon and assistant similar views. The venous coupler is an adjunct that does speed up the time taken for end-to-end venous anastomosis and is relatively simple to use, but it cannot be used for true end-to-side anastomosis.

Skin grafting for donor site

When a split-skin graft is harvested for donor site coverage, this should be harvested using the air-powered dermatome at a thickness of between 0.008 and 0.016 inches. Split-skin grafts should be fenestrated or 'pie crusted' (fewer larger holes than in fenestration). Full-thickness skin grafts do not require fenestration. Pressure must be applied and maintained to the grafted area to prevent haematoma and shearing. This can be achieved by the use of sterile sponge secured with either staples or suture bolsters or by using fluffed gauze with overlying suture bolsters.

Drain placement

Drains can be placed entering either high or low in the neck. If they enter low, care must be taken to avoid the external jugular vein. If they enter high, for instance through the skin overlying level 5b, they can be passed posterior to the accessory nerve and cervical plexus branches, thereby preventing the drain from migrating anteriorly and sucking on the flap pedicle, or worse, a microvascular anastomosis, which tend to lay lower in the neck.

▌ Postoperative care

The first 48 hours after free flap surgery are the most crucial. It is common practice for free flap patients to be nursed in the intensive care unit (ICU) or surgical high-dependency unit (SHDU), because of the enhanced facility for patient monitoring, higher nursing ratios and an increased burden of postoperative checks that nursing staff are required to undertake. Some advocate keeping the patient intubated in the intensive care unit (ICU) for a period of at least 12 hours to allow for the careful monitoring and maintenance of haemodynamic stability and regular flap checks, but this is by no means universal [14].

Immediate postoperative care should include the following [15]:

- Continued sedation and ventilation as per the ICU/SHDU team.
- Avoidance of circumferential neck ties securing the tracheostomy.
- Avoid inotropes/vasopressors.
- The head of the bed should be elevated at 30°.
- The patient's head should be kept in a neutral position and turning the patient's head away from the side of the vascular anastomosis should be avoided.
- Flap checks should be every 15 minutes for the first hour, every 30 minutes for the following 2 hours and then houtrly for the next 24 hours.
- Nasogastric (NG) feeds should be started the following morning, pending radiographic verification of nasogastric tube tip position. For deep circumflex iliac artery (DCIA) or jejunal free flaps, this should be delayed until the surgical team has confirmed the presence of borborygmi after abdominal examination.
- Patients should have at least two doses of postoperative intravenous antibiotics.
- Deep venous thrombosis (DVT) prophylaxis should be maintained as per local protocol. This will commonly be a combination of low molecular weight heparin and thromboembolic deterrent stockings (TEDS).
- If vasopressor use is unavoidable in order to keep the systolic blood pressure above 100 mmHg, the judicious use of metaraminol is best tolerated in head and neck free flap patients [16].
- Blood transfusion is controversial. Ideally haemoglobin should be maintained above 80 g in order to ensure good perfusion of the flap. However, concern has been raised over transfusion increasing risk of haematogenous metastasis and recurrence, as well as increasing risk of thrombosis and flap failure [17].

When to remove items

1 In tracheal stoma patients – tracheostomy tubes out ideally on day 1 postoperatively
2 Tracheotomy patients – tube out day 7 after 24 hours of capping

3 Removal of sutures on day 7–9 (day 10–14 for previously irradiated patients)
4 Remove implantable Doppler day 7–9
5 Removal of NG tube once oral intake established by medical team and dietetic team satisfied with nutritional intake orally
6 Encourage early mobilisation and physiotherapy, but avoid weight bearing on leg plaster casts for 1 week
7 Plaster cast/dressings from any skin grafted donor site to be removed on day 9

Implantable Doppler

It is now commonplace to use an implantable Doppler for free flap cases. This consists of a silastic sleeve with an attached electronic flow sensor which is wrapped around the vascular pedicle. This can be arterial or venous, or both. Use of the implantable Doppler has revolutionised the postoperative monitoring of free flaps. Whilst the implantable Doppler is not a replacement for good regular clinical examination postoperative free flaps, it is an extremely useful adjunct, especially for those not very familiar with the aftercare of free flaps and for flaps without a visible skin paddle. Should the Doppler signal be lost, the surgical team must be immediately informed and, after careful corroborating clinical evaluation of both the patient and flap, an emergency return to theatre for flap salvage planned.

Pedicled flap postoperative care

The postoperative care of pedicled flaps in contrast to free flaps is far less onerous. Where a skin paddle or flap muscle is visible, flap health can be assessed by warmth, turgor and skin capillary refill. Pressure or constriction of the vascular pedicle must be avoided (e.g. from tracheostomy ties around the neck). Should the patient develop a significant neck haematoma, this must be drained early to prevent risk to the vascular pedicle. No routine flap observation is required by nursing staff. If non-absorbable skin sutures or staples are used to close the donor site, they are generally removed after 7–9 days.

Flap examination and what to document on rounds

At each of the nursing/medical staff flap checks for the first 24 hours and thereafter, the following should be interrogated, examined and documented:

1 Observe the patient's heart rate, respiratory rate, blood pressure, temperature and oxygen saturations.
2 The implantable Doppler should be connected if not already on. This can be connected intermittently after 48 hours.
3 The neck should be observed and palpated to ensure that it is soft with no sign of haematoma or fistula.
4 Where possible, the flap skin paddle should be observed for colour, bearing in mind what it looked like immediately postoperatively. The flap should be palpated for warmth, turgor and capillary refill (press for 5 seconds, refill <2 seconds). The wound edges between the inset of the skin paddle and native tissue should be inspected for dehiscence, predisposing to fistula.
5 Observe whether the patient is being ventilated or breathing spontaneously, and check the ventilator settings.
6 Urine output.
7 Use of any vasopressors.
8 Examine donor sites, and skin grafts. Distal donor limbs should be examined for warmth, capillary refill (<2 seconds), and movement where appropriate.
9 Check the patient's drug chart, and ensure all appropriate medication has been prescribed, including regular medications. Discontinue inappropriate medications.

▌ Flap salvage

The standard quoted flap failure rate in the literature is up to 5% [16,18]. Although problems with the venous anastomosis are more common than those of the arterial anastomosis, patient factors also play a key role, such as hypotension, anaemia and the effect of pre-existing co-morbidities including intraoperative events that have occurred as a result of these.

Should the Doppler signal be lost, especially within the first 48 hours following surgery, and this corroborated by the clinical examination, an emergency return to theatre should be organised including perioperative work-up including group and save. Intraoperatively, any neck haematoma must be removed, and the arterial and venous anastomoses scrutinised. Problems with the arterial inflow or venous outflow from the flap must be identified and addressed. This can involve taking down the existing microvascular anastomoses and revising them. Consideration should also be given to the use of tissue plasminogen activator (TPA), which can either be given systemically intravenously or flushed through only the flap via a cannula [19].

CONCLUSION

Reconstruction in head and neck surgery requires insight from all members of the multidisciplinary team in order to provide the best oncologic, functional and aesthetic outcomes for the patient.

REFERENCES

1 Venkatramani H, Rodrigues JN, Sabapathy SR. Revisiting the reconstructive surgery framework: The reconstruction supermarket. *J Plast Reconstr Aesthet Surg.* 2019;72(4):529–31.

2 Howard BE, Nagel TH, Donald CB, Hinni ML, Hayden RE. Oncologic safety of the submental flap for reconstruction in oral cavity malignancies. *Otolaryngol Head Neck Surg.* 2014;150(4):558–62.

3 Van Lierop AC, Fagan JJ. Buccinator myomucosal flap: Clinical results and review of anatomy, surgical technique and applications. *J Laryngol Otol.* 2008;122(2):181–7.

4 Brown JS, Shaw RJ. Reconstruction of the maxilla and midface: Introducing a new classification. *Lancet Oncol.* 2010;11(10):1001–8.

5 Menick FJ. Practical details of nasal reconstruction. *Plast Reconstr Surg.* 2013;131(4):613e–30e.

6 Gal TJ, Kerschner JE, Futran ND et al. Reconstruction after temporal bone resection. *Laryngoscope.* 1998;108(4 Pt 1):476–81.

7 Chu PY, Chang SY. Reconstruction of the hypopharynx after surgical treatment of squamous cell carcinoma. *J Chin Med Assoc.* 2009;72(7):351–5.

8 Kamhieh Y, Fox H, Hallett E, Berry S. Routine use of salivary bypass tubes in laryngectomy patients: Systematic review. *J Laryngol Otol.* 2018;132(5):380–4.

9 Haller JR. Concepts in pharyngoesophageal reconstruction. *Otolaryngol Clin North Am.* 1997;30(4):655–61.

10 Patel RS, Goldstein DP, Brown D, Irish J, Gullane PJ, Gilbert RW. Circumferential pharyngeal reconstruction: History, critical analysis of techniques, and current therapeutic recommendations. *Head Neck.* 2010;32(1):109–20.

11 Mehta SA, Sarkar S, Mehta AR, Mehta MS. Mortality and morbidity of primary pharyngogastric anastomosis following circumferential excision for hypopharyngeal malignancies. *J Surg Oncol.* 1990;43(1):24–7.

12 Hamoir M, Schmitz S, Suarez C et al. The current role of salvage surgery in recurrent head and neck squamous cell carcinoma. *Cancers (Basel).* 2018;10(8):267.

13 Sayles M, Grant DG. Preventing pharyngocutaneous fistula in total laryngectomy: A systematic review and meta-analysis. *Laryngoscope.* 2014;124(5):1150–63.

14 Arshad H, Ozer HG, Thatcher A et al. Intensive care unit versus non-intensive care unit postoperative management of head and neck free flaps: Comparative effectiveness and cost comparisons. *Head Neck.* 2014;36(4):536–9.

15 Salgado CJ, Chim H, Schoenoff S, Mardini S. Postoperative care and monitoring of the reconstructed head and neck patient. *Semin Plast Surg.* 2010;24(3):281–7.

16 Fang L, Liu J, Yu C, Hanasono MM, Zheng G, Yu P. Intraoperative use of vasopressors does not increase the risk of free flap compromise and failure in cancer patients. *Ann Surg.* 2018;268(2):379–84.

17 Chau JK, Harris JR, Seikaly HR. Transfusion as a predictor of recurrence and survival in head and neck cancer surgery patients. *J Otolaryngol Head Neck Surg.* 2010;39(5):516–22.

18 Las DE, de Jong T, Zuidam JM, Verweij NM, Hovius SE, Mureau MA. Identification of independent risk factors for flap failure: A retrospective analysis of 1530 free flaps for breast, head and neck and extremity reconstruction. *J Plast Reconstr Aesthet Surg.* 2016;69(7):894–906.

19 Novakovic D, Patel RS, Goldstein DP, Gullane PJ. Salvage of failed free flaps used in head and neck reconstruction. *Head Neck Oncol.* 2009;1:33.

INDEX